The Cerebellum, Epilepsy, and Behavior

The Cerebellum, Epilepsy, and Behavior

Edited by

Irving S. Cooper and Manuel Riklan

St. Barnabas Hospital
Bronx, New York

and
Ray S. Snider

Center for Brain Research
University of Rochester
Rochester, New York

PLENUM PRESS   NEW YORK-LONDON

Library of Congress Cataloging in Publication Data

Main entry under title:

The Cerebellum, epilepsy, and behavior.

"Proceedings of the symposium 'The Cerebellum, Epilepsy and Behavior,' held at
St. Barnabas Hospital, Bronx, New York, from August 6-10, 1973."
Includes bibliographies.
1. Epilepsy–Congresses. 2. Cerebellum–Congresses. 3. Brain stimulation–Con-
gresses. I. Cooper, Irving Spencer, 1922–   ed. II. Riklan, Manuel, ed. III. Snider,
Ray Solomon, 1911–   ed. IV. New York. St. Barnabas Hospital for Chronic
Diseases.
[DNLM: 1.   Cerebellum–Physiology–Congresses. 2. Epilepsy–Congresses. WL320
C414 1973]
RC372.AlC47   616.8'53   73-21971
ISBN 0-306-30775-8

Proceedings of the symposium "The Cerebellum, Epilepsy and Behavior,"
held at St. Barnabas Hospital, Bronx, New York, from August 6-10, 1973.

1974 Plenum Press, New York
A Division of Plenum Publishing Corporation
227 West 17th Street, New York, N.Y. 10011

United Kingdom edition published by Plenum Press, London
A Division of Plenum Publishing Company, Ltd.
Davis House (4th Floor), 8 Scrubs Lane, Harlesden, London, NW10 6SE, England

Printed in the United States of America

Dedicated to the memory of

Sir Victor Horsley,

Explorer of the physiology and surgery of
the cerebellum

INTRODUCTION AND ACKNOWLEDGMENTS

These proceedings incorporate all of the formal papers presented at a Symposium entitled "The Cerebellum, Epilepsy and Behavior", held at St. Barnabas Hospital, Bronx, New York, from August 6 to 10, 1973. The primary purposes of this Symposium were (1) to review the existing experimental literature in the area, (2) to present more recent experimental data, (3) to permit an exchange of views among the various experimental disciplines represented, (4) to present clinical data and results derived from techniques of stimulating the human cerebellum, and (5) to permit discussion and exchanges of views between the laboratory and clinical investigators present. It has been pointed out that physiologic functions, as well as gross and microscopic structure of the cerebellum have been as well understood as virtually any other part of the central nervous system. However, neither neurosurgical nor neuropharmacological therapeutic measures of significance have yet evolved from this basic knowledge. One of the speculations and hopes that stimulated the organization of this Symposium was the belief that the time for therapeutic surgery and medicine of the cerebellum has come.

Over one year ago cerebellar stimulation was first applied to an individual with a previously intractable seizure disorder. During the ensuing year 7 other patients with a variety of intractable seizure disorders were subjected to cerebellar cortex stimulation, designed to relieve such seizures. This therapeutic approach was developed on the basis of existing anatomic and electrophysiologic studies which indicated that the cerebellar cortex modulates a wide variety of sensory-motor functions. From the clinical investigations data have now been accumulated in relevant physiological, neurological, and behavioral areas which seem to bear very much upon the role of the cerebellum in man not only in seizure disorders but in the modification and modulation of sensory-motor functions more generally.

The Symposium participants will be presenting recent data, derived from various laboratories, which pertain to the anatomy, electrophysiology, and biochemistry of the cerebellum and its influences on various levels of the neuraxis. Such data will be derived largely from laboratory studies utilizing the rat, cat and monkey. With respect to the clinical data to be presented and general efficacy of the technique of cerebellar cortex stimulation in man, it has always been the practice of the Neurosurgical Department of St. Barnabas to demonstrate clinical results to interested colleagues from both the clinical and laboratory sciences. It is hoped that actual patient presentation, accompanied by accumulated physiological, neurological, and psychological data will provide significant feedback for the various laboratory investigators present, so that new insights may be developed with respect to cerebellar function in man. The Symposium is multidisciplinary in nature, based upon the concept that only such studies can lead to more meaningful understanding of the many manifestations of cerebellar function.

It is hoped that as a result of the formal presentations and discussions which will ensue during the Symposium, that practical and significant plans will be made for continuing relevant laboratory and clinical investigations, and for developing collaborative programs in this respect.

The editors of this Symposium are very pleased to acknowledge the collaboration and assistance of many individuals who have contributed generously of their time and effort in the planning, execution and publication of these proceedings. First, appreciation is expressed to all of the individual contributors whose investigations form the basis for this Symposium, and for their prompt preparation of manuscripts to provide rapid publication. Gratitude is also expressed to Mr. Charles M. Bliss, President of the Board of Managers of St. Barnabas Hospital, and Mr. John T. Kolody, Executive Director, for generously making available the necessary hospital facilities. We are also grateful to Rose Marie Spitaleri, medical photographer, and Mary Lorenc, medical artist, for their contribution during the Symposium and in the publication of the manuscript. We particularly acknowledge the efforts of Anne David for her careful and conscientious typing of the manuscript, and to Mrs. Janet Dowling for editing and proofreading of the various manuscripts. Thanks are also offered to The John A. Hartford Foundation, Inc., New York City, for its many years of research support to the Department of Neurologic Surgery of St. Barnabas Hospital, support which led to the development of the clinical techniques described. Finally, we are appreciative of the very close cooperation of

Mr. Seymour Weingarten, Senior Editor, and Mr. Thomas Lanigan, Editor of Plenum Press, for their cooperation in a speedy and effective production of these proceedings.

I. S. C.
M. R.
R. S. S.

CONTENTS

CONTRIBUTORS

THE ST. BARNABAS HOSPITAL SYMPOSIUM ON "THE CEREBELLUM, EPILEPSY AND BEHAVIOR" AUGUST 6-10, 1973, BRONX, NEW YORK

ISMAIL M. AMIN, M.D.
Department of Neurologic Surgery
St. Barnabas Hospital
Bronx, New York

FRUCTUOSO AYALA, M.D.
Institute of Biomedical Investigations, UNAM
Cuidad Universitaria
Mexico 10, D.L., Mexico

THOMAS L. BABB, Ph.D.
Assistant Research Neurophysiologist
Division of Neurologic Surgery
UCLA Center for the Health Sciences
Los Angeles, California

A. J. BERMAN, M.D.
Clinical Professor of Neurosurgery
Mt. Sinai School of Medicine
New York, New York

DOREEN BERMAN, Ph.D.
Assistant Professor of Psychology
Queens College, City University
Jamaica, New York

REGINALD BICKFORD, M.D.
Professor of Neuroscience
University of California
San Diego Department of Neurosciences
La Jolla, California

SIMON BRAILOWSKY, M.D.
Institute of Biomedical Investigations, UNAM
Cuidad Universitaria
Mexico 10, D.L., Mexico

JOSE M. CALVO, M.D.
Institute of Biomedical Investigations, UNAM
Cuidad Universitaria
Mexico 10, D.L., Mexico

D. CARR, B.S.
Department of Neurology
Columbia University
New York, New York

CARLOS M. CONTRERAS, M.D.
Institute of Biomedical Investigations, UNAM
Cuidad Universitaria
Mexico 10, D.L., Mexico

IRVING S. COOPER, M.D., Ph.D.
Director, Department of Neurologic Surgery
St. Barnabas Hospital, Bronx, New York
Research Professor of Neuroanatomy
New York Medical College
New York, New York

PAUL H. CRANDALL, M.D.
Professor of Neurological Surgery
UCLA Center for the Health Sciences
Los Angeles, California

G. W. DAUTH, Ph.D.
Research Associate
Department of Neurology
Columbia University
New York, New York

ROBERT S. DOW, M.D.
Head, Department of Neurology
Director, Department of Neurophysiology
Good Samaritan Hospital & Medical Center
Portland, Oregon

AUGUSTO FERNANDEZ-GUARDIOLA, M.D.
Research Professor of Neurophysiology
Institute of Biomedical Investigations, UNAM
Cuidad Universitaria
Mexico, D.L., Mexico

SID GILMAN, M.D.
Professor of Neurology
Columbia University
New York, New York

ROBERT GRIMM, M.D.
Director of Neurological Education
Good Samaritan Hospital & Medical Center
Portland, Oregon

ROBERT M. JULIEN, Ph.D.
Assistant Professor, Department of Medicine,
Pharmacology and Therapeutics
University of California Medical School
Irvine, California

KAREN MARISAK, M.A.
Research Assistant
St. Barnabas Hospital
Bronx, New York

BLAINE S. NASHOLD, Jr., M.D.
Associate Professor of Neurosurgery
Duke University Medical School
Durham, North Carolina

JAMES W. PRESCOTT, Ph.D.
National Institute of Child Health
and Human Development
Bethesda, Maryland

DOMINIC PURPURA, M.D.
Chairman, Department of Anatomy
Albert Einstein College of Medicine
Bronx, New York

MANUEL RIKLAN, Ph.D.
Chief Psychologist, St. Barnabas Hospital
Bronx, New York
Adjunct Professor, Fordham University
Bronx, New York

DONALD S. RUSHNER, Ph.D.
Associate Director, Laboratory of Neurophysiology
Good Samaritan Hospital & Medical Center
Portland, Oregon

ALFONSO SALGADO, M.D.
Institute of Biomedical Investigations, UNAM
Cuidad Universitaria
Mexico 10, D.L., Mexico

HARMON L. SMITH, Ph.D.
Professor of Moral Theology
The Divinity School, Duke University
Durham, North Carolina

RAY S. SNIDER, Ph.D.
Professor, Center for Brain Research
University of Rochester
Rochester, New York

HUGO SOLIS, M.D.
Institute of Biomedical Investigations, UNAM
Cuidad Universitaria
Mexico 10, D.L., Mexico

CARLO TERZUOLO, M.D.
Director, Laboratory of Neurophysiology
University of Minnesota Medical School
Minneapolis, Minnesota

PAOLO VIVIANI, Ph.D.
Laboratory of Neurophysiology
Department of Physiology
University of Minnesota Medical School
Minneapolis, Minnesota

JOSEPH M. WALTZ, M.D.
Associate Neurosurgeon
Department of Neurologic Surgery
St. Barnabas Hospital
Bronx, New York

CEREBELLAR MODIFICATIONS OF ABNORMAL DISCHARGES

IN CEREBRAL SENSORY AND MOTOR AREAS

Ray S. Snider

Center for Brain Research
University of Rochester Medical School
Rochester, New York

Thirty years have passed since Snider and Stowell's (1942, 1944) descriptions of the cerebellar sensory areas. The significance of these observations is not yet known; however, they introduced me to a new cerebellar physiology. No longer were functions limited to reflex motor activity. New questions could be asked and new experiments proposed. To cite an early one: What relationships, if any, existed between these areas and the cerebrum?

Henneman, Cooke and Snider (1950) discovered discrete projections extending between cerebellar tactile, auditory and visual areas to similar ones in the cerebrum. Whiteside and Snider (1953) described two ascending cerebellar systems: one by way of sensory relay thalamic nuclei and the other through the ascending reticular formation. Additional questions were asked: What influence or influences did the cerebellum exert on these cerebral areas? We are still trying to answer that one and indeed that question may prove to be a central theme of this conference. Early electrophysiological studies on the intact anesthetized brain furnished no answers. Cooke and Snider (1955) circumvented some difficulty by asking a different question, namely, What happens to abnormal cerebral activity when the cerebellum is stimulated in an animal with minimal anesthesia? Electro-shock was used to induce seizure activity in various cerebral areas and the influences of cerebellar excitations studied. The results in some instances were startling since seizure discharges could be abruptly terminated while in others the discharges were modified and there was gradual cessation of the abnormal high voltage activity.

Four years later (1959) Iwata and Snider extended the studies to the hippocampus and observed that cerebellar excitation could stop seizure patterns and prolonged after discharges which had been established by electrical stimulation. In the non-seizuring hippocampus, cerebellar stimulation could induce slow waves while activation-like patterns (low voltage, fast) simultaneously appeared in the cerebrum. For the first time a functional interaction had been established between these two widely separate structures and indeed, if temporal lobe epilepsy involves paratemporal areas, then this work may prove to be a very fundamental contribution. Fundamental not only because of changes in EEG activity but because of future studies which may involve subtle corrections in abnormal behavioral patterns. These observations were confirmed by Fanardjian and Donhoffer, 1963. In 1962, Dow, Fernández-Guardiola and Manni published two papers which showed that cerebellar stimulation could alter EEG activity in the rat made abnormal by cobalt powder. Of additional interest was the observation that cerebellar ablation enhanced the electrocortical manifestations of the experimental epilepsy. Five years later (1967) this work was extended to the cat. Rucci, Ginetti and La Rocca (1968) demonstrated the inhibitory role of the cerebellum in hyperoxic seizures.

The effects of cerebellar stimulation on the human EEG as reported by Snider and Wetzl (1965) is relevant to the present study. In 26 awake individuals the pial surface of anterior and posterior folia were electrically stimulated and EEG alterations noted, care being taken to avoid the effects of unwanted current spread. When posterior cerebellar structures were activated, the usual response was a change from low voltage alpha-like or fast frequencies to high voltage slow ones. When anterior structures were activated a low voltage fast record usually resulted although an alpha rhythm could result if the prestimulatory record was a low voltage fast one. Muscular movements, disturbances of consciousness and epileptiform discharges were never seen. The prominent alterations in EEG frequencies were such a consistent finding that it was a surprise to observe no changes in awareness or behavior of the patient.

A series of single unit studies were done following the original ones by Brookhart, Moruzzi and Snider (1951). In an attempt to determine what was happening at thalamic and cerebral levels when the cerebellum was stimulated, Snider, Sato and Mizuno (1964) reported that reactional interference occurred in the medial geniculate nucleus when conditioning and test stimuli were applied to the vermal folia of the middle lobe. Cohen, Housepian and Purpura (1962) had shown that intrathalamic activity especially in rostral ventralis lateralis was an important factor in the genesis of rhythmic discharges in corticospinal neurons. Mitra and Snider

(1969) in a detailed single unit study of the cerebral auditory area and medial geniculate nucleus noted that combined click and fastigial stimulation (10/sec) produced 10/sec bursts in the ectosylvian cortex while faster frequencies (100–300/sec) depressed the number of active ectosylvian units in the early post–stimulatory period. This was followed by rebound facilitation. Of special interest in this study was the observation that cerebellar stimulation in the the 8 to 12/second range not only imposed these frequencies on cerebral units but they often continued for seconds and even minutes into the post–stimulatory period despite their absence in the pre–stimulatory tracings. If such studies can be confirmed in the human, then our understanding of the mechanisms involved in the cerebellar control of seizure discharges may be closer than we realize. It must be remembered that long after effects have been considered a peculiar characteristic of cerebellar function for more than four decades and, indeed, if this organ proves to be the strong modulator of neurological activity which we consider it to be, then with confidence I will indicate that each of you is attending a more significant meeting than you realize.

Snider, Mitra and Sudilovsky (1970) reported on cerebral and thalamic units responding both to tactile and to cerebellar stimulation. Inhibition of activity in ventralis posterior thalami and tactile receiving area of the cerebrum was the characteristic result although when stimulation frequencies faster than 10/sec were used facilitation was observed occasionally. Post–stimulatory inhibition and facilitation were observed more frequently in the cerebrum than in the thalamus.

Snider and Sinis (1973) have done a detailed study on units in cerebral visual areas, the activities of which have been modified by cerebellar stimulation. Both extracellular and intracellular records were taken and analyzed. The most characteristic findings were: 1) stereotyped EPSP's and excitation in area 17 occurring simultaneously with IPSP's and inhibition in area 18 following stimulation of the cerebellar visual area or nucleus fastigii. Since these same units also responded to photic stimulation there can be little doubt about their identity. Such data are difficult to interpret without parallel behavioral studies. However, the fact that the cerebellum can simultaneously produce excitation in a primary sensory receiving area and inhibition in a sensory associational area can be used as additional support for the thesis that subtle regulations and/or modulations are being imposed on a higher sensory system for functional purposes yet to be accurately defined. While motor ataxia is a well accepted term, sensory ataxia is not and, thus far, this field has attracted very few experimental psychologists even in the light of interactions with the limbic system as shown by Fox et al. (Fox, Liebeskind, Obrien, & Dingle, 1967) and recent proposals on autism by Prescott (1971) and others.

However, promising studies have been made with some of the anti-epileptic drugs. Merritt and Putnam (1939) in their pioneering studies on Dilantin (DPH), a drug of choice for grand mal attacks, were the first to point out that toxic doses can produce signs of cerebellar deficiency. Utterback, Ojeman and Malek (1958) reported neuropathological signs of cerebellar degeneration following DPH intoxication. Kokenge, Kutt and McDowell (1965) observed severe Purkinje cell loss in a patient following DPH overdose. del Cerro and Snider have published two papers (1967, 1972) on ultrastructural changes in Purkinje cells resulting from chronic Dilantin toxicity. These cells pass through the stages of increased production of ribosomes, increased production of cellular membranes, and with continued overdosage there is first mild, then severe loss of cells. The bizarre action of this commonly used anti-epileptic drug is unknown. However, Woodbury (1969) has suggested an effect of DPH on nucleic acid metabolism and the enhancement of active Na transport. In additon, there is a decrease of glutamic acid and an increase in brain gamma-amino-butyric acid. Recently, Julien and Halpern (1972) have demonstrated that DPH given systemically causes a prominent increase in Purkinje cell unitary discharges, amounting to tripling and quadrupling the resting activity. Diazepam (Valium) has a similar effect but trimethadione and acetozola-mine has no effect. Hutton, Frost and Foster (1972) were able to inhibit cortical penicillin foci by cerebellar stimulation, while Julien and Halpern (1972) have shown that there is abrupt cessation of P cell discharges during penicillin induced generalized cortical seizures which Dilantin can reverse with an increase of P cell discharges. This should be considered as strong supporting evidence for electrical cerebellar stimulation inducing suppression of cerebral seizures.

The present report is an extension of our cerebellar studies to seizure control in the monkey.

METHODS

Eleven Macaca mulatta monkeys have been used in these experiments six of which form the basis of this report. The cerebrum and cerebellum was quickly exposed under ether anesthesia. Then the animal was placed in a stereotaxic instrument, a tracheal cannula was inserted, the animal was given I.P. Flaxedil (10-20 mg/Kg), 1% Novocain was carefully in-jected adjacent to incised areas and the animal was attached to a positive and negative pressure respirator. Four bipolar, concentric recording stain-less steel electrodes were placed either unilaterally or bilaterally into thalamic areas. A bipolar side-by-side stimulating electrode was placed in nucleus fastigii and in posterior hippocampus. Bipolar silver-silver chloride surface stimulating electrodes were placed on pial surface of cerebral hemisphere and cerebellar vermis. In some experiments it was necessary to use silver-silver chloride surface recording electrodes on the cerebellar and cerebral corticles. The animal's rectal temperature was kept between 35° and 38° C and warm mineral oil was dripped over the surface of exposed neural structures. Supplemental IP injections of Flaxedil were given when muscular twitchings appeared. Subcutaneous injections of normal saline and 5% glucose were usually given at hourly intervals. Care was taken to maintain good aeration of the animal, good circulation, and to avoid subpial hemorrhages in the cerebellar cortex.

Seizure induction was accomplished via biphasic pial surface 40 to 60/second biphasic electrical pulses ranging between 60 and 90 volts applied to various cerebral sensory and motor areas (see legends of figures for additional details). Side by side stereotaxic electrodes were oriented into the posterior hippocampus and 5 to 20 volts at 50 to 100 pulses per second were used to induce seizure discharges. In all cases, we attempted to limit stimulation to 5 seconds in order to have seizures which consistently endured for an average of 30 seconds. This is an essential requirement if seizure shortening times are being measured. In addition, we have found that long enduring seizures (over two minutes) are difficult to stop by cerebellar stimulation and indeed early death of the animal can result.

Four groups of cerebellar stimulations were used: a) 8-12 per second, and b) 150-300 per second biphasic pulses applied to cerebellar cortex, c) 8-12 per second and d) 150-300 per second biphasic pulses applied to a cerebellar nucleus, usually nucleus fastigii. From 0.5 to 3.0 milliamperes applied for 5 seconds were used. The usual value was 2.0 ($\pm$ 0.5) milliamperes. Higher values were commonly employed on cortical as compared with nuclear areas. Care was taken to remove dura mater from the area being stimulated and control stimulations were applied to such nearby structures as occipital lobe, tectum, and regions around the fourth ventricle in order to monitor for unwanted spread of current.

In all cases of depth recordings, for example, in diencephalic structures and depth stimulations, for example in cerebellar nuclei and hippocampus, histological verification of electrode sites were made via Nissl stained sections.

RESULTS

The following data have been taken from young adult <u>Macaca</u> mulatta monkeys of both sexes. In each figure the prestimulatory records are
shown on the left, then 5 seconds of electrical stimulations are given to
either the hippocampus (Hipp.) or the pial surface of the cerebral hemisphere (CBR) (not shown) then 4 to 5 seconds of seizure activity is shown.
If no cerebellar stimulation is used the record is labelled "O" or "NO";
however, if the cerebellar cortex or nucleus is stimulated, the 5 second
interval is labelled "CBL". If the record is too long to include conven-
iently in an illustration, then the removed area is labelled (-10 sec,
example).

Figure 1 shows representative tracings taken from thalamic nuclei
before, during and after a seizure which was triggered by electrical
stimulation of the hippocampus. Such seizures tend to show more high
voltage fast activity (12 to 15/sec) in the initial phases than do seizures
triggered by neocortical stimulation. In the later phases there is an increased amount of high voltage 4 to 6 per second slow waves. In this
experiment the recording site in the caudal part of ventralis lateralis
showed higher voltage activity than that in the cephalic part, although
this is not always the case. It has not been possible to record seizure
activity in one part of nucleus ventralis without finding it throughout although there is considerable variability in amplitude. The fact that the
post seizure record after cerebellar stimulation and after spontaneous seizure stoppage resembles the preseizure one may be one indication that the
mechanisms involved are similar.

Figure 2 shows recordings taken from a different animal but from
similar recording sites to those shown in Figure 1 before, during and after
seizure activity induced by electrical stimulation of neocortex. The 2 to
3 per second slow waves, usually more than 100 microvolts in amplitude
and occasionally accompanied by spikes are characteristic of these types of
discharges. This record was taken 8 hours after the start of the experiment
and shows more slow waves in the pre- and post-stimulatory periods than
is usually found. However, there were prompt alterations of the discharges
associated with bilateral fastigial stimulation without selective influences on
nucleus ventralis lateralis when compared with ventralis anterior and ventralis posterior.

Figure 3 illustrates some influences of stimulation of cerebellar cortex on seizure activity in cerebral cortex and ventral nuclei of thalamus.
As shown in series B tracings the seizure continued for 23 seconds before

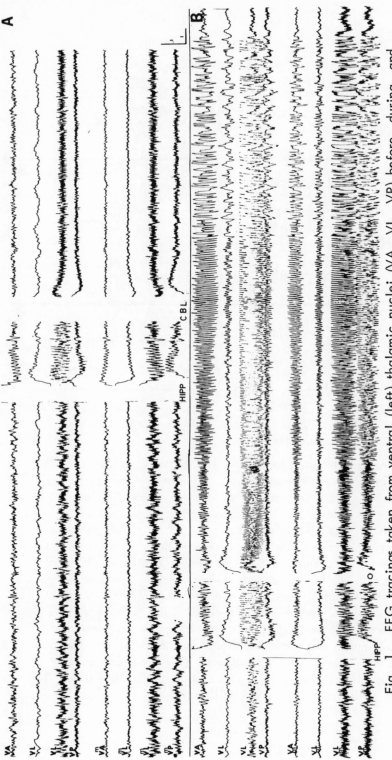

Fig. 1. EEG tracings taken from ventral (left) thalamic nuclei (VA, VL, VP) before, during, and after electrically induced seizure (9 volts, 40/second for 5 seconds) discharges were produced by stimulation of left hippocampus (HIPP). Both monopolar (m) and bipolar recordings were used to obtain data on animal under Flaxedil medication. In series B the seizure discharges continued for 35 seconds before stopping spontaneously. However, if the nucleus fastigii (CBL) is stimulated (8 per second 0.8 milliampere for 5 seconds) bilaterally the seizure activity is stopped within the 5 second period of stimulation. Calibration values: Horizontal = 1 second, Vertical = 0.1 Millivolt.

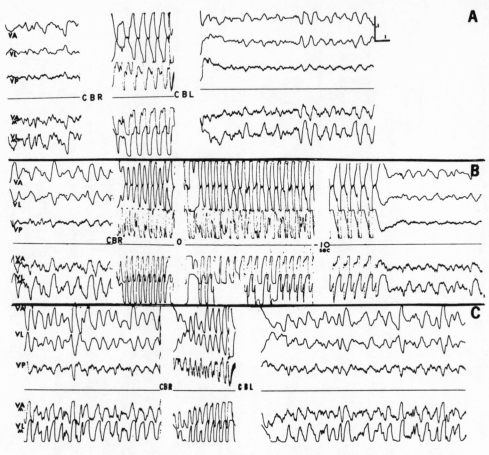

Fig. 2.   EEG tracings taken from left ventral thalamic nuclei (VA, VL, VP) of monkey under Flaxedil medication.   Bipolar and monopolar (m) recording was used.   Prestimulatory, stimulatory and poststimulatory trac- ings are shown.   In series A, B, C seizure activity was induced by elec- trical stimulation of (CBR) left precentral gyrus at 60 pulses per second with 65 volts for 5 seconds.   Series B represents the control records since the cerebellum was not stimulated and the seizure continued (10 seconds of record removed. -10) for 20 seconds before stopping spontaneously. In series A the nuclei fastigii were stimulated bilaterally at 10 pulses per second with 0.8 milliamperes for 5 seconds (CBL) and the seizure activity disappeared.   In series C the nuclei fastigii were stimulated bilaterally at 300 pulses per second with 1.0 milliamperes for 5 seconds (CBL) and there was seizure stoppage although there was considerable slowing in the poststimulatory period.   Horizontal calibration line = 1.0 second, vertical calibration line = 0.1 millivolt.

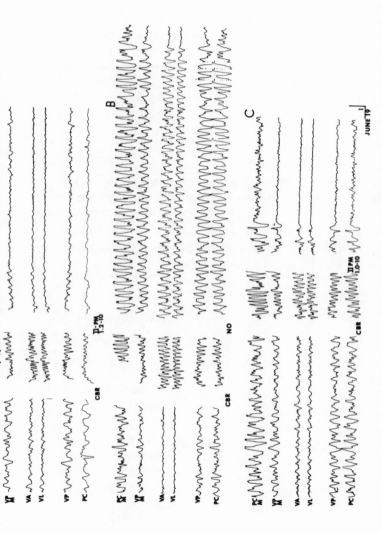

Fig. 3. EEG tracings taken from left postcentral gyrus (PCm and PC) and left ventral thalamic nuclei (VA, VL, VP) before, during and after seizure stoppage. The left area 6 and 4 were surgically removed five months previous. For 5 seconds (CBR) 75 volts (50/second) were applied to left temporal lobe to induce seizure activity. As shown in series B the seizure lasted for 23 seconds before stopping spontaneously. By comparison series A shows that the seizure can be stopped (questionable post central gyrus) within 5 seconds by applying 1.2 milliamperes at 10 pulses per second to left crus II – paramedian lobule. Series C shows that 1.0 milliamperes (at 10/second) will stop the seizure within 2 seconds. Not shown in this series is the observation that 2% Xylocaine locally applied blocks the effects of cerebellar stimulation. Horizontal calibration line = 1 second; vertical line = 0.1 millivolt.

stopping spontaneously. On the other hand (see series A) if the left posterior cerebellum (bipolar-medial crus II to anterior paramedian lobule) was electrically stimulated for 5 seconds with 1.2 milliamperes (10 biphasic pulses per second) the abnormal activity disappeared except for some questionable slow waves in the left postcentral gyrus. When the stimulating current was reduced from 1.2 to 1.0 milliamperes (see series C) the seizure activity lasted about three seconds longer. When such small stimulating currents are used, there is no evidence of unwanted representative spread to adjacent tissues. Additional precautions were taken by surgically removing the nearby dura and applying for 10 seconds a cotton pellet soaked with 2% Xylocaine to the area and blocking the cerebellar influence. Forty minutes later suppression of seizure activity could be obtained by crus II paramedian stimulation although the threshold had increased by almost 20%.

Figure 4 gives additional support to the concept that cerebellar activation can suppress seizure activity activated by electroshock to the cerebrum. In this series A tracing 10/second pulses (2.6 milliamperes) for 5 seconds applied to caudal folia of anterior lobe stops seizure activity which as shown in the control series B tracings would have continued for 22 seconds. These records with anterior lobe stimulation are to be compared with those shown in Figure 3 which were obtained following posterior lobe stimulations.

DISCUSSION

The foregoing experiments indicate that under these experimental conditions, electrical excitation of either the cerebellar nuclei or cortex can either alter or stop seizure discharges which have been initiated in the neocortex or hippocampus by overt electrical stimulation. The term "seizure discharge" is arbitrarily defined as: abnormal repetitive discharges, both spontaneous and induced, which show marked alterations in the amplitude, frequency and wave form. If the animal is lightly anesthetized and not medicated with a curare-like drug there are prominent periodic muscular contractions resembling the so-called convulsive contractions observed in man during a clinically diagnosed grand mal episode. The periodic slow waves resemble those described by Gibbs and Gibbs (1952) as characteristic of grand mal epilepsy. Nevertheless, it is emphasized that we are reporting upon electrical activity and not clinical epilepsy in the monkey.

This study on the monkey is a continuation of the earlier research by

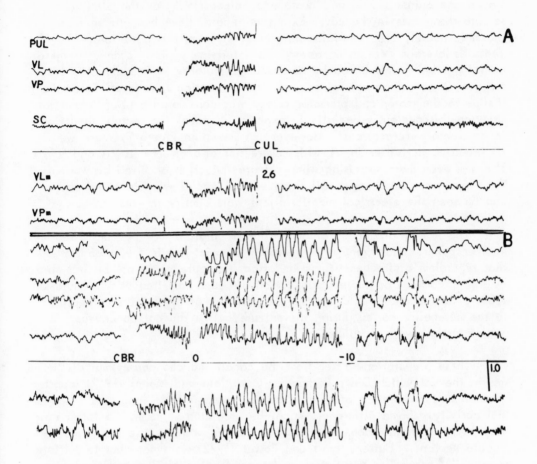

Fig. 4. EEG tracings taken from left pulvinar (PUL), ventralis lateralis (VL), ventralis posterior (VP) and superior colliculus (SC) of monkey under ether and Flaxedil medication. Both monopolar (m) and bipolar recordings were made of preseizure, seizure and postseizure activity. The seizures were induced by applying 70 volts, 50 pulses per second to left postcentral-superior temporal gyri (CBR). As shown in control series B the seizure continued for 22 seconds before stopping spontaneously. Series A records show that 10/second pulses (2.6 milliamperes) applied for 5 seconds to posterior folia of culmen (CUL) stop the seizure discharges. Horizontal calibration line = 1 second; vertical line = 0.1 millivolt.

Cooke and Snider (1955) and Iwata and Snider (1959) on the alteration of seizure discharges in the cat. Extensive records have been taken from thalamic nuclei, i.e. ventralis anterior (VA), ventralis posterior (VP) and ventralis lateralis (VL) in an attempt to determine which, if any, of these nuclei are being influenced by cerebellar stimulation. The almost univer- sal acceptance of an extensive cerebellar projection to ventralis lateralis thence to the motor and premotor cortex was considered a prior reason for studying this nucleus especially in experiments involving seizure induction in the sensory-motor areas. However, as shown in Figure 2, there were no selective activities in VL which were not also present in VA and VP. This was even more surprising when seizure induction occurred by way of the hippocampus. Clearly, all three ventral nuclei were involved and as can be seen the electrical manifestations were similar in each area.

The role of frequency of cerebellar stimulation will be considered in another paper. However, it is desirable to point out in the present study that regardless of frequency of stimulation a seizure could not be initiated by either cortical or nuclear stimulation although fast frequency stimulation (100 to 300/second) would prolong the duration of the seizure if applied to the cerebellar cortex during the seizure. This did not occur when the nuclei fastigii were stimulated.

These preparations differ from the cobalt induced paroxysmal dischar- ges in the cat which Dow, Fernández-Guardiola and Manni (1967) reported upon in that stimulation of midline cortex could initiate long runs of abnor- mal activity. Some differences might be predicted since in the latter case very little is known about membrane alterations which cause the hyperex- citable neurons. Hutton, Frost and Foster (1972) were not able to initiate seizures by cerebellar stimulation following focal penicillin application to the cerebral cortex and in unpublished work we have never been able to initiate seizures following focal penicillin treatment except near the end of a long experiment when there are evidences of cerebellar deterioration.

These results cannot be due to unwanted spread of current to brain stem structures because: 1) The dura mater was always removed from the site of stimulation and the area flooded with warm mineral oil. 2) Per- iodically, adjacent structures such as occipital lobe, dura mater, tectum and dorsal surface of brain stem were stimulated electrically to determine the effects of such stimulation. 3) Insulating material, such as used photo- graphic acetate, was inserted between cerebellum and tectum or caudal brain stem when spurious activity was suspected. 4) Movement of face or neck musculature is such a common sign of current spread that I am sur- prised it is not used oftener. 5) Currents used for fastigial stimulation were not high enough to spread to brain stem as shown by deliberate deeper placement of the stimulating electrode to control for the effects.

The distinct suppression and stoppage of cerebral and thalamic seizure activity in the monkey by cerebellar stimulation has strong and consistent support from previous studies. Cooke and Snider (1955) made similar observations on the cat. Iwata and Snider (1959) were able to stop hippocampal seizures by cerebellar stimulation. Kreindler (1962) arrested penicillin induced cortical spikes by paleocerebellar activation. Dow, Fernandez-Guardiola and Manni (1962) were able to alter cobalt induced seizure discharges in the rat by cerebellar stimulation, but Reimer et al (Reimer, Grimm, & Dow, 1967) had difficulty doing so in the cat. Mutani, Bergamini and Donguzzi (1967) stopped cobalt induced rhinencephalic seizures in unrestrained cats by electrical stimulation of caudal anterior lobe. Hutton, Frost and Foster (1972) were able to suppress penicillin cortical focal discharges by vermal stimulation. And even more recently seizure control by cerebellar stimulation has been extended to man by Cooper et al (Cooper & Gilman, 1973).

The mechanisms involved in such a prominent effect appear to be more complex than had been indicated by our earlier work. Iwata and Snider (1959) in studies on hippocampal seizures were impressed by the post seizure activation-like patterns which occurred after threshold stimulation of the cerebellum and suggested that the reticular activating system might be desynchronizing the slow wave discharges but such patterns are not always seen. Eccles and associates (Eccles, Ito, & Szentagothai, 1967) in the past decade have emphasized the prominent inhibition which Purkinje cells exercise on efferent systems but there is widespread agreement that this means inhibition of cerebellar nuclear excitation to projections to thalamus, ascending reticular formation and diencephalic tegmentum. The present work shows that there is no selective action on the ventral nucleus of the thalamus. Nevertheless, the pharmacological studies of Julien and Halpern (1972) clearly implicate increased Purkinje cell discharges with seizure suppression and the recent single unit study by Mitra and Snider (1973) shows an unequivocal increase in Purkinje cell discharges during the early stage of penicillin focal cortical activity but not in the late stage when the seizures become generalized and cannot be stopped by cerebellar stimulation. At present, it appears that we have to accept the phenomenon and believe that we can resolve in the future the mechanisms whereby it is accomplished.

SUMMARY

A short review is given of the relevant literature related to cerebellar influences on seizure discharges in higher centers.

Electrical stimulation of the cerebellar cortex or nuclei can shorten and/or stop seizure discharges initiated in the cerebrum of monkey by electroshock.

Electrically induced cerebral seizures in the monkey have spread to and involved the ventral thalamic nuclei can also be stopped by cerebellar stimulation. Such abnormal discharges resemble those seen in the cortex and stop simultaneously with them.

It is proposed that the well known inhibitory functions of the cerebellum can be recruited by electrical stimulation for the control of abnormal cerebral and thalamic paroxysms and that there is substantial basic neuroscience data which can be used for extending the studies to the human.

REFERENCES

BROOKHART, J.M., MORUZZI, G., & SNIDER, R.S. Origin of cerebellar waves. J. Neurophys. 14:181-190, 1951.

COHEN, D., HOUSEPIAN, E.M., & PURPURA, D.P. Intrathalamic regulation of activity in a cerebello-cortical projection pathway. Exp. Neurol. 6:492-506, 1962.

COOKE, P.M. & SNIDER, R.S. Some cerebellar influences on electrically induced cerebral seizures. Epilepsia (Amst) 4:19-28, 1955.

COOPER, I.S. & GILMAN, S. The effect of chronic cerebellar stimulation upon epilepsy in man. 98th Annual Meeting, American Neurological Association, July 11-13, 1973, Montreal.

del CERRO, M.P. & SNIDER, R.S. Studies in Dilantin intoxication. I. Ultrastructural analogies with the lipoidoses. Neurology, 17: 452-462, 1967.

del CERRO, M.P. & SNIDER, R.S. Cerebellar alterations resulting from dilatnin intoxication: An ultrastructural study. In Fields, W. & Willis, Jr., W. (Eds.) "The Cerebellum in Health and Disease". St. Louis: W.H. Green, 1972.

DOW, R.S., FERNANDEZ-GUARDIOLA, A., & MANNI, E. The influence of the cerebellum on experimental epilepsy. Electroenceph. Clin. Neurophysiol. 14:383-398, 1962.

ECCLES, J.C., ITO, M., & SZENTAGOTHAI, J. "The Cerebellum as
    a Neuronal Machine". New York: Springer-Verlag, 1967.
FANARDJIAN, V.V. & DONHOFFER, H. An electrophysiological study
    of cerebello-hippocampal relationships in the unrestrained cat.
    Acta Physiol. Acad. Sc. Hung. 24:321-333, 1963-4.
FOX, S.S., LIEBESKIND, J.C., OBRIEN, J.H., & DINGLE, R.
    Mechanisms for limbic modification of cerebellar and cortical
    afferent information. Prog. Br. Res. 27:254-280, 1967.
GIBBS, F.A. & GIBBS, E.L. "Atlas of Electroencephalography Vol. II".
    Cambridge: Addison-Wesley Press, 1952.
HENNEMAN, E.M., COOKE, P., & SNIDER, R.S. Cerebellar projec-
    tions to the cerebral cortex. Res. Publ. Ass. Nerv. Ment. Dis.
    30:317-333, 1950.
HUTTON, J.T., FROST, J., & FOSTER, J. The influence of the
    cerebellum in cat penicillin epilepsy. Epilepsia (Amst) 13:401-
    408, 1972.
IWATA, K. & SNIDER, R.S. Cerebello-hippocampal influences on the
    electroencephalogram. Electroenceph. Clin. Neurophysiol. 11:
    439-446, 1959.
JULIEN, R.M. & HALPERN, L. Effects of diphenylhydantoin and other
    antileptic drugs on epileptiform activity and Purkinje cell discharge
    rates. Epilepsia (Amst) 13:387-400, 1972.
KOKENGE, R., KUTT, H., & McDOWELL, F. Neurological sequelae
    following Dilantin overdose in a patient and in experimental anim-
    als. Neurology, 15:823-829, 1965.
KREINDLER, A. Active arrest mechanisms of epileptic seizures.
    Epilepsia, 3:329-337, 1962.
MERRITT, H.H. & PUTNAM, T. Sodium diphenyl hydantoinate: Toxic
    symptoms and their prevention. Arch. Neurl, Psych. 42:1053-
    1064, 1939.
MITRA, J. & SNIDER, R.S. Cerebellar modification of unitary dischar-
    ges in auditory system. Exp. Neurol. 23:341-352, 1969.
MITRA, J. & SNIDER, R.S. Effects of cerebral seizure activity on
    single unit activity in cerebellum. Fed. Proc. 32:420, 1973.
MUTANI, R., BERGAMINI, L., & DONGUZZI, T. Experimental
    evidence for the existence of an extrarhinencephalic control of the
    activity of the cobalt rhinencephalic epileptogenic focus. Effects
    of the paleocerebellar stimulation. Epilepsia, 10:351-362, 1967.
PRESCOTT, J.W. Early somatosensory deprivation as an ontogenetic
    process in the abnormal development of the brain and behavior.
    2nd Conf. on Exp. Medicine. New York: S. Karger, 1971.
REIMER, G.R., GRIMM, R., DOW, R.S. Effects of cerebellar stimulation
    on cobalt induced epilepsy in the cat. Electroenceph. Clin.
    Neurophysiol. 23:456-462, 1967.

RUCCI, F.S., GIRETTI, M., & La ROCCA, M. Cerebellum and hyper-
    baric oxygen. Electroenceph. Clin. Neurophysiol. 25:359-371,
    1968.
SNIDER, R.S. & STOWELL, A. Evidence of a projection of the optic
    system to the cerebellum. Anat. Rec. 82:448-449, 1942.
SNIDER, R.S. & STOWELL, A. Receiving areas of the tactile, auditory
    and visual systems in the cerebellum. J. Neurophys. 7:331-357,
    1944.
SNIDER, R.S., SATO, K., & MIZUNO, S. Cerebellar influences on
    evoked cerebral responses. J. Neurol. Sci. 1:325-339, 1964.
SNIDER, R.S. & WETZEL, N. Electroencephalographic changes induced
    by stimulation of the cerebellum of man. Electroenceph. Clin.
    Neurophysiol. 18:176-183, 1965.
SNIDER, R.S., MITRA, J., & SUDILOVSKY, A. Cerebellar effects on
    the cerebrum: A microelectrical analysis of somatosensory cortex.
    Int. J. Neurol. 7:141-151, 1970.
SNIDER, R.S. & SINIS, S. Cerebellar influences on cerebral units in
    visual cortex. Exp. Neurol. 39:449-460, 1973.
UTTERBACK, R., OJEMAN, R., & MALEK, J. Parenchymatous cerebel-
    lar degeneration with Dilantin intoxication. J. Neuropath. Exp.
    Neurol. 17:516-521, 1958.
WHITESIDE, J.A. & SNIDER, R.S. Relation of cerebellum to upper
    brain stem. J. Neurophys. 16:397-413, 1953.
WOODBURY, D.M. Mechanisms of action of anticonvulsants. In
    Jasper, H., Ward, A., & Pope, A. (Eds.) "Basic Mechanisms of
    the Epilepsies". New York: Little Brown & Co., 1969.

CHANGES IN SPONTANEOUS NEURONAL FIRING IN CEREBELLUM RED NUCLEUS AND RAPHE NUCLEAR COMPLEX DURING CONVULSIVE ACTIVITY

Augusto Fernández-Guardiola, Carlos M. Contreras, Jose M. Calvo, Fructuoso Ayala, Simon Brailowsky, Hugo Solis, and Alfonso Salgado

Instituto de Investigaciones Biomedicas, U.N.A.M. Ciudad Universitaria, Mexico 20, D.F.

It has been shown in experimental epilepsy models that the concomitant cortical and subcortical recordings of a tonico-clonic seizure reveal fast activities which develop at the end of the clonic phase and persist during electrocortical postcritical "silence". In regard to the significance of these subcortical activities at the end of the seizure, and due to the fact that they have often been considered as "propagation" of the cortical convulsive activities to subcortical structures (Fig. 1) a doubt arises as to the accuracy of this assumption.

Though we do not deny the subcortical propagation of clonic waves, we have postulated that the subcortical rhythmic rapid activities mentioned before and recorded in the Cerebellum, Nucleus Ruber, Ventral Reticular formation and Raphe Nuclei, reflect a progressive inhibitory process which acts upwards and downwards, and is responsible for the seizure arrest. Hypotheses aducing that neuronal fatigue is mainly responsible for the seizure arrest were refuted first by Rosenblueth and Cannon (1942) and recently by Caspers et al. (Caspers & Speckmann, 1972) who concluded that the degrees of hypoxia and hypercapnia found during prolonged convulsive activity do not reach the critical levels enough to depress it.

Efforts directed to the topographic localization of depressor mechanisms have included structures as the nucleus caudatus (Jung, 1949; Gastaut et al., 1959; la Grutta et al., 1971); the mesencephalic reticular formation (Arduini & Lairy-Bounes, 1952; Lairy-Bounes, Parma, & Zanchetti, 1952;

19

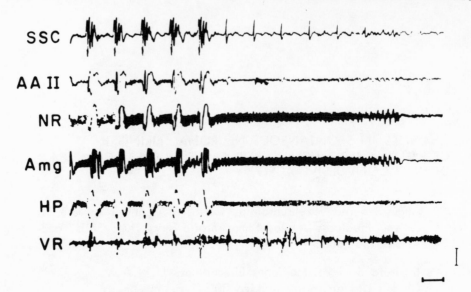

Fig. 1. Clonic Phase and Seizure Arrest - SSC, Sensory Motor Cortex; AA II, Secondary Auditory Area; NR, Nucleus Ruber; Amg., Amygdala; Hp., Hippocampus; VR, Spinal Monosynaptic Reflex recorded in a lumbar ventral root. Curarized Cat.

Fernandez-Guárdiola, Alcaraz, & Guzman-Flores, 1956, 1961; Fernández-Guardiola, Okujava, & Guma, 1968) and the cerebellum (Snider & Cooke, 1954; Dow, Fernández-Guardiola, & Manni, 1962a, b; Dow, 1965; Fernández-Guardiola, Manni, & Wilson, 1962; Raimer, Grimm, & Dow, 1967). The Red Nucleus (RN) receives important connections coming from the cerebellum that have been thoroughly studied (Massion, 1967; Bachman & Choh-Luh-Li, 1969; King, Schwyn, & Fox, 1971). On the other hand, the electrical stimulation of RN induces inhibition of the spinal intrinsic electrical activity (Appelberg, 1962; Appelberg & Kosary, 1963). The spinal monosynaptic reflex (SMR) is a good index of spinal excitability and may be modified by spinal and supra spinal influences. These facilitatory or inhibitory influences are reflected by the amplitude of the monosynaptic reflex. During the convulsive activity induced by cortical stimulation, facilitatory and inhibitory processes are developed in the Central Nervous System. These processes are not limited to the stimulated area, but they influence other brain structures determining the temporal course and propagation of the seizures.

Fernández-Guardiola et al. (Fernández-Guardiola, Alcaraz, & Gus-
mán-Flores, 1961; Fernández-Guardiola, Muñoz-Martinez, & Velasco,
1964; Fernández-Guardiola & Ayala, 1971) studied the temporal development of spinal facilitation and inhibition during convulsive activity, establishing the relationship between the monosynaptic reflex amplitude and the
different phases of seizures (Fig. 2). The electrical activity of several
subcortical structures was simultaneously analyzed. In all the experiments
a depression of the monosynaptic reflex amplitude was observed, which
coincided with the end of the seizure and the electrocortical "silence".
During the clonic period of the seizure, the facilitation and inhibition of
the monosynaptic reflex took place. The greatest facilitation was present
20 milliseconds after the peak of clonic wave (Fig. 3) and a more

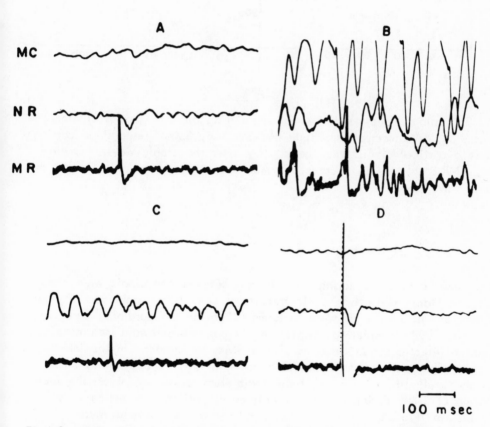

Fig. 2. MR, Spinal Monosynaptic Recording; NR, Nucleus Ruber; MC,
Motor Cortex – A, control; B, generalized seizure; C, seizure arrest;
D, recovery phase. Notice the maximal depression of MR and the con-
comitant fast sinusoidal activity in NR.

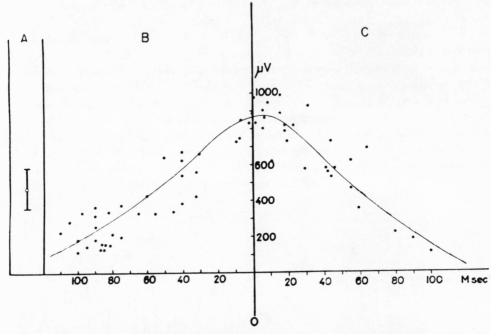

Fig. 3. Spinal monosynaptic variability during the last periods of clonic phase. A, SMR control amplitude and SD. B, Spinal responses occurring before a cortical clonic wave peak. C, after the clonic wave. Ordinates, SMR amplitude in microvolts. Abcissae, time in msec. O marks the clonic wave peak.

conspicuous inhibition, during the intervals between the clonic waves and during the tonic phase of the electrocortical convulsive discharge. Partial sections of the brain stem were performed (Fernandez-Guardiola, Okujava, & Guma, 1968) in order to investigate the possible pathways mediating the effects of electrocortical seizures on the SMR, as recorded in the intact animal. The results showed that in animals in which the pyramids were sectioned, all other structures of the brain stem remaining intact; the facilitation of SMR during seizure as well as its postictal depression were still present (Fig. 4). On the other hand, when the pyramids were left intact (Fig. 5), and a section of the remaining brain stem was performed, no postictal depression of SMR was observed and only a slight facilitation was present during the clonic phase of the seizure. These results demonstrate that the inhibitory descending influences which appear at the final

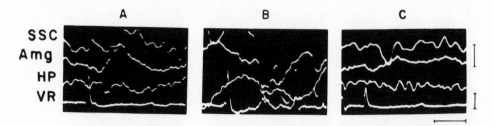

Fig. 4. Sectioned pyramids. Intact Brain-stem. A, control; B, clonic phase; C, seizure arrest; SSC, Sensory-motor cortex; Amg. Amygdala; Hp. hippocampus; VR, spinal monosynaptic reflex.

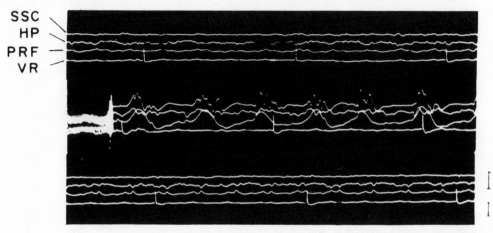

Fig. 5. Sectioned brain stem. Intact pyramids. SSC, sensory motor cortex; Hp, hippocampus; PRF, Pontine reticular formation; VR, spinal monosynaptic reflex.

stages of a seizure and during its extinction are mediated by extrapyramidal pathways, most probably throughout the rubro spinal bundle.

As we have shown, the maximal inhibition of SMR occurs during the interclonic intervals. The recording during these periods of nucleus ruber's activity shows the increasing frequency and amplitude of the sinusoidal characteristic activity of this structure. Figure 6 shows this relationship; the enhancement of recruiting activity in NR during the longest interclonic intervals is significant. A similar relationship of enhanced activity and cortical depression was observed in the cerebellum, both in anoxia and megimide or electrically induced seizures in the rat (Fernandez-Guardiola, Manni, & Wilson, 1962). The above mentioned results seem

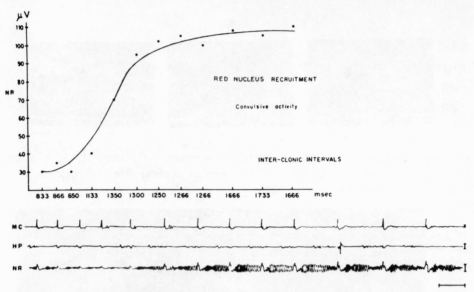

Fig. 6. Last stages of clonic activity. Ordinates, RN discharge amplitude; Abcisae, interclonic-intervals in milliseconds. MC, motor cortex; Hp., hippocampus; NR. nucleus ruber. Notice the increasing frequency and amplitude in NR.

to reaffirm the hypothesis of an inhibitory role of the cerebellum and Red Nucleus upon convulsive activity.

Other experiments of lesion procedures have also been conclusive in this respect. Both lesions or reversible inactivation of the cerebellum enhanced seizures in cobalt epileptic rats (Dow, Fernández-Guardiola, & Manni, 1962a). Cats with chronic partial lesions of the cerebellum and bilaterally NR lesionated cats which survived for more than one year, showed a significant lowering of photometrazolic threshold (Fig. 7). These animals, particularly the NR lesionated, had spontaneous myoclonic jerks and persistent alterations of muscle tonus. When long lasting EEG recordings were done for these lesionated animals, a noticeable diminution of REM phase of sleep was observed. It was very tempting to correlate the low threshold for convulsions with the REM deprivation since it has been repeatedly demonstrated that REM deprived animals can develop convulsive states. On the other hand, the fast subcortical activity concomitant with spinal monosynaptic reflex depression detected in rombencephalic structures, and progressively developing at the end of clonic activity, is manifested in other circumstances, particularly in anoxia and in the REM phase of sleep.

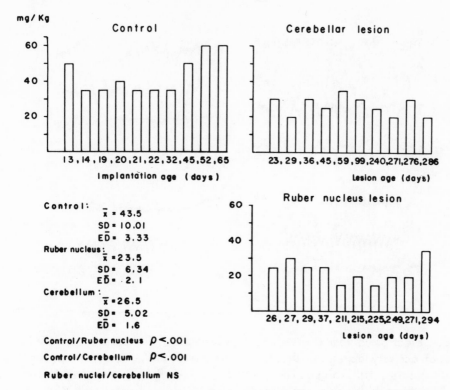

Fig. 7. Effect of cerebellar and N. Ruber lesions on the photometrazolic convulsive threshold.

Keeping in mind the facts mentioned before, we performed experiments in order to look for other signs of REM phase of sleep, namely,
neck and jaw muscle tonus depression and Rapid Eye Movements (REMs)
appearing in the late periods of clonic activity. The results were clearcut. The neck depression of the muscle tonus was maximal, REMs similar
to those described during the paradoxical or REM phase of sleep were
developed. Both phenomena, the muscle tonus depression and REMs coincided with the increased activity in the cerebellar cortex and Red Nucleus
and theta hippocampal discharges. These results observed during the extinction of a long generalized seizure are illustrated in Figures 8 and 9.
In other experiments we recorded the sleep phases in the chronic implanted
cat, before and after experimental convulsions. As expected, and due to
the appearance of prolonged REM signs at the end of the clonic phase,
the post convulsive sleep was REM deprived. The cat sleeps in slow waves
(SW) phase during a long period that lasts depending on the strength and
duration of the seizure (Fig. 10).

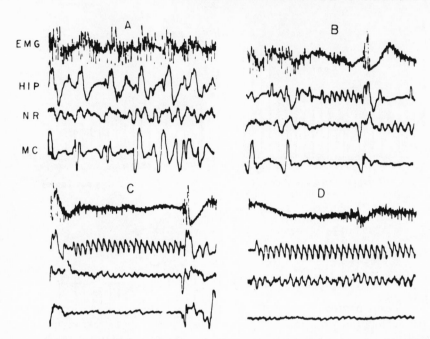

Fig. 8. Electromyogram depression, hippocampal theta activity and RN sinusoidal activity appearing during seizure arrest EMG, electoymyogram of neck muscles; HIP, hippocampus; NR, Nucleus Ruber, MC, motor cortex. Low encéphale-isolé cat's preparation.

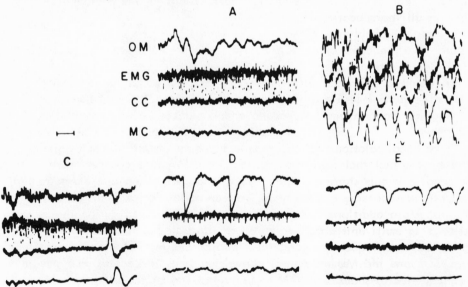

Fig. 9. Electromyogram depression, REMs and cortical cerebellar activation appearing during seizure arrest. OM, Ocular movements; EMG, electromyogram; CC, cerebellar cortex, MC, motor cortex.

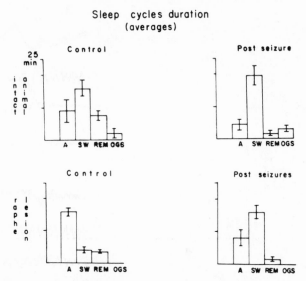

Fig. 10. Sleep phases distribution histograms of the cat of intact animal and raphe lesionated animals before and after electrically induced seizures. A, awakening periods; SW, slow wave sleep; REM, paradoxical sleep; OGS, occipito-geniculate spiking phases.

One of the subcortical structures more closely related to the sleep mechanisms is probably the Raphe nuclear complex. These nuclei receive afferents from the deep cerebellar nuclei (fastigii, dentate and interpositus) N. reticularis lateralis, the olive, vestibular nucleus and sensory motor cortex; and send efferents to the nucleus ruber and cerebellum (Brodal, 1960). The partial lesion of Raphe also results in a lowering of convulsive threshold both in acute (short-term) and in chronic cats (Fig. 11).

Functional relationships between Raphe and nucleus Ruber is confirmed by the fact that Raphe destruction induces spontaneous NR activity depression. At this state and judging the available information from the gross activity recording and the lesion experiments, it was considered useful to obtain additional information through microelectrode extracellular recordings of multi unit activity (MUA) of the subcortical structures which show progressive frequency acceleration in the tardive stages of seizures. Figure 12 shows the MUA activity in the red nucleus before and after a convulsant electro-shock applied to the ipsilateral sensory motor cortex (MC). During the clonic phase, the RN MUA activity is depressed, and accelerates again when the interclonic intervals gradually increase.

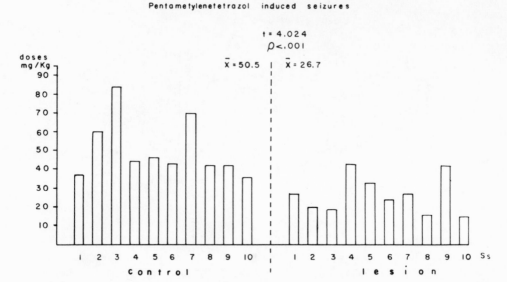

Fig. 11. Lowering of convulsive threshold in Raphe lesionated animals.

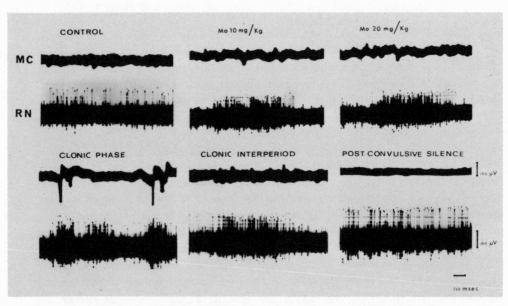

Fig. 12. MUA recording of RN during seizures and seizure arrest.
MC, motor cortex, RN, Nucleus Ruber.

During the seizure arrest these oscillating RN bursts of MUA activity prevail with a recruiting aspect due to the appearance of additional high voltage units discharge.

The Raphe nuclear complex also shows a great variance in relation to the clonic waves and the electrical behavior of these nuclei during seizure arrest displays oscillating bursts with a periodicity similar to the late clonic waves. The periodic oscillating Raphe burst morphology clearly reveals the activation of big sized neurons during the cortical post-seizure silence that were relatively silent in control condition (Fig. 13).

The MUA recorded in the superior olive shows a conspicuous voltage increase with deacceleration of frequency, interrupted by bursts of acceleration noticeable during the seizure arrest (Fig. 14).

The electrical behavior of nucleus Dentatus during seizure was somewhat different from the changes described for RN, Raphe and Olive. The clonic waves appearing in this structure precede the cortical clonic discharges. MUA activity shows a notorious rhythmicity and frequency depression during the seizure (Fig. 15).

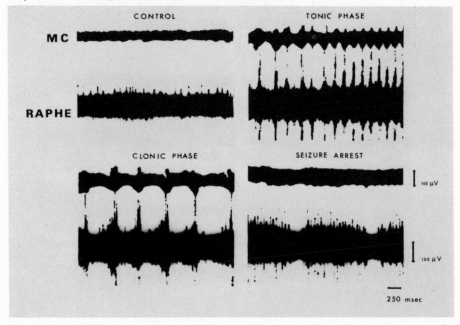

Fig. 13. MUA recording of Raphe nuclear complex during tonic and clonic phases and seizure arrest. Notice the oscillating and recruiting bursts of raphe activity during cortical post-convulsive "silence".

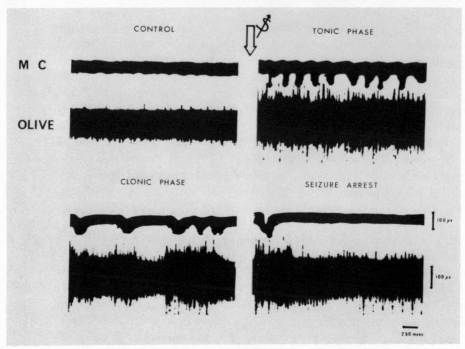

Fig. 14.   MUA recording of superior olive during electrically induced seizures.   MC, motor cortex.

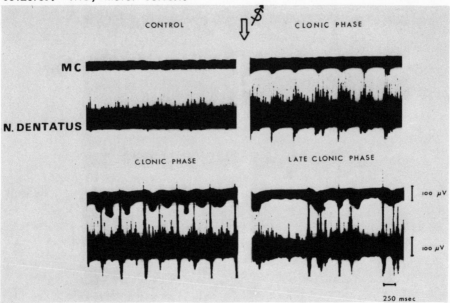

Fig. 15.   MUA activity of nucleus dentatus during electrically induced seizures.   The clonic waves in this structure seem to precede those of the cerebral cortex.   MC, motor cortex.

The MUA activity was processed throughout operational amplifiers and fed to an electronic counter. Frequency was measured every second and frequency distribution hystograms were constructed.

Figure 16 shows the temporal course of frequency changes in motor cortex and subcortical structures in control situation and under somatic stimulation, asphictic anoxia and electrically induced seizures.

Somatic stimulation induces RN frequency enhancement while anoxia effect is more clearly seen in Olive. During the clonic phase of cortical seizure a notorious depression takes place in RN, Olive and Dentatus. During seizure arrest, Dentatus quickly recovers its rhythmicity and Red Nucleus shows its characteristic high frequency bursts activity.

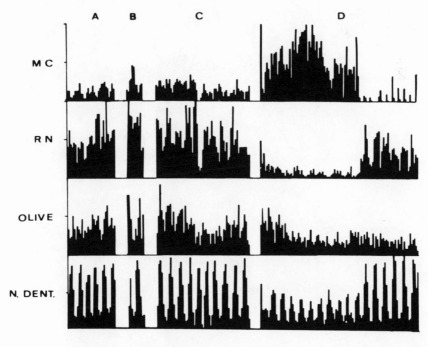

Fig. 16. Standardized frequency distribution histograms of MUA activity of cortical and subcortical structures in control (A), under somatic stimulation (B), under light asphixia (C), and during seizure arrest (D).

The lesion of dentate nucleus in the cat is followed by 50% cell degeneration of the red nucleus (Brodal & Gogstod, 1954). The rubro-cerebellar connections in cats have been shown by Courville and Brodal (1966). Rubro olivar fibres exist and also olivo cerebellar connections. Then a cerebellum-rubro-olivo-cerebellar circuit is structured. This circuit can be activated by the cortico-ponto-cerebellar pathways (Fig. 17). During the development of cortical seizures signals that elicit a continuous and progressively increasing reverberating activity in this circuit, arrive to the cerebellum. This activity is inhibitory in nature and tends to suppress the convulsive activity throughout a feed-back mechanism. In addition to the neurophysiological data we have already exposed, this hypothesis is supported by several facts.

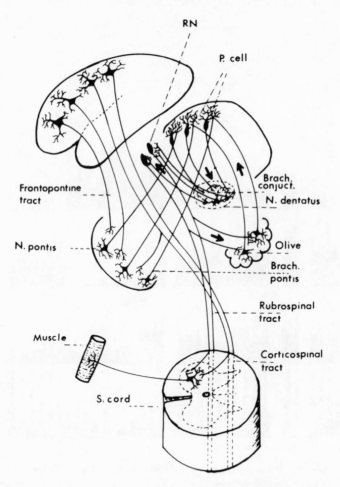

Fig. 17.   Cerebellum-rubro-olivo-cerebellar circuit.

Pharmacological experiments have shown that diphenylhydantoin and phenobarbital administration is followed by MUA acceleration in NR (fig. 18). Julien and Halpern (1972) have shown a similar effect of anticonvulsants on the Purkinje cell discharge in the cerebellar cortex.

The relation between cerebellar lesions and myoclonic epilepsy should also be considered. In addition to the well known dyssinergia – cerebellaris – myoclonica other cerebellar symptoms are found in a substantial number of epileptic patients (Dow & Moruzzi, 1958).

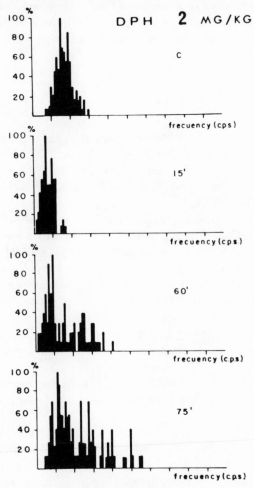

Fig. 18. Standardized frequency distribution histograms of MUA in Nucleus Ruber. Effect of diphenylhydantoin (I.V.). Notice the frequency acceleration and enhancing variance 75 min. after the drug administration.

The postseizure REM diminution is worthy of special discussion. As we have demonstrated, there are signs of REM sleep appearing during the seizure arrest. REM sleep is integrated in rombencephalic structures, probably in locus coeruleus and Raphe nuclear complex.

It is very likely that the subcortical activation in the last stage of seizure and seizure arrest induces a neurotransmitter depletion that is reflected in the peculiar post-seizure sleep phase distribution. Thus, it is postulated that the same neurotransmitter that elicits REM phase of sleep is involved in the general processes of seizure arrest. Bergamasco et al. (Bergamasco, Bergamini, & Mutani, 1967) findings about the lack of paradoxical (REM) phase of sleep in patients suffering from dyssynergia cerebellaris myoclonica support this hypothesis.

REFERENCES

APPELBERG, B. The effect of electrical stimulation of nucleus ruber on the gamma motor system. Acta Physiol. Scand. 55:150–154, 1962.

APPELBERG, B. & KOSARY, I.Z. Excitation of flexor fusimotor neurones by electrical stimulation in the red nucleus. Acta Physiol. Scand. 59:445–453, 1963.

ARDUINI, A. & LAIRY-BOUNES, G.C. Action de la stimulation électrique de la formation réticulaire du bulber et des stimulation sensorielles sur les ondes strychniques corticales chez le chat encéphales isolé. Electroenceph. Clin. Neurophysiol. 4:503–512, 1952.

BACHMAN, D. & CHOH-LUH-LI. The effect of dentate and rubral stimulation on neuronal activity in the nucleus ruber. Exp. Neurol. 23:58–66, 1969.

BERGAMASCO, B., BERGAMINI, L., & MUTANI, R. Spontaneous sleep abnormalities in a case of Dyssynergia cerebellaris myoclonica. Epilepsia, (Amst) 8:271–281, 1967.

BRODAL, A., TABER, E., & WALBERG, F. The Raphe nuclei of the Brain Stem in the cat efferent connections. J. Comp. Neurol. 114:239, 1960.

BRODAL, A. & GOGSTOD, A.C. Rubro-cerebellar connections: An experimental study in the cat. Anat. Rec. 118:455–485, 1954.

CASPERS, N. & SPECKMANN, E.J. Cerebral PO_2 POC_2 and Ph, changes during convulsive activity and their significance for spontaneous arrest of seizures. Epilepsia, (Amst) 13:699–725, 1972.

COURVILLE, J. & BRODAL, A. Rubro-cerebellar connections in the cat. J. Comp. Neurol. 126:471–486, 1966.

DOW, R.S. Extrinsic regulatory mechanisms of seizure activity.
     Epilepsia (Amst.) 6:122–140, 1965.
DOW, R.S., FERNANDEZ-GUARDIOLA, A., & MANNI, E. The in-
     fluence of the cerebellum in experimental epilepsy. Electroenceph.
     Clin. Neurophysiol. 14:383–398, 1962a.
DOW, R.S., FERNANDEZ-GUARDIOLA, A., & MANNI, E. The pro-
     duction of cobalt experimental epilepsy in the rat. Electroenceph.
     Clin. Neurophysiol. 14:399–407, 1962b.
DOW, R.S. & MORUZZI, G. "The Physiology and Pathology of the
     Cerebellum". Minneapolis: University of Minnesota Press, 1958.
FERNANDEZ-GUARDIOLA, A., ALCARAZ, M., & GUZMÁN-FLORES,C. .
     Modificácion de la descarga convulsiva cortical por la estimulacion
     mesencefálica. Boletin del Instituto de Estudios Medicos y Biolog-
     icos. (Mexico) 14:15–21, 1956.
FERNÁNDEZ-GUARDIOLA, A., ALCARAZ, M., & GUZMÁN-FLORES,C.
     Inhibition of convulsive activity by the reticular formation. Acta
     Neurol. Lat. Amer. 7:30–36, 1961.
FERNÁNDEZ-GUARDIOLA, A., MANNI, E., WILSON, J.H., & DOW,
     R.S. Microelectrode recording of cerebellar and cerebral unit ac-
     tivity during convulsive after discharge. Exp. Neurol. 6:48–69,
     1962.
FERNÁNDEZ-GUARDIOLA, A., MUÑOZ-MARTINEZ, F., & VELASCO,M.
     Facilitatory and inhibitory influences on the spinal activity during
     the cortical tonic-clonic post-discharge. Boletin del Instituto de
     Estudios Medicos y Biologicos (Mexico), 22:205–215, 1964.
FERNÁNDEZ-GUARDIOLA, A., OKUJAVA, V.M., & GUMA, E.
     Peripheral and central phenomens of post-epileptic extinction.
     Epilepsia (Amst), 9:303–310, 1968.
FERNANDEZ-GUARDIOLA, A. & AYALA, F. Red nucleus fast activity
     and signs of paradoxical sleep appearing during the extinction of
     experimental seizures. Electroenceph. Clin. Neurophysiol. 30:547–
     555, 1971.
GASTAUT, H. & FISCHER-WILLIAMS, M. The physiopathology of epil-
     eptic seizures. In Field & Magoun (Eds.) "Handbook of Physiology".
     Washington, D.C.: American Physiological Society, 1959, pp. 329–
     363.
JULIEN, R.M. & HALPERN, M.L. Effect of Diphenylhydantoin and
     other antiepileptic drugs on epileptiform activity and Purkinje cell
     discharge rates. Epilepsia (Amst.) 13:387–400, 1972.
JUNG, R. Hirnelektriche Untersuchungen uber den Elektrokrampf., die
     Erregungsablaufe in cortical en Hirnregionen bei Katze und Hund.
     Arch. Psychiat. Nervenkr. 183:206–244, 1949.

KING, J.S., SCHWYN, R.C., & FOX, C.A. The red nucleus in the monkey (Macaca Mulatta): A Golgi and electron microscopic study. J. Comp. Neurol. 142:75-108, 1971.

La GRUTTA, V., AMATO, G., & ZAGUMI, M.T. The importance of the caudate nucleus in the control of convulsive activity in the amygdaloid complex and the temporal cortex of the cat. Electroenceph. Clin. Neurophysiol. 31:57-59, 1971.

LAIRY-BOUNES, G.C., PARMA, M., & ZANCHETTI, A. Modifications pendant la reaction "d'arrest" de Berger de l'activité convulsive produite par l'application locale de strychnine sur le cortex cérébral du lapin. Electroenceph. Clin. Neurophysiol. 4:495-502, 1952.

MASSION, J. The mammalian red nucleus. Physiol. Rev. 47:383-436, 1967.

RAIMER, G.R., GRIMM, R.J., & DOW, R.S. Effects of cerebellar stimulation cobalt induced epilepsy in the cat. Electroenceph. Clin. Neurophysiol. 23:456-462, 1967.

ROSENBLUETH, A. & CANNON, W.B. Cortical responses to electrical stimulation. Amer. J. Physiol. 135:690-741, 1942.

SNIDER, R.S. & COOKE, P.M. Cerebral seizures as influenced by cerebellar stimulation. Trans. Amer. Neurol. Assn. 79:87-89, 1954.

CEREBELLAR INFLUENCES ON THE HIPPOCAMPUS

T. L. Babb, A. G. Mitchell, and P. H. Crandall

Division of Neurological Surgery
UCLA Center for the Health Sciences
Los Angeles, California 90024

INTRODUCTION

The finding of cerebellar influences on forebrain electrical activity was established very early by experiments demonstrating changes in the EEG after cerebellar stimulation (Walker, 1938). That such influences may be largely inhibitory was indicated later by findings that cerebellar stimulation suppressed electrically-induced cortical seizures (Snider & Cooke, 1953), chemically-induced motor cortex epilepsy (Dow, Fernandez-Guardiola, & Manni, 1962; Hutton, Frost, & Foster, 1972), or limbic seizures (Iwata & Snider, 1959; Mutani, Bergamini, & Doriguzzi, 1969; Zaitsev, 1969). Recent findings have indicated a cerebellar site of action for certain anti-convulsants (Julien & Halpern, 1972).

One unanswered question generated by these various studies is which cerebellofugal pathway is involved in these inhibitory influences. Reimer et al. (Reimer, Grimm, & Dow, 1967) tried to answer this question by comparing midline versus hemispheric cerebellar stimulation in cats in order to differentially influence the deep nuclei and hence the efferent path. However, they reported that all the surface stimulations were generally ineffective in blocking the cobalt motor cortex seizure activity. Grimm et al. (Grimm, Frazee, Bell, Kawasaki, & Dow, 1970) found no effect of direct fastigial or dentate stimulation on the average number of cobalt motor cortex spikes in monkeys. On the other hand, Snider and Cooke (1953) have reported cessation of neocortical electrical seizures with fastigial stimulation. Zaitsev (1969) has shown transient interruption of hippocampal seizures with stimulation of nucleus

37

tentorii cerebelli (sic), and Hutton et al. (Hutton, Frost, & Foster, 1972) found that dentate stimulation blocked motor cortex penicillin spikes. In the present study we have used direct electrical stimulation to cerebellar roof nuclei to assess their influence on the cat ventral hippocampus before, during and between cobalt seizures. We have found some evidence which suggests the existence of a fastigiobulbar inhibitory pathway to hippocampus and other evidence which indicates a dentatothalamic excitatory pathway to hippocampus.

In all studies using electrical stimulation of the brain, unintended stimulation of adjacent structures or fibers of passage is a problem that can be only partly managed by controlling voltage and limiting electrode tip exposure. For this reason we have stimulated the nuclear regions to which the cerebellar nuclei project as the first relay in the putative pathway and tested for similarity of action on hippocampus. Hence, the fastigiobulbar pathway, in our experience, involves cells and fibers of the left fastigial nucleus which traverse the resitform body (fasciculus uncinatus) to terminate in the right medial reticular formation of the medulla (nucleus reticularis gigantocellularis). It is known that only about 10-15 per cent of fastigial fibers pass out the brachium conjunctivum (Flood & Jansen, 1966) and a majority of the fibers of the uncinate fasciculus terminate in gigantocellularis (Thomas, Kaufman, Sprague, & Chambers, 1956). The dentatothalamic pathway originates in cells and fibers of the left dentate (lateral) nucleus which project exclusively in the brachium conjunctivum, mostly contralaterally, and terminate in the right ventralis lateralis of the thalamus.

METHOD

Bipolar stimulating and recording electrodes were implanted in 20 adult cats fully anesthetized with sodium pentobarbital (30 mg/kg i.p.). Each electrode was made with two .005 inch diameter stainless steel wires insulated except for 0.5 mm. at the tips which were separated by one mm. All cats were implanted in both somatosensory cortices (Som. Ctx.), both ventral hippocampi (V.Hippo) and right ventralis anterior (V.A.: A 10.5, L 5.5, H 4.5; Snider & Niemer, 1961). A 20 gauge spinal needle was placed in the right ventral hippocampus (A 8.0, L 11.0, H-5.0) to serve as a cannula for injection of a cobalt solution from a 26 gauge microsyringe. Two microliters of a solution of hexahydrate cobalt chloride[1] (2.3 mg per microliter) was sufficient to reliably establish epileptiform activity. Electrical stimuli consisted of biphasic pulses

---

[1] Mallinckrodt Chemical Works

generated by a Grass S-4 stimulator, isolated through a transformer, and
the voltage and current were monitored.   Stimulation was delivered to the
vermis, fastigial nucleus (P 9.0, L 1.5, H + 1.0), nucleus reticularis
gigantocellularis (P 9.0, L 1.5, H - 7.5) or dentate (lateral) nucleus
(P 8.0, L 7.0, H - 0.5) and ventralis lateralis (A 8.5, L 4.7, H + 2.2).

Conventional EEG recordings were taken at least one week after
surgery with the cat suspended in a canvas bag.   Three cats were studied
unrestrained to view all the motor effects of the electrical stimulation as
well as of the cobalt seizures.   Seizure activity was studied for up to 12
hours after cobalt injection and then controlled by anti-convulsants (usually phenobarbital, 10 mg./kg. i.m.).   Several cats were studied the day
after injection while seizures were controlled by phenobarbital.   The cats
were sacrificed with i.p. sodium pentobarbital followed by successive in-
tracarotid perfusion with heparinized normal saline, potassium ferrocyanide,
and 10 per cent formalin.   The fixed brains were cut serially at 40 mic-
rons and stained with cresylviolet or thionin.   The electrode placements
were verified by light microscopy of electrode tracks and the Prussian blue
reaction with iron deposited during stimulation.

RESULTS

Pathophysiology of the Cobalt Hippocampal Epilepsy

The first clinical seizure occurred with an average latency of 90
minutes after injection of 4.6 mg. of cobalt salt.   Focal paroxysmal events occurred as early as 50 minutes after and in some cases EEG flattening was detected as early as 20 minutes after cobalt injection.   In many
cases hippocampal spikes occurred and with time often developed after-
discharges which remained localized to the right hippocampus.   Eventually
these after-discharges developed into the tonic phase of a clinical seizure
which was clearly indicated by bilateral spread to other brain structures
(Fig. 1A) and by behaviors such as "staring", head-turning (tonic phase)
and ear twitching, eye blinking, and masticating (clonic phase as indicated in Fig. 1B).

The average duration of seizures in different animals varied widely
but was somewhat reliable for a given animal for periods as long as two
hours.   Beyond that, seizure severity and its duration in seconds increased
with time.   In Figure 2 is shown the evolution of seizure durations (ordinate) as a function of time elapsed since first seizure (abscissa) in three
unstimulated control cats.   Note that the baseline in all three plots rises;

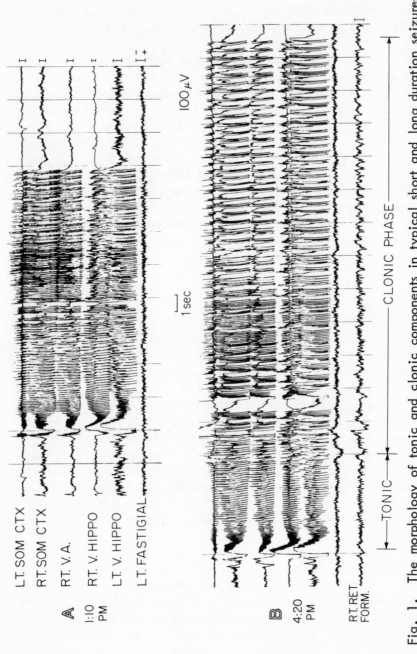

Fig. 1. The morphology of tonic and clonic components in typical short and long duration seizures recorded from the same cat. In A is shown a short 16 second seizure with a tonic phase of a little over 6 seconds. In B, 190 minutes later, the seizure durations are as long as 31 seconds, but the tonic phase remains about 6 seconds long. This indicates that the duration of the clonic phase alone increases with time. (Reprinted from Babb et al. (1974) with permission from the author and publisher).

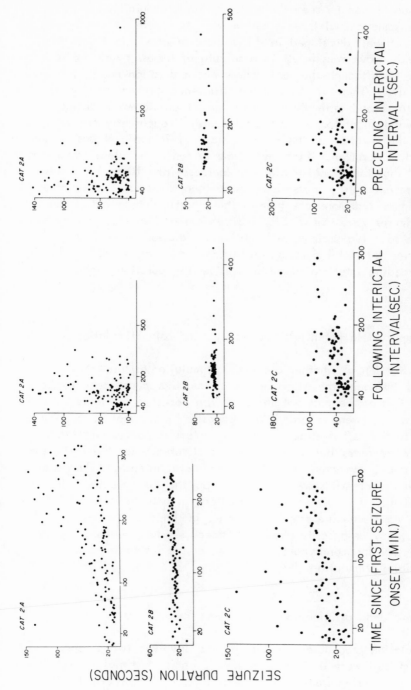

Fig. 2. Two co-ordinate plots are shown based on three unstimulated cats in order to characterize certain features of cobalt hippocampal epilepsy. In the first column, on the left, seizure durations (ordinate) are plotted as a function of time (abscissa). In the middle and right hand columns seizure durations (ordinate) are shown as not reliably related to following interictal interval (middle column) or to preceding interictal interval (right hand column).

although there is a good deal of short-term stability of the seizure durations. In Figure 1 can be seen the different seizure durations which occurred in the same animal three hours apart. In Figure 1A clonic waveforms are not well developed in this second seizure. In Figure 1B pronounced clonic waveforms result in a seizure of almost twice the duration of Figure 1A although the tonic phase has a duration nearly identical to Figure 1A. There is virtually no difference between the two seizures until 16 seconds after onset, when slower clonic waves appear in 1B. The evolution of longer duration seizures is apparently due to a lengthening of the duration of the clonic phases while tonic phases remain relatively fixed in duration. Plots over time of tonic and clonic durations have confirmed that the clonic phase may increase from 10 to 100 times while tonic durations rarely increase by more than three-fold. The other two plots of Figure 2 demonstrate that in these unstimulated controls the durations of seizures were statistically independent of the interictal activity and vice-versa. No positive or negative correlations were found between following interictal duration and seizure duration (middle column) or between preceding interictal duration and seizure duration (right column).

Hippocampal Field Potentials Evoked by Hindbrain Stimulation

As an indication of whether electrical stimulation of hindbrain structures might influence the hippocampus we calculated averaged evoked potentials in a few of the cats not injected with cobalt. In Figure 3, the top pair of potentials were recorded from opposite hippocampi in response to 100 stimuli to the left dentate. There are clear responses, similar to each other in wave-form, but with an ipsilateral latency for the first peak being about 5 msec. compared with the contralateral latency of 11 msec. The bottom pair of potentials were recorded from the same electrode in response to 100 stimuli to either right reticularis gigantocellularis of left fastigial. The waveforms are somewhat similar in shape and latency, with the reticular latency being only about one msec. shorter, which is approximately the latency for monosynaptic EPSPs in bulbar reticular neurons evoked by fastigial stimulation (Ito, Udo, Mano, & Kawai, 1970).

Vermis and Fastigiobulbar Effects on Hippocampus

The stimulation procedures used in all cats involved two phases. In phase one, stimuli were delivered to either vermis, fastigial, or reticular formation at differing frequencies and currents and their effects on

STIM. (0.1 msec 50 μA) IN LT. DENTATE

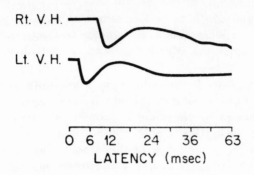

Rt. V. H.

Lt. V. H.

0 6 12   24   36   63
LATENCY (msec)

RECORD FROM RT. V.H.

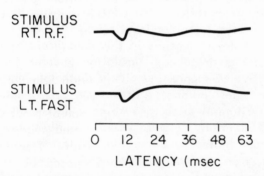

STIMULUS
RT. R.F.

STIMULUS
LT. FAST

0   12   24   36   48   63
LATENCY (msec

Fig. 3. Four averaged field potentials each evoked by 100 stimuli to either left dentate (top two potentials), right bulbar reticular formation (third potential), or left fastigial bottom potential. The top two potentials are recorded from opposite hippocampi while the bottom two potentials are recorded from the same electrode in a different cat. Pulse duration 0.1 msec., current 50μA, 1c/s.

the EEG were observed between or during seizures. From these observations one structure was chosen for repeated stimulation at a given frequency and current in phase two. The timing of onset and duration of all stimuli in both phases were at the discretion of the experimenter and they were given both between and during seizures. Since it was shown earlier that seizure durations tend to increase with time, stimulations in phase two were alternated with periods of no stimulation in order to get statistical estimates of seizure durations and interictal intervals unaffected by brain stimulation. At the end of phase two, average seizure durations and average interictal intervals were computed with or without stimulation in order to determine whether the stimulus effects were statistically reliable.

During phase one tests for stimulus effects on hippocampal seizure activity it was found that stimulation of vermis, fastigial, or reticular formation often coincide with cessation of seizure activity. When it occurred, it was always during the clonic phase, never during the tonic phase, and usually in the later stage of the clonic phase when wave periods were 200 msec. or longer. Figure 4 illustrates this point. Stimulation of the vermis was repeatedly ineffective throughout the seizure until clonic waveforms appeared at a frequency of about four per second.

Figure 5 A, B and C show a variety of instances of apparent seizure cessation due to fastigial or reticular stimulation. Note that a wide range of frequencies have been effective (10 Hz, 45 Hz, 100 Hz). We were not able to study stimulus parameters in this experiment; nevertheless it was our impression that high frequency stimulation (greater than 20 Hz) was generally more effective at suppressing clonic discharges and altering interictal waveforms. In a few instances in the same cats stimulation was followed by the onset of bilateral discharges which were usually anomolous types of seizures of short duration. Figure 5 D and E illustrates two such seizures from the same cat elicited by either high or low frequency reticular stimulation. Other, more typical seizures were observed, though rarely. Despite these occasional findings of epileptogenesis, interictal stimulation of vermis, fastigial, or reticular formation reliably resulted in modification of ongoing hippocampal waveforms, usually a dramatic desynchronization of large slow waves or occasional suppression of focal spiking. The desynchronizing effects, like the large slow waves, were recorded in all forebrain structures simultaneously, suggesting that the influence may be transmitted by diffuse projection paths.

Several cats were studied the day following the cobalt injection while medicated with phenobarbital which effectively suppressed the development of ictal discharge. Periodic interictal discharge, with a morphology similar to barbiturate spindles, were reliably altered or abolished by bulbar reticular stimulation, as shown on Figure 6, as well as by fastigial stimulation (Figure 7) in the same cat. This finding was the most reliable effect in our experiments, as it was observed in all cats tested under anticonvulsant medication. Again, the stimulus effects appear to have a diffuse influence on the EEG and ECoG.

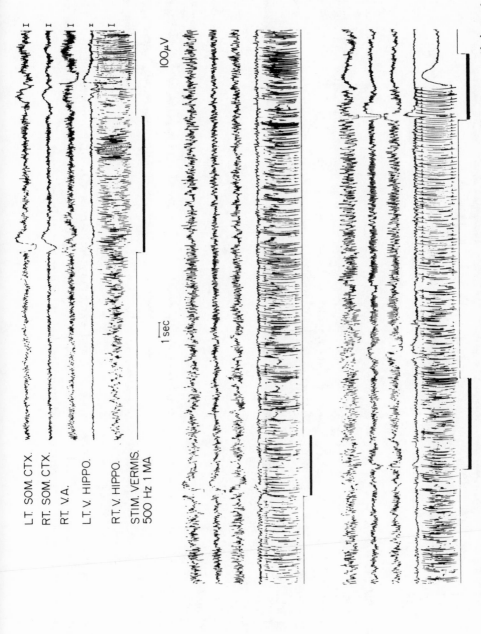

LT. SOM. CTX.
RT. SOM. CTX.
RT. V.A.
LT. V. HIPPO.
RT. V. HIPPO.
STIM. VERMIS.
500 Hz 1 MA

100 μV

1 sec

Fig. 4. Record of a complete seizure during which vermis stimulation was ineffective until late in the clonic phase during large amplitude slow waves.

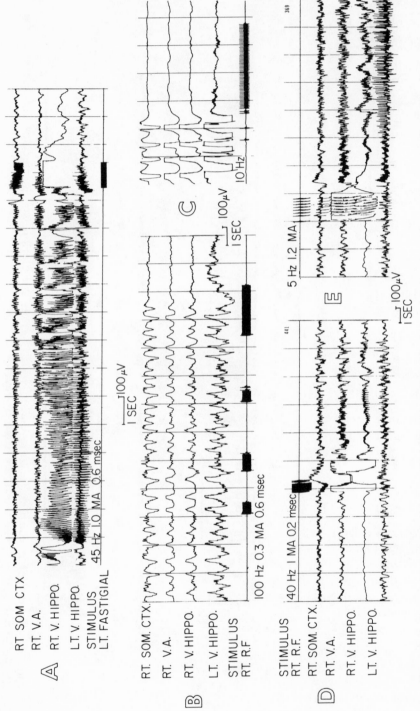

Fig. 5. Examples of inhibitory (A, B, C) and excitatory influences (D, E) in different cats. Note that inhibition occurs only in the late clonic phase in A, B, and C. In D and E, in the same cat, low (E) or high (D) rate reticular stimulation led to anomalous seizure onset.

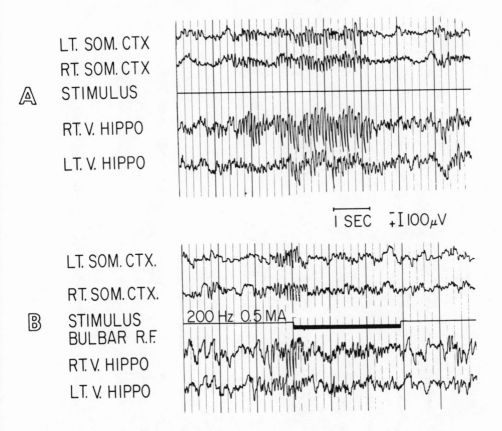

LT. SOM. CTX
RT. SOM. CTX
A STIMULUS

RT. V. HIPPO

LT. V. HIPPO

1 SEC   ∓I 100μV

LT. SOM. CTX.

RT. SOM. CTX.

B STIMULUS
BULBAR R.F.

200 Hz 0.5 MA

RT. V. HIPPO

LT. V. HIPPO

Fig. 6. Suppression of epileptiform activity by reticular stimulation in a cat with seizures controlled by phenobarbital (10 mg./kg. i.m.).

The overall impression gained from these phase one stimulation procedures was that vermis, fastigial, and bulbar reticular areas exert some degree of inhibition on hippocampus. However, these results are not unequivocal because most of the observed inhibitory effects were somewhat variable, not always predictable by the experimenter, and most importantly similar or identical effects occurred spontaneously. For example, seizure termination spontaneously at the end of the clonic phase was followed by a post-ictal depression which was indiscriminate from the seizure termination coinciding with brain stimulation. In order to test whether, in fact, the stimulus-related inhibitory effects were coincidental, difference tests were computed on average seizure durations with or without stimulation,

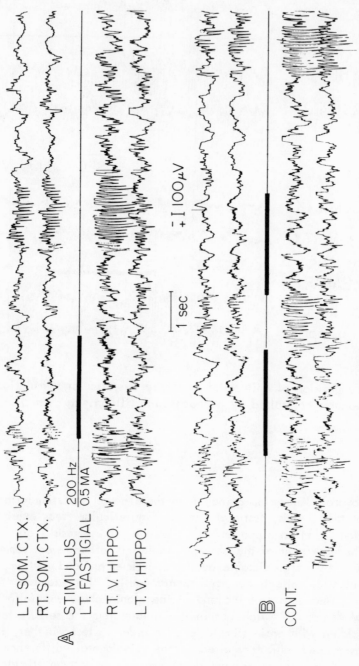

Fig. 7. Suppressing effect of fastigial stimulation on phenobarbital-controlled epileptiform discharges in the same cat as Fig. 6.

during phase two stimulation.   In each cat only one structure was stimulated during and between seizures, alternating with periods of no stimulation.   Table 1 shows, in the upper section, that on the average seven
of eight cats had shorter seizure durations with vermis-fastigiobulbar
stimulation.   In only three (I, J, K) of these seven, however, was this
statistically significant.   Note that in all three of these cats the average
seizure durations (without stimulation) were very long, which is indicative
of a pronounced clonic phase.   This, then, would support an earlier observation that stimulation is effective in terminating seizures only in the
later part of the clonic phase, during pronounced slow waves.

Whether or not hindbrain stimulation might postpone the onset of
a seizure has been tested by comparing average interictal intervals in
which stimulation has been given with those without stimulation.   Note
that in the bottom section of Table 1 seizures, on the average, were
postponed in five of nine cats, two being statistically significant (I, Z).
In one cat stimulation reliably shortened the average time between seizures.   These results, then, appear to discount the idea that interictal
stimulation might suppress those mechanisms which control the timing of
or lead to the onset of seizures.

In summary, stimulation of vermis, fastigial or reticularis gigantocellularis often resulted in EEG phenomena which could be interpreted
as inhibitory in nature (e.g. spike suppression, cessation of clonic activity).   However, these effects were statistically reliable in only a few
cases.

Dentatothalamic Effects on Hippocampus

In phase one stimulation of dentate (lateral) nucleus and ventralis
lateralis many effects, both inhibitory and excitatory, were observed.
Many of the effects just reported for fastigiobulbar stimulation were found
(e.g. seizure termination during the clonic but not tonic phase and spike
suppression).   Figure 8A illustrates seizure termination well into the clonic
phase during dentate stimulation.   In many other cases dentatothalamic
stimulation appeared to activate a typical seizure (see, e.g., Figure 8B).
Such activation was seen more frequently than with fastigiobulbar stimulation.   In cats with active spiking, which usually lasted only for a few
hours after injection, dentatothalamic stimulation usually blocked the
spikes for as long as 10-20 seconds.   For example, Figure 8C illustrates
suppression of focal spiking with a 30 Hz pulse train to left dentate, with
spiking reappearing 13 seconds later.   In Figure 8D, right V.L. stimulation suppressed the spikes for over 12 seconds.

TABLE 1

Statistical Analysis and Significance Levels for Vermis, Fastigial, and Reticular Formation Effects on Seizure Duration (top section) and on Interictal Interval Length (bottom section).

AVERAGE SEIZURE DURATION (SEC.)

STIM	CAT	ICTAL STIM WITHOUT	WITH	
Lt. Fastigial	I	96.05	74.66	(p < .05)
	W	32.03	28.25	(n.s.)
	Y	24.69	20.12	(n.s.)
	Z	20.09	50.41	(n.s.)
Rt. Ret. Form.	J	92.22	39.40	(p < .05)
	K	63.26	28.27	(p < .025)
	X	16.50	15.50	(n.s.)
Vermis	N	77.00	60.95	(n.s.)

AVERAGE INTERICTAL INTERVALS (SEC.)

STIM	CAT	INTERICTAL STIM WITHOUT	WITH	
Lt. Fastigial	I	390.73	536.00	(p < .05)
	W	244.70	163.92	(p < .01)
	Y	129.18	116.61	(n.s.)
	Z	140.98	186.63	(p < .01)
Rt. Ret. Form.	J	203.05	365.87	(n.s.)
	K	1,073.50	1,081.50	(n.s.)
	X	468.52	508.16	(n.s.)
Vermis	N	116.87	114.18	(n.s.)

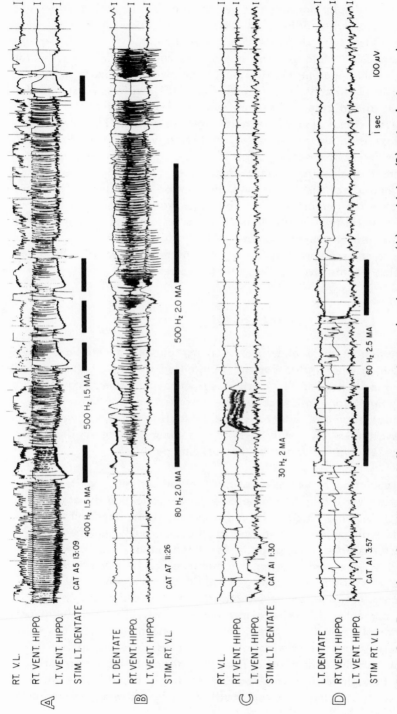

Fig. 8. Examples of excitatory influences on seizures by dentate (A) or V.L. (B) stimulation and other examples of inhibitory influences on spiking by dentate (C) and V.L. (D) stimulation. (Reprinted from Babb et al. (1974) with permission from the author and publisher).

Phase two stimulation consisted of repeatedly stimulating either dentate or V.L. or withholding stimulation. Comparison of average seizure durations under these different conditions indicated that both dentate and V.L. stimulation prolonged the average seizure duration (see the top of Table 2). This apparent facilitation of the ongoing seizure activity was statistically significant in only one case (A5), with V.L. stimulation. However, five of ten cases were significant at less than the .10 level. Dentate or V.L. stimulation between seizures resulted in longer average interictal intervals in six of ten cases, statistically significant in only one case (see the bottom section of Table 2, Cat A3). These findings would indicate that dentatothalamic stimulation, like fastigiobulbar stimulation, does not affect the timing and distribution of seizures. In summary, stimulation of dentate or V.L. produces varied effects on hippocampal seizure activity. While it appears to reliably suppress spiking it may apparently initiate seizure onset. Also, while there appear to be instances where seizures are terminated by dentatothalamic stimulation, such stimulation on the average lengthens seizures.

DISCUSSION

The findings in these experiments do not provide a clear-cut answer to the question of what influences are transmitted by way of the cerebellar peduncles to the hippocampus. Certain evidence, however, suggests a predominantly inhibitory influence by the fastigiobulbar pathway while dentatothalamic influences tend to excite or facilitate the epileptic hippocampus. Nevertheless, in many cases it was clear that cerebellar stimulation had no reliable influence on the seizure patterns.

With stimulation of vermis, fastigial, or bulbar reticular formation seizure cessation was often found; seizure precipitation rarely occurred. Mutani et al. (Mutani, Bergamini, & Doriguzzi, 1969) reported similar results in cats with cobalt foci in ventral hippocampus when they were given cerebellar surface stimulation. As Mutani et al. found, we were able to affect seizures only during the clonic phase. If this influence were reliable in shortening seizures, it would be a beneficial mode of treatment for epileptics in whom prolonged clonus would result in injury. However, in our cats, this seizure arrest was statistically reliable in only three of eight cats. In those three cases the long clonic durations were apparently more susceptible to incoming influences. We would like to conclude that such influences arise from activation of fibers originating in or passing through fastigial and/or reticularis gigantocellularis which then project to hippocampus through multi-synaptic pathways, as indicated

TABLE 2

Statistical Analysis and Significance Levels for Dentate and V.L. Effects on Seizure Duration (top section) and on Interictal Interval Length (bottom section).

AVERAGE SEIZURE DURATION (SEC.)

STIMULUS	CAT	ICTAL STIM WITHOUT	WITH	
Left Dentate	A1	25.71	25.33	(n.s.)
	A3	25.15	31.25	(n.s.)
	A5	31.66	51.40	(p < 0.1)
	A6	42.14	48.00	(n.s.)
	A7	38.27	51.50	(p < 0.1)
Rt. Vent. Lateralis	A1	25.71	31.66	(p < 0.1)
	A3	25.15	31.25	(n.s.)
	A5	31.66	55.76	(p < 0.05)
	A6	42.14	48.00	(n.s.)
	A7	38.27	25.85	(p < 0.1)

AVERAGE INTERICTAL INTERVALS (SEC.)

STIMULUS	CAT	INTERICTAL STIM WITHOUT	WITH	
Left Dentate	A1	570.00	679.80	(n.s.)
	A3	624.60	919.80	(n.s.)
	A5	660.00	705.00	(n.s.)
	A6	798.00	744.00	(n.s.)
	A7	574.20	714.60	(n.s.)
Rt. Vent. Lateralis	A1	570.00	519.60	(n.s.)
	A3	624.60	900.00	(p < .001)
	A5	660.00	486.60	(n.s.)
	A6	798.00	870.00	(n.s.)
	A7	574.20	436.80	(n.s.)

by the long-latency evoked potentials. Grantyn and Grantyn (1972) have recorded long-latency IPSPs in hippocampal pyramids following stimulation of mesencephalic reticular formation, which would lie in the ascending path of fibers from reticularis gigantocellularis.

The answer to why such influences do not have a uniformly reliable effect on hippocampus is probably due in part to the technique of gross stimulation. Despite attempts to control stimulus parameters, successive stimulations are probably not equivalent in the amount and location of tissue excited. This may be largely a result of varying states of refractoriness in neurons and fibers in the current path from time to time. But perhaps the most important factor is fluctuating excitability within the hippocampus (as indicated by the ineffectiveness of stimulation during tonic discharge) or earlier at relay synapses.

Facilitation of hippocampal seizures during dentatothalamic stimulation was evident from observations of prolonged seizures as well as of activation of seizure onset. On the average, four of five cats had longer seizures when given dentatothalamic stimulation, a result opposite from those given fastigiobulbar stimulation. Between seizures, however, dentatothalamic stimulation often inhibited focal spiking. Such a result perhaps underlines the notion of differing stimulus effects with different excitability levels in hippocampus. Perhaps both of the effects, seizure activation and spike suppression are mediated by the same set of excitatory fibers, with spike suppression resulting from cathodal block or de-synchronization of the neuronal population. On the other hand, it is possible that inhibitory fibers project to hippocampus and are activated by dentatothalamic stimuli. Li (1956), for example, has demonstrated the existence of occassional long-latency inhibition in motor cortex neurons following V.L. stimulation, whereas most reports have emphasized short-latency EPSPs (Klee & Offenloch, 1964; Amassian & Weiner, 1966).

In conclusion, we want to reiterate that the most reliable influence on hippocampal activity occurred while tonic seizure onset was controlled by phenobarbital. Under these conditions hippocampal discharges were readily altered, usually attenuated into a non-rhythmic pattern. Perhaps from this we can conclude that the altered responsivity of the hippocampus would be more susceptible to hindbrain influences. If so, then cerebellar stimulation for seizure control in epileptics partially-controlled by anti-convulsants may be more feasible than we would predict from the statistical results of this study using experimental epilepsy.

ACKNOWLEDGMENTS

Supported by USPHS Grant NS02808

REFERENCES

AMASSIAN, V.E. & WEINER, H. Monosynaptic and polysynaptic activation of pyramidal tract neurons by thalamic stimulation. In Purpura, D.P. & Yahr, M.D. (Eds) "The Thalamus". New York: Columbia University Press, 1966, pp. 255-286.

BABB, T.L., MITCHELL, A.G.,Jr., & CRANDALL, P.H. Fastigiobulbar and dentatothalamic influences on hippocampal cobalt epilepsy in the cat. Electroenceph. Clin. Neurophysiol., 1974 (in press).

DOW, R.S., FERNANDEZ-GUARDIOLA, A., & MANNI, E. The influence of the cerebellum on experimental epilepsy. Electroenceph. Clin. Neurophysiol. 14:383-398, 1962.

FLOOD, S. & JANSEN, JAN. The efferent fibers of the cerebellar nuclei and their distribution on the cerebellar peduncles in the cat. Acta Anat. 63:137-166, 1966.

GRANTYN, A.A. & GRANTYN, R. Postsynaptic responses of hippocampal neurons to mesencephalic stimulation: Hyperpolarizing potentials. Brain Res. 45:87-100, 1972.

GRIMM, R.J., FRAZEE, J.G., BELL, C.C., KAWASAKI, T., & DOW, R.S. Quantitative studies in cobalt model epilepsy: The effect of cerebellar stimulation. Int. J. Neurol. 7:126-140, 1970.

HUTTON, J.T., FROST, J.D., & FOSTER, J. The influence of the cerebellum in cat penicillin epilepsy. Epilepsia, 13:401-408, 1972.

ITO, M., UDO, M., MANO, N., & KAWAI, N. Synaptic action of the fastigiobulbar impulses upon neurons in the medullary reticular formation and vestibular nuclei. Exp. Brain Res. 11:29-47, 1970.

IWATA, K. & SNIDER, R.S. Cerebello-hippocampal influences on the electroencephalogram. Electroenceph. Clin. Neurophysiol. 11: 439-446, 1959.

JULIEN, R.M. & HALPERN, L.M. Effects of Diphenylhydantoin and other anti-epileptic drugs on epileptiform activity and Purkinje cell discharge rates. Epilepsia, 13:387-400, 1972.

KLEE, M.R. & OFFENLOCH, K. Postsynaptic potentials and spike patterns during augmenting responses in cat's motor cortex. Science, 143:488-489, 1964.

LI, C-L. The inhibitory effect of stimulation of a thalamic nucleus on neuronal activity in the motor cortex. J. Physiol. (Lond.) 133: 40-53, 1956.

MUTANI, R., BERGAMINI, L., & DORIGUZZI, T. Experimental evidence for the existence of an extrahinencephalic control of the activity of the cobalt rhinencephalic epileptogenic focus. Epilepsia, 10:351-362, 1969.

REIMER, G.R., GRIMM, R.J., & DOW, R.S. Effects of cerebellar stimulation on cobalt-induced epilepsy in the cat. Electroenceph. Clin. Neurophysiol. 23:456-462, 1967.

SNIDER, R.S. & NIEMER,W.T. "A Stereotaxic Atlas of the Cat Brain". Chicago: University of Chicago Press, 1961.

THOMAS, D.M., KAUFMAN, R.P., SPRAGUE, J.K., & CHAMBERS, W.W. Experimental studies of the vermal cerebellar projections in the brain stem of the cat (fastigiobulbar tract). J. Anat., London, 90:371-385, 1956.

WALKER, A.E. An oscillographic study of the cerebello-cerebral relationships. J. Neurophysiol. 1:16-23, 1938.

ZAITSEV, Iu.V. Influence of paleocerebellum on the excitability of midbrain reticular formation and some structure of the limbic system. Fiziol. Zh. SSSR. 55:777-782, 1969.

EXPERIMENTAL COBALT EPILEPSY AND THE CEREBELLUM

Robert S. Dow

Laboratory of Neurophysiology and Department of Neurology
Good Samaritan Hospital and Medical Center
Portland, Oregon

For over half a century there have been some clinical observations of a relationship between epilepsy and cerebellar pathology (Hodskins & Yakovlev, 1930) and a number of acute experiments which demonstrated seizures being arrested by cerebellar stimulation (Moruzzi, 1941a, b, c; Cooke & Snider, 1953, 1955; Iwata & Snider, 1959). However, no one had studied the influence of the cerebellum on a model of chronic epilepsy in the awake unanesthetized animal prior to work in our laboratory over 10 years ago. This work was done in collaboration with Dr. Fernandez-Guardiola and Prof. Ermanno Manni (Dow, Fernández-Guardiola, & Manni, 1962a, b).

Cobalt application to the cerebral cortex was the method chosen to induce a chronic form of epilepsy and the rat was the animal selected for this initial study. It had previously been shown that this animal was relatively resistant to the epileptogenic effects of aluminum cream but Kopeloff in 1960 had produced seizures in both rats and mice by the application of cobalt powder to the cortex.

We induced chronic epileptic foci in every one of 40 rats used in this study and described in detail the sequential electrical and histological changes as the lesion progressed. A recording technique was employed which in itself did not induce any seizure activity for over 2 months of recording prior to cobalt application (Figure 1). Neither photic or audio stimulation resulted in any kind of epileptic activity in these normal preparations. The details of the methods employed are fully described in the original papers and will not be repeated here (Dow, Fernández-Guardiola, and Manni, 1962a, b).

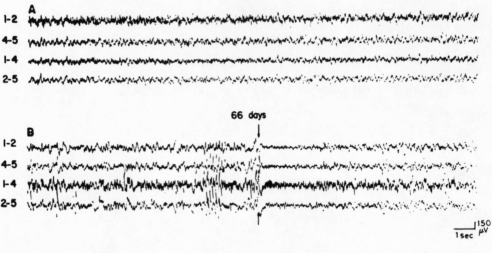

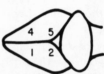

Fig. 1. A: Electrocorticogram of rat #10 during alert wakefulness 27 days after placement of cortical electrodes. B: Arousal reaction from natural sleep provoked by a hand clap (arrows) in the same animal 66 days after placement of the cortical electrodes. Electrode placements noted on the diagram and the same numbers used in all subsequent figures. (EEG & Clin. Neurophysiol. 14:399-407, 1962.

When approximately 30 mg of commercially available (200 mesh) cobalt powder was applied to the right frontal lobe 37 of the 40 rats became hypersensitive and restless and attempted to escape from their cage within the first few days and fifty percent of those in whom the powder was applied to the motor area of forelimb and face demonstrated clonic movements of the contralateral corresponding body parts by the second week following cobalt application. These focal seizures only lasted 1 or 2 days and generalized seizures were seen in only a few animals.

It is, of course, possible that clinical signs were missed in some animals. However, all showed a very constant electrical effect. On the first few days following cobalt application high voltage delta waves were seen followed by a regression of this slow activity to a more normal pattern (Figure 2). The spike activity which also developed gradually was later in onset and was fully developed only after the background activity had returned to a more normal pattern. Spikes and poly spikes were seen usually 10 to 20 days after cobalt was first applied. A mirror focus on the contralateral cortex was also observed in some instances.

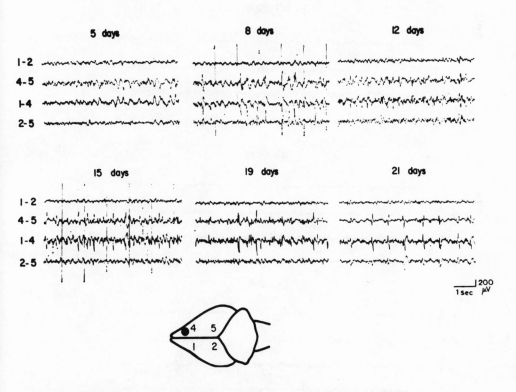

Fig. 2. Development of cobalt epilepsy. Rat #63. The days refer to the interval after application of cobalt. Note the development of spikes following a period of delta activity. The abnormality in this animal was restricted to the right frontal area, near the site of application shown in the accompanying diagram. (EEG & Clin. Neurophysiol. 14:399-407, 1962).

Many animals showed these electrical manifestations without clinical seizures but there was always a good correspondence between the clonic jerks and the ECoG. After continuing in some animals for as long as 2 months (Figure 3) it gradually abated and was replaced by low voltage activity as the destructive lesion became more extensive. Both repetitive photic and audio stimulation were effective in enhancing the spike activity at any stage of the evolution of this epileptic focus and at its height focal or generalized convulsions could be precipitated. It should be noted that when seizures were induced they never outlasted the stimulus and usually stopped before the repetitive stimulation was terminated.

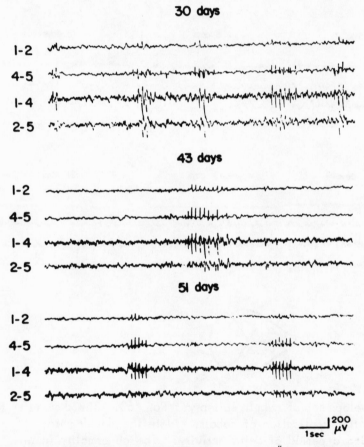

Fig. 3. Development of cobalt epilepsy. Rat #91. This illustrates a later phase of the effect of cobalt applied to the right frontal lobe. Note the more widespread changes as well as a more prolonged effect than was the case in animal #63 illustrated in Figure 2. (EEG & Clin. Neurophysiol. 14:399-407, 1962).

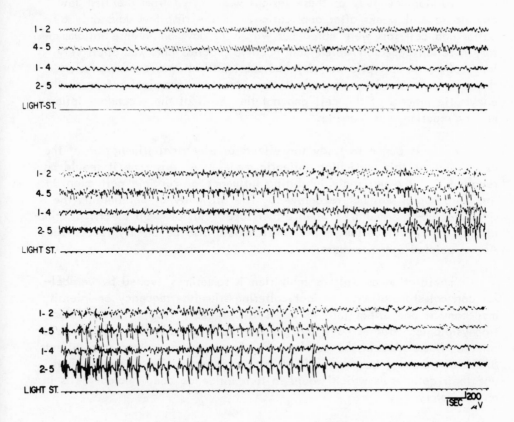

Fig. 4. A continuous record of a generalized electrocortical seizure provoked by photostimulation in rat #58, 5 days after cobalt application on
the right frontal lobe. Note the lack of epileptic activity prior to onset
of photostimulation whose onset and frequency is recorded on channel 5.
The spikes first appeared in the right occipital leads (lead 5) 15 sec
after the beginning of the photostimulation. (EEG & Clin. Neurophysiol.
14:399-407, 1962).

The effects of intraperitoneal Megimide was compared in normal and
cobalt epileptic rats. In normal rats subconvulsant doses 6.25 mg/kg resulted in a slowing and increase in voltage of the ECoG with bursts of
sharp waves and spindles. The rats with previous cobalt application always showed a lower threshold for Megimide induced seizures. The spiking of the cobalt focus was consistently enhanced by the drug in subconvulsant doses and clonic movements were easily induced with low doses.

Histological study of these lesions was carried from the first few
days to several weeks after application.   In the first few days only a
pallor and cell loss were noted but within 11 days an intense inflamma-
tory reaction appeared which continued to progress and was often very
large after all epileptic activity had subsided.   It was our conclusion
that effects induced by the cobalt were due to a chemical effect on the
enzymatic process of the cell and not the result of the secondary inflam-
matory reaction and scarring.

We next began to study the effects of electrical stimulation of the
cerebellum on this particular epileptic model.   At this time it should be
recalled that the uniformly inhibiting influence of Purkinje cell axon on
the deep nuclei was not recognized.   The difficulty of determining the
structures being stimulated when either superficial or deep electrical stimulation of the cerebellum is performed should also be clearly recognized.
As we pointed out elsewhere:

"Facilitation as well as inhibition is sometimes evoked by cerebellar cortical stimulation.   In fact, altering stimulus frequency or intensity
may convert one effect into its opposite (Moruzzi, 1950).   Recent electrophysiological studies have brought out the large role that collaterals of
afferent fibers play in the cerebellum.   Some of the contradictory effects
of stimulation may be the result of retrograde activation of mossy fibers
and their collaterals which would in turn influence deep nuclear cells in
an excitatory way.

"It is not surprising that great variability in the effects of stimulation of the white matter and deep nuclei are found among various investigators and even by the same investigators in a series of individual experiments (Manni, Henatsch, & Dow, 1964).   This is particularly under-
standable in the case of the fastigial nucleus and its surrounding white
matter.   The rostral and caudal parts of the fastigial nucleus have opposite effects on posture and tone.   Furthermore, both the fibers of entry and
exit traverse the nuclei and those from the caudal half of one fastigial
nucleus pass rostral to the opposite fastigial nucleus in leaving the cerebellum.   Direct cortical-fugal fibers also traverse the nuclei.   Any stimulus within the area of the deep nuclei will result in a composite of many
different and often opposite effects.

"Following stimulation of either the medial or intermediate cortex
on their underlying nuclei there is a post stimulating rebound in which an
effect opposite to that produced by the stimulus occurs....The rebound
effect may be maintained for a prolonged period and at times is more
prominent than the movement seen during the stimulation." (Dow, 1969).

That the results of stimulation have been variable in ours and other hands is therefore not at all unexpected. It is rather remarkable that in the particular model we first studied the results of electrical stimulation were as constant as they proved to be. In 24 rats one or two bipolar stimulating electrodes were chronically implanted into the cerebellum. Lobules V, VI, VIIA, VIIB, HVIIA, HVIIB, the interpositus and dentate nucleus were stimulated. The points of electrical stimulation were verified by histological control. Pulse frequencies from 20 to 50 or 200 to 400/sec were employed. In normal rats high frequency stimulation (300/sec, 1 mil sec duration 1-5V for 1 second) did not provoke any noticeable effect on the ECoG or motor behavior aside from occasional short arousal response. With higher voltages (5-20V) it was occasionally possible to observe the slow reactions (turn of the head and lifting of the forelimbs, etc.) first described by Clark (1939a, b) in unrestrained cats.

In the cobalt epileptic rats cerebellar stimulation provoked different effects depending on the stage of development of the cobalt focus. When only paroxysmal slow waves were present short trains (1-3 sec) of low voltage (1-4V) high frequency (300/sec) cerebellar stimulation uniformly blocked this activity. This effect was obtained from all the cerebellar points explored (Figure 5). Later when sharp waves appeared the cerebellar influence was similarly suppressant. Afterward when the spikes were present, the cerebellar stimulation usually resulted in their suppression as well (Figure 6) but facilitation occasionally occurred (Figure 7). At times lower voltages of stimulation produced this facilitatory effect and sometimes it was seen when lower frequencies were employed. If the cerebellar stimulation was prolonged more than 2 sec an "escape" phenomena was sometimes observed. After the initial reduction in spike activity a clearly evident rebound of the epileptic activity would occur in many cases. The inhibitory effect of cerebellar stimulation consisted of an interruption or decrease in the cortical spiking and an arrest of the clonic jerking. The rebound effect consisted of the reappearance of voltage and frequency of the spiking after a variable latency of 1 to 3 seconds.

High frequency (300/sec) cerebellar stimulation usually inhibited the slow waves and spindles induced by subconvulsant doses of Megimide but lower frequencies did not give consistent results. Megimide induced generalized seizures were not stopped by cerebellar stimulation although sometimes the duration of the seizures appeared to be shortened. The spiking of the cobalt focus induced by Megimide might be either suppressed (Figure 8) or facilitated by the cerebellar stimulation (Figure 9). While these varying effects seemed at times to be related to the site of stimulation a review of all the experiments demonstrated that no consistent pattern emerged which would indicate location of points of maximal effect.

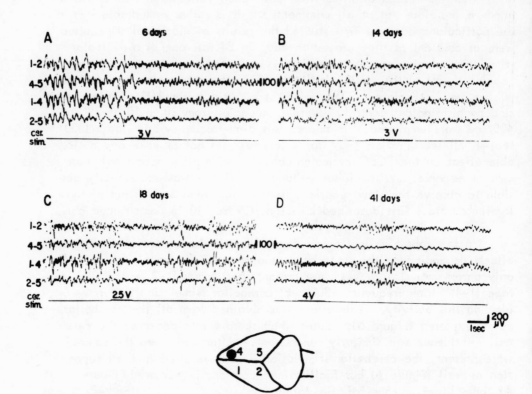

Fig. 5.   Inhibition of the cobalt epileptic activity by electrical stimulation of the lobules H VI (simplex) and H VIIA (crus I) of right cerebellar hemisphere in rat #88, 6, 14, 18 and 41 days after cobalt powder
application on the right frontal lobe.   In A and in D the predominant
abnormality is slow wave activity while in B and in C fast potentials
are also inhibited.   Note that the gain on channel 2 is double that of
the other leads.   The progressive lower voltage of the activity of the
involved hemisphere is commonly seen as the lesion increases in size.
The location of the cobalt application is shown in the diagram.   Its
location as well as the position of ECoG leads are the same in all
illustrations.   (EEG & Clin. Neurophysiol. 14:383-398, 1962).

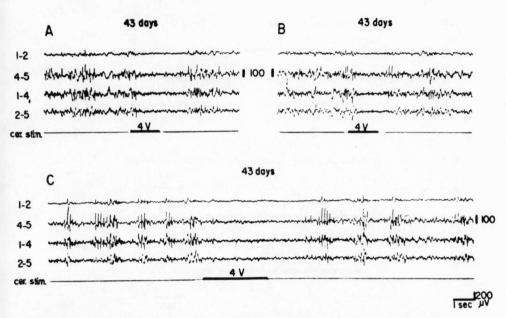

Fig. 6. Inhibition of cobalt epileptic activity by electrical stimulation
of lobule HVII A (Crus II) of right cerebellar hemisphere in rat #91, 43
days after application of cobalt powder on the right frontal cortex.
Note that the gain on channel 2 is double that of the other three
channels. The latency of the effect was somewhat variable. (EEG &
Clin. Neurophysiol. 14:383-398, 1962).

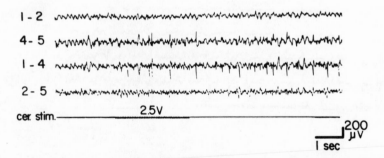

Fig. 7. Facilitation of spiking provoked by stimulation of lobule VI
(declive) of cerebellum in rat #63, 5 days after application of cobalt
powder on the right frontal cortex. Note the increase in spiking during
and after the stimulation which is limited to the electrode near the
cobalt focus. At other times the same animal showed inhibition of the
activity. (EEG & Clin. Neurophysiol. 14:383-398, 1962).

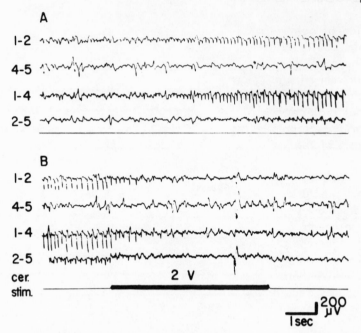

Fig. 8. Cerebellar inhibition of electrocortical seizure induced by the
intraperitoneal injection of Megimide in rat #57. 10 days after application of cobalt powder on the right frontal area. Electrical stimulation
of lobules V-VI (culmen-declive). A and B are a continuous record.
Note the seizure is located in the mirror focus. (EEG & Clin. Neurophysiol. 14:383-398, 1962).

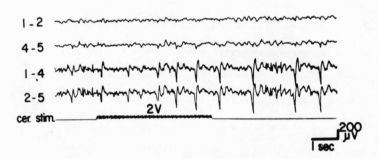

Fig. 9. Facilitation of the Megimide induced spiking and inhibition of
the background activity by stimulation of left interpositus nucleus in rat
#54, 22 days after cobalt application on the right frontal cortex. Every
spike corresponded to a clonic jerk of the left forelimb. Although the
spike activity is originating in the right hemisphrere, it is so synchronized
by the Megimide as to be barely discernible in the recording from the
right side. (EEG & Clin. Neurophysiol. 14:383-398, 1962).

Stimulation of points in the hemisphere or vermis of the anterior or posterior lobe could result in modification of the seizures in this cobalt model in the rat. The best inhibition of clonic movements were generally obtained from stimulation of the rostral part of the cerebellum. It was our expectation that with a larger animal and particularly in primates where the spinal projection had been found to be more limited and functional localization was presumed to be better developed it could be determined which part of the cerebellum would be responsible for these effects.

Before embarking on studies in primates in order to bring added evidence to our conclusion that stimulation of the cerebellum in all areas exhibits a predominantly inhibitory effect on cobalt experimental epilepsy in the rat, experiments of cerebellar ablation and temporary cooling were employed. Total cerebellar ablation in the normal rat resulted in a slowing and synchronization of the ECoG. Beginning in the first week there appeared spindle-like bursts of high voltage 6 to 8 per sec waves (Figure 10). These changes occurred without any behavior suggestive of sleep but like sleep activity the spindles could be totally blocked by audio or photic stimulation. Histological control after 3 months of observation in two animals with particularly striking spindling showed the cerebellectomy had been complete and there was no lesion of the reticular formation of the brain stem.

The effects of cerebellectomy on the cobalt epileptic rats were tested in two different experimental conditions. In a first group of 4 rats the cerebellectomy was carried on 7, 8, 11, and 12 days after the cobalt application when epileptic manifestations were not present or had only just begun.

In a second group of nine rats the cerebellum was removed 13, 14, 15, 17, 19, 23, 26, 70, and 114 days before the cobalt application. In several of these the cobalt was applied when the dynamic phenomena of Luciani was still present. In others stabilized cerebellar deficiency as defined by Dow and Moruzzi (1958) had already been reached. Cerebellar symptoms were always more striking than was the case in normal rats in the first group. There was a return of cerebellar deficiency symptoms for which varying degrees of compensation had already occurred when cobalt lesions were made in the second group. Spontaneous generalized seizures were common in this group; one animal died in status epilepticus and in two a clonus of the forelimb lasted for more than two weeks until the rats were sacrificed.

BEFORE CEREBELLECTOMY

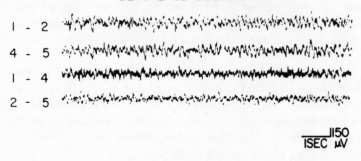

I - 2

4 - 5

I - 4

2 - 5

150
ISEC µV

41 DAYS AFTER CEREBELLECTOMY

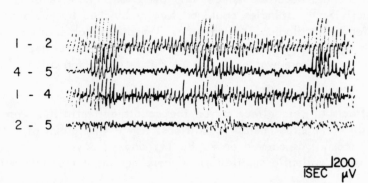

I - 2

4 - 5

I - 4

2 - 5

200
ISEC µV

Fig. 10. An illustration of the marked hypersynchronization of cerebral cortical activity occasionally seen after total cerebellectomy, before and 41 days after the cerebellectomy. This rat began to show these outbursts of spindles 10 days after the cerebellectomy and the pattern lasted more than 3 months until the rat was sacrificed because it lost its electrodes. (EEG & Clin. Neurophysiol. 14:383-398, 1962).

The ECoG modifications in the cerebellectomized rats were characterized by an increase in voltage and frequency of the spikes and sharp waves, and by irradiation of the focal activity to other cerebral regions to a degree not seen in the intact animal. The response to sensory stimulation was changed significantly (Figure 11). The cerebellectomized cobalt epileptic rats showed striking after-effects, often lasting for more than 15

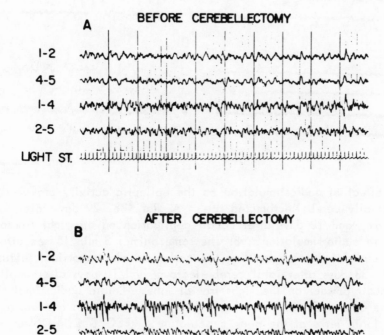

Fig. 11. The effect of cerebellectomy on the flicker activation in rat #67. A: 7 days after the application of cobalt powder on the right frontal cortex and immediately before cerebellectomy. B: 5 days after cerebellectomy. Note the spiking has spread to areas remote from the site of application. (EEG & Clin. Neurophysiol. 14:383-398, 1962).

minutes, following the cessation of stimulation, consisting of spikes and
sharp waves and often generalized or focal seizures with clinical manifestations (Figure 12). Such failures to recover promptly from activation
procedures were never seen in these animals with intact cerebelli.

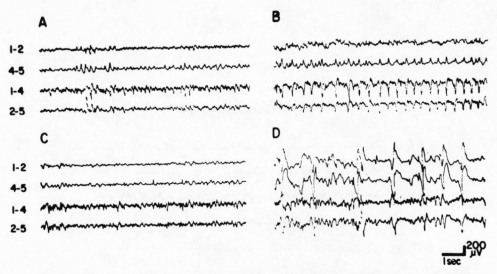

Fig. 12. Effect of audiostimulation on the epileptic activity provoked by
cobalt in totally cerebellectomized rats. A: Rat #78, 29 days after total
cerebellectomy and 13 days after cobalt application on the right frontal
lobe. Before audiostimulation. B: The same animal 3 min 15 sec after
the end of audiostimulation showing the prolonged electrocortical seizure.
C: Rat #73, 33 days after total cerebellectomy and 10 days after application of cobalt powder on the right frontal lobe. Before audiostimulation.
D: The same animal 5 min after the end of audiostimulation and during
prolonged clonic jerks of the neck musculature. (EEG & Clin. Neurophysiol. 14:383-398, 1962).

In order to further control the effect of removal of the cerebellar
influence on experimental epilepsy, a technique for temporary cooling of
the cerebellum was devised. This produced a rapidly reversible affect
which eliminated the inherent difficulties of observing the influence of
cerebellar ablation on a continuously changing process of epileptic activity. A thin sheet of platinum foil was applied over lobules VI, VII,
and VIII. Part of the foil was brought to the surface, and a small

cubicle was fashioned into which dry ice could be placed. In the first days after cobalt application when the ECoG did not yet show epileptic activity, cooling of the cerebellum provoked generalized low waves. During the development of the epileptic activity when sharp waves and spikes were present, cooling of the cerebellum provoked facilitation of spiking and the appearance of a clonus of the forelimb and irradiation of the paroxysmal activity resulting in repeated generalized seizures. Figure 13 shows the effect of temporary cooling of the dorsal cerebellar

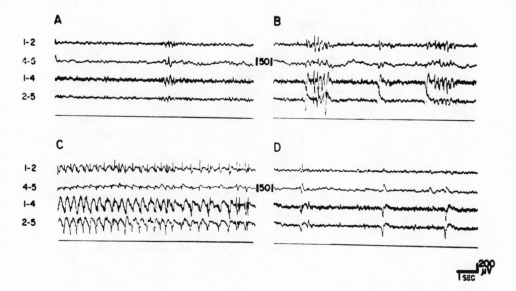

Fig. 13. Effect of temporary cooling of the dorsal cerebellar surface on the development of cobalt epilepsy in rat #93, 8 days after cobalt applic-ation on the right frontal cortex. A. Before cooling, control record. B: 15 min after the beginning of the cooling showing an increase in the spiking. C: 16 min after the beginning of the cooling during the first of two spontaneous seizures; a second occurred 15 min after the cooling was stopped. D: 55 min after the end of the cooling period with a re-turn to activity more nearly like that in A, although occasional clonic activity was still seen. The gain of channel 2 is increased. Control of temperature changes induced in the cerebellum by similar cooling at the time of sacrifice under pentobarbital anesthesia showed that the temper-ature of the cerebellum 3.5 mm below the surface dropped from 35.25°C to 30°C within 3 min of the application of dry ice and to 27°C in 15 min. (EEG & Clin. Neurophysiol. 14:383-398, 1962).

surface on the development of cobalt epilepsy 8 days after cobalt application of the right frontal cortex. These effects were seen within 15
minutes after the beginning of cooling. The ECoG responses to single
and repetitive photo and audio stimulation were also more striking during
cooling (Figure 14). The effect of cooling which also included cerebellar
deficiency symptoms for about 1 hour after the dry ice was removed from
the platinum foil box. When a clinically evident epileptic state resulted
from the cooling the convulsion occasionally had to be stopped by the injection of small doses of pentabarbital. As a control the frontal poles
were cooled in 2 animals on two occasions with either a slightly depressing or no effect on the epileptic activity.

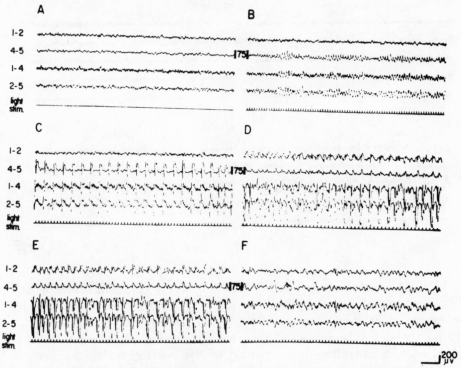

Fig. 14. Effect of the temporary cooling of the dorsal cerebellar surface
on the photoactivation of the cobalt epilepsy. Rat #93 the day after the
cobalt was placed on the right frontal area. A: Before the cooling,
control record. B: Photostimulation before the cooling. C, D and E:
Electrocortical seizure induced by the photostimulation during cooling.
F: Control photostimulation 45 min after the end of cooling. Interval
between C and D is about 40 sec and D and E are continuous. The
gain in channel 2 is increased. (EEG & Clin. Neurophysiol. 14:383-
398, 1962).

Finally the threshold to both electrical and clinical manifestations of Megimide were lowered significantly by cerebellectomy. In one of the animals where the excessive spindling of ECoG activity was occurring as described above, the dose of Megimide necessary to produce generalized seizure was only one-half that required to produce the slightest clinical signs of seizures in the intact animals.

Our conclusion that the cerebellum exerts an inhibitory influence on cobalt experimental epilepsy in the rat was further strengthened by other observations on the reciprocal relation of cerebellar and cerebral activity during convulsions. The same team of investigators working in our laboratory studied the activity of single units of the cerebellar cortex and nuclei before, during, and after convulsive seizures by electrical stimulation of the brain, by intraperitoneal injection of convulsant drugs (Megimide and Metrazol) and by anoxia in curarized rats under local anesthesia. Cerebral activity was studied simultaneously with a recording by either microelectrode or macroelectrodes of the sensory motor cortex. The changes tended to be reciprocal between the cerebrum and cerebellum. These observations have been described already in this symposium and will not be repeated now.

We interpreted reciprocal relationship to be another evidence that the cerebellum may actively suppress cerebral seizure activity from a variety of causes. At the conclusion of these experiments in the rat the results seemed consistent in all respects and the conclusion that the cerebellum had a predominantly inhibitory influence on the cobalt model in this species seemed inescapable.

On beginning to study this model in the cat and later the monkey the first observation was that in both the cat and the monkey the effect of cobalt application began earlier and lasted a shorter time. In the monkey experiments Halothane anesthesia was probably an important contributor to the fact that some epileptic manifestations in these experiments could be seen within minutes after the application of cobalt. In both species, both clinical and electrical effects had subsided within a few days. (Henjyoji (Henjyoji & Dow, 1965) confirmed the prolonged time course in the rat using the same technique he had employed in the cat and the quantity of cobalt used was not responsible for this species difference. It is possible that in the rat the chemical effect could have spread more widely because of the small brain. Mutani (1967a, b) has subsequently shown that cobalt application in the amygdala and hippocampus was capable of producing long duration epileptic activity even in the cat. However, no histological changes were found in the hippocampus in the rat material. Acutally we still have no good explanation for the species differences in the cobalt model. The fact that they exist makes it important that if one wishes to make an application of this model to human epilepsy primates should be the animal chosen for studies in the future.

The results of electrical stimulation of the cerebellum in the cobalt epileptic cat were disappointingly variable in our laboratory. Reimer (Reimer, Grimm, & Dow, 1967) studied 9 awake cats in which he stimulated the cerebellum 864 times at 13 different sites during either spontaneous or induced seizures. Unlike the rat, seizures were not induced by photic or audio stimulation but could readily be activated by touching the affected limb.

If the cerebellum was stimulated in an animal which had not yet developed seizure activity or after activity had ceased no effect beyond an arousal response was noted at low intensity stimulation. If volleys were raised to 5 to 7.5 V the slow tonic movements first described by Clark (1939a, b) were noted. These bore no resemblance to the cobalt epileptic seizure seen in the same animal at different times and, unlike the cobalt seizures, were not accompanied by any change in the ECoG as had been found by Clark and Ward (1949). The 7 vermian sites were in Larsell's lobule VI, VIIA, and VIIIA and the 6 hemisphere sites were in HVIA and HVIIA Crus I and HVIIA Crus II. Only in (HVIIA) Crus I did cerebellar stimulation fail completely to influence cerebral activity in all trials. In all the other sites the results were variable even in the same animal from time to time without any change in the parameter of stimulation. Unlike our experience in the rat, stimulation was usually ineffective; when an effect was seen it was usually excitatory and the activation of the seizure might occur during stimulation or more frequently as a rebound effect beginning 10 to 20 mil sec after the end of the stimulation (Figure 15). A seizure might be initiated from the same site either during or after the stimulation without any consistent difference in the parameters. The majority of such effects were at stimulus rates of 100-300/sec. During interictal phases this activation occurred less than 15% of the trials from all sites except the pyramis VIII. Here evoked seizure activity occurred in 159 out of 350 trials or 45% of the time. When cerebellar stimulation was given during a spontaneous seizure or one induced by touching the contralateral forepaw no effect was seen on the duration of the seizure, nor on the amplitude of the epileptiform activity in most instances. Prolongation of the seizure was rarely observed during stimulation in HVIIA Crus II, VIIA, and VIIIA (less than 10% of the trials). However, when lobulus VI was stimulated such an effect was

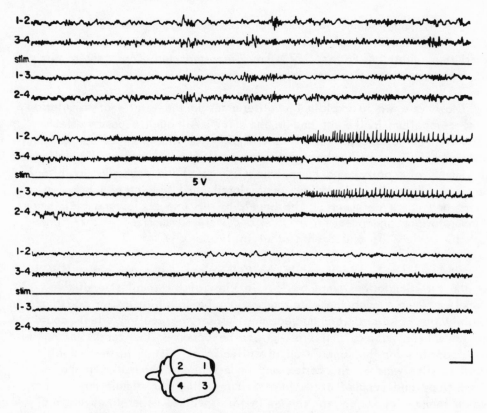

Fig. 15. "Rebound" epileptic activity following random electrical stimulation of pyramis (VIIA) with 5 V at a frequency of 100/sec, 0.1 msec
pulse. Calibrations: 20 uV, 1 sec. (EEG & Clin. Neurophysiol. 23:
456-462, 1967).

noted in 9 of 15 trials or 60% of the time. In all instances when prolongation of a seizure was seen stimulation rates less than 10/sec were
used. Faster frequencies were uniformly ineffective in modifying an ongoing seizure in the cat regardless of the site stimulated. The volleys of
stimulation required to produce these effects on seizures were 4-5V which
was below the threshold for the tonic movements of Clark.

One conclusion which seemed valid was that stimulation of sites
near the mid-line were more effective than those in the hemispheres.
This had been the only conclusion which could be drawn from some work
by Barton (Barton & Dow, 1965) in our laboratory on the effect of stimulation of the cerebellum in penicillin induced seizures in the cat.

Because this model seemed in most instances not to be affected by cerebellar stimulation the work was never published. We now know that others (Hutton, Frost, & Foster, 1972) have reported more consistent results
with this model than we were able to achieve.

How were we to explain the differences in the effects of stimulation
of the cerebellum in the rat and in the cat? Although opposite effects
of ablation of cortex and nuclei were known from the work of Sprague and
Chambers (1953) and Chambers and Sprague (1955a, b) and of stimulation
experiments of Moruzzi and Pompeiano (1957a, b) the exclusive inhibitory
role of the Purkinje cell was not appreciated until the interval between
our rat and cat experiments. The papers by Ito and Eccles and their many
collaborators began appearing in 1964 and were summarized in the monograph by Eccles, Ito and Szentagothai in 1967.

We tentatively concluded in the Reimer and associates paper (1967)
that the rat stimulations were nuclear in view of the small size of the
cerebellum even though the electrodes might be in white matter and that
certainly the ablations were nuclear and further the cooling effects could
well have been nuclear. If this were to be accepted the cerebellar nuclei
are responsible for the suppression of epileptic activity. In the cat all
electrode sites were in the cortex and underlying white matter in the
Reimer study and because of its larger size we thought stimulation did not
involve the nuclei by current spread in this species. Therefore, cortical
stimulation most often produced activation in this species.

As the result of this reasoning and in order to clearly separate the
dentate n. outflow from the fastigial n. outflow Grimm & Frazee, 1970a;
Grimm, Frazee, Bell, & Kawasaki, 1970b; Grimm, Frazee, Kawasaki, &
Savic, 1970c; Grimm, Frazee, & Ozbay, 1973, began studying cobalt
epilepsy and the effects of dentate stimulation on evoked potentials on
the cerebral cortex in the squirrel monkey. In their initial study (Grimm,
Frazee, Bell, & Kawasaki, 1970b) it was established for the first time in
primates that small amounts of cobalt powder applied to the surface of
cerebral cortex eccentric to the motor area will produce an acute, but
self-limited epileptogenic process resulting in focal motor jerks on the
contralateral limbs. By using halothane anesthesia (Grimm, Savic,
Petersen, & Griffith, 1969) it was possible to show that the cobalt response begins very early. It also provided the opportunity to study the
evolution of this form of model epilepsy and to establish clearly different
stages. It was evident, for example, that a buildup in amplitude and
duration of the initial epileptogenic event preceded the clinical manifestations, and that when they occur an afterdischarge component is added to

the preceding spike or sharp wave. At times the onset of the afterdischarge per se clearly decreased the frequency of epileptogenic events
which followed (Grimm, Frazee, & Ozbay, 1973).

To study the question of cerebellar control over cortical epileptogen-
isis, as provided by the cobalt model in the primate, Grimm (Grimm,
Frazee, Bell, & Kawasaki, 1970b) then used quantitative techniques to
test the hypothesis that fastigial or dentate n. stimulation in the awake
monkey alters the discharge characteristics of a small cobalt lesion in
cortex. Stimulating electrodes were implanted in both dentate and fastigial n. prior to cobalt placement, stimulus parameters for arousal (fastigial n.) or evoked cortical potentials (dentate n.) were identified and
set at 3x threshold. The effort here was to activate these efferent systems
at above known physiologic levels in order to test their effect on a discharging cobalt focus.

Squirrel monkeys were then lesioned with small amounts of cobalt
and the cerebellar stimulation parameter previously established were then
automatically programmed such that over the ensuing hours, the effect of
dentate n. and fastigial n. stimulation and no stimulation periods could
be compared with regard to the number of epileptogenic events arising
from the focus. Stimulations were presented in a set pattern of 3 minutes
of fastigial stimulation, 3 minutes off, 3 minutes of dentate stimulation
followed by three minutes off. The paroxysmal events were counted elec-
tronically and checked by manual counts.

Using this paradigm the results were entirely negative. Neither fastigial or dentate stimulation, so programmed, diminished, or augmented the
number of epileptogenic events produced by the focus during its major period of activity. This kind of approach is complicated by the fact that if
the animals become drowsy they inactivate the dentothalamic cortical pathway (Grimm & Frazee, 1970a) to greater than 9x threshold for dentate
stimulus, and sleep itself, in addition to raising arousal thresholds also
profoundly alters various thalamic mechanisms important in the control of
cortical activity. The results of the studies of Grimm and his colleagues,
while negative, raise two possibilities: 1) cerebellar circuits must be stimulated in some other manner (e.g. supramaximal) to achieve the effect,
or 2) that it is not the electrical activity per se that is crucial but some
biochemical alteration induced by cerebellar stimulation that is occurring.

It will be remembered that in both the rat and cat experiments stimulus strengths of 1.0 to 5V were required to see an effect on seizures.
3X threshold to be sure seemed more physiologic and more easily compared

from animal to animal for the quantitative studies with which these experiments were concerned. However, actual voltages were only 0.6-0.9
volts for fastigial stimulation which was uniformly delivered at 200 to
250 Hz. The voltages used for dentate stimulation was 0.6 to 1.2 volts
and because it had been determined that cerebral evoked potential to
dentate stimulation would not follow at faster frequencies, only frequencies
at 10 Hz were used in this site. It was anticipated that this stimulus site
would be excitatory to the epileptic activity as it is to the threshold of
electrical stimulation of the cortex.

The fact is, as stated above, these parameters of stimulation at these
sites in this species was ineffective in modifying the number of paroxymal
events in any statistically significant way.

In the light of the positive effects of cerebellar stimulation in cases
of clinical epilepsy in man, to be reported later at this symposium, it is
not the fact that these experiments were performed in primates that no influence on the cobalt model could be shown. As stated above, perhaps
the cerebellar stimulation required to produce a change in epilepsy exceeds
that which could be related to some physiological function in normal man
or an intact animal (i.e. supramaximal stimulation). Neither a patient
with epilepsy nor an epileptic model in an animal is in a normal state.
Certainly drug therapy is not physiologic and there are many instances in
which the therapeutic effects of naturally occurring compounds may only
be achieved when they are given in nonphysiological quantities.

Species differences while important do not appear to be the main
reason that those working in our laboratory were unsuccessful in duplica-
ting our earlier observations in the rat when they were attempted in the
cat and monkey. Others have been more successful than we were in the
cat and a number of workers in other laboratories have been able to show
cerebellar inhibition on various epileptic models in rabbits, rats, and cats.

Payan and associates (Payan, Levine, & Strebel, 1966) had shown
that in rats a cobalt implant in the homolateral cerebellar hemisphere
counteracts the epileptogenic effects of cobalt applied to the frontal lobe.
They ascribed this to a chronic irritation and stimulation of the cerebellum.
However, cobalt applied to the cerebellum alone produced no significant
alteration in seizure threshold as determined by other methods of seizure
production.

Cereghino (Cereghino & Dow, 1970) in our laboratory attempted to
duplicate this work and to define by this method which part of the

cerebellum was responsible for this effect. The findings of previous workers in our laboratory concerning the cobalt model in the cat were confirmed. Adversive spontaneous seizures not previously noted were described.
No significant differences in the duration, frequency, spread, or ECoG
manifestations depending on whether the lesion was placed in the pre-
cruciate gyrus or post-cruciate gyrus were found.

This study, which involved 32 cats, failed to detect any difference
in the pattern of cobalt epilepsy in those animals where cobalt had been
applied simultaneously to the homolateral or contralateral cerebellar hemisphere. When applied to the vermis it seemed to enhance the susceptab-
ility as measured by Megimide induction but on statistical analysis this
tendency could not be demonstrated with certainty. The histological control showed that the cerebellar lesions in all instances were confined to
the cortex and none penetrated to involve the deep cerebellar nuclei.
We assumed that in the rat, due to its small size, the chronic stimulatory
effect of cobalt cerebellar implantation affected the nuclei and that explained the difference in the Cereghino study compared to that of Payan
and associates (Payan, Levine, & Strebel, 1966). To reiterate we were
of the opinion that the explanation for the differences between the rat and
the cat, so far as the effect of stimulation was concerned, was because
that in the rat we were stimulating in most instances the nuclei while in
the cat it was a cortical stimulation which had an inhibitory effect upon
the nuclei. This, of course, is different than Julien's conclusion to be
expressed shortly in this symposium and does not fit with the results of
Mutani's studies to be reported below.

Let us now turn to the experience elsewhere than at the Laboratory
of Neurophysiology at Good Samaritan Hospital and Medical Center. The
cobalt epilepsy model has become widely used in the last 10 years as the
following references will document. If no attempt was made to influence
the model by cerebellar stimulation or ablation they will not be discussed
in detail in this presentation. As indicated above, Kopeloff described its
effect in the rat and mouse in 1960. Extensive work on cobalt epilepsy
in the rabbit has been described by Atsev and associates (Atsev, Arutyunov,
Dimov, &Chavdarov, 1966). Chusid and Kopeloff induced seizures in monkeys in cobalt application in 1967 though these authors reported unsuccessful attempts in this species in 1962. Fischer, Holuber and Malik (1967)
modified the techniques by introducing cogelatin sticks and reported that
a more uniform cortical lesion was produced. Dawson and Holmes (1966)
used cobalt in different cortical sites in both anesthetized and unanesthetized rats and applied it to various parts of the motor cortex in rats.
Holuber and Fischer (1967) observed the coincident development of

gliomesenchymal scar at the primary focus with the appearance of spiking
in the electrophysiological records. Fischer and associates (Fischer,
Holuber, & Malik, 1968) described in great detail the histological features of the lesion studied in 77 rats examined at various stages of development with a variety of histological methods including electron microscopic studies. On the basis of these investigations they felt that the
effect was not exclusively chemical as we and others had suggested, but
the scar formation also played a significant role. Fischer (1968, 1969)
also made important observations on the electron microscopic features of
the cobalt lesion and Holuber and Fischer (1967) studied the mirror focus
in comparison with the primary focus and pointed out methods by which
it could be modified.

Mancia and Lucioni (1966) observed the effect of cobalt introduced
into the mesencephalic reticular formation and intralaminar thalamic nuclei
in cats. This work was extended by Cesa Bianchi and associates (Cesa
Bianchi, Mancia, & Mutani, 1967) to involve lower brainstem structures
and midline thalamic nuclei. Mutani (1967a, b) introduced cobalt in the
amygdala and later that year described the effects in the hippocampus.
Cobalt lesions at these sites produced a long lasting epileptic disorder in
the cat in contradiction to its short term effect on the sensory motor cortex in cats and monkeys in our laboratory. Needham and Dila (1969)
implanted cobalt in the mesencephalic reticular formation and applied a
suspension of cobalt powder in Elliott's solution diffusely over the cortex
in acute experiments. Mutani and his collaborators have used their cobalt
epilepsy model to study the effect of stimulation of the caudate nucleus
and the paleo cerebellum and their results will be described in some detail
(Mutani, 1969; Mutani, Bergamini, & Doriguzzi, 1969).

The animals were observed during sleep and waking and when activated by Metrazol with a careful measurement of convulsive thresholds preoperatively and post-operatively. In addition, photic stimulation, acoustic
stimulation, and olfactory stimulation were used in the post-operative period in all animals. EEG recording was initiated 48 hours after cobalt
implantation when the EEG effects on the cortex were already manifest.
They lasted for about one to two months. After about a week's delay a
mirror focus appeared on the opposite temporal lobe. In the animals with
amygdala implants, as long as the discharge remained relatively unilateral,
so-called "psychomotor seizures" were described consisting of a sudden onset of apparent anxiety, rapid respiration and dilated pupils. This was
followed by clonic jerks of the right side of the face, sniffing, chewing,
and salivation followed by a period of unresponsiveness. Occasional de-
viations and turning to the left occurred and at the end urination and

defecation occurred.   The entire attack lasted 30 to 60 seconds.   In those
with hippocampal implants the attack started with an attitude of fear with
dilated pupils, ears flattened back and hyperventilation.   The animal re-
acted to any approach as if in fear and often tried to get out of its cage
at the slightest approach.   When the abnormal epileptic activity spread to
the entire cortex either directly from the hippocampus or following a period when it was confined to the temporal lobe, the animal became mo-
tionless, spell-bound, eyes staring with dilated pupils and hyperventilating.
There was a complete unresponsiveness to external stimuli.   This was followed by a post-ictal state during which the animal appeared confused,
with automatic movements of walking, digging, licking, purring, followed
by sleep.   Attacks from hippocampal implants were of longer duration
lasting 1-2 minutes.   At these times seizures might terminate with a generalized 10 to 20 sec duration episode of myoclonic jerks of facial, cer-
vical and upper limb muscles.   Metrazol and photic, auditory and olfactory stimulation could activate the amygdala seizures but in the hippocampal seizures olfactory stimulation was ineffective in activating the epileptic process while other methods were effective.   Histological controls

CAT Cd 1

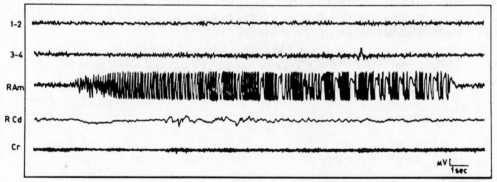

Fig. 16.   Cobalt epileptogenic lesion in the right ventral amygdala.
Cat Cd 1,4 days after cobalt introduction.   Recording of a seizure dis-
charge strictly localized to the amygdala, without neocortical involve-
ment.   No significant changes of the bioelectric caudate activity occur.
R Am, right ventral amygdala; Cr, paleocerebellar corticogram.
(Epilepsia, 10:337-350, 1969).

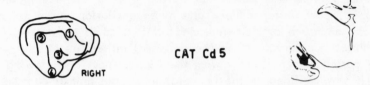

CAT Cd 5

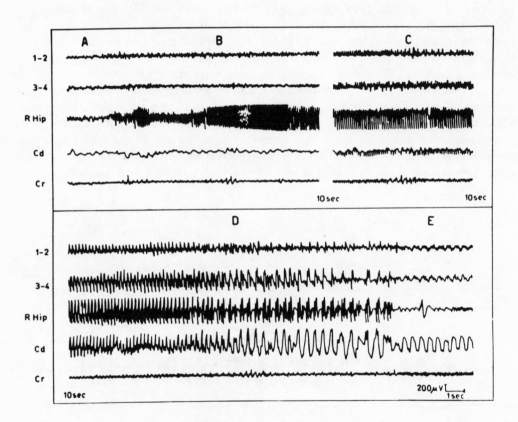

Fig. 17. Cobalt epileptogenic lesion in the right ventral hippocampus. Cat Cd5, 22 days after cobalt introduction. Recording of a hippocampal seizure discharge. A: pre-ictal pattern. B: onset of the hippocampal seizure discharge. C: diffusion of the discharge to the neocortex and caudate nucleus. D: the change-over is rhythmically interrupted by a slower activity and, at the caudate level, slow high voltage activity appears. The caudate activity persists after the end of the attack (E). (Epilepsia, 10:337–350, 1969).

showed that in each instance the lesions were limited to the target area. In both the amygdala and hippocampal series control lesions of electrylytic type failed to produce any part of the syndrome. Many times the seizure discharge remained confined to the amygdala or hippocampus in which case no behavioral change was noted (Figure 16). At other times these discharges spread to the caudate nucleus or the cortex (Figure 17) with the behavioral changes as described above.

The caudate activity (Mutani, 1969) mirrored that of the cerebral cortex when activity spread from the hippocampal or amygdala sites but usually outlasted that on the cortex. When the caudate nucleus was stimulated the effect on the hippocampal discharge was excitatory regardless of whether given between or during a spontaneous discharge. If the stimulating electrode was in the internal capsule the excitatory effect was more marked and could be elicited at a lower voltage. Mutani was of the opinion that this was therefore a truly internal capsule effect produced by current spread from the caudal nuclear electrode to the capsular fibers (Figure 18). If, however, the hippocampal or amygdal focus had entered

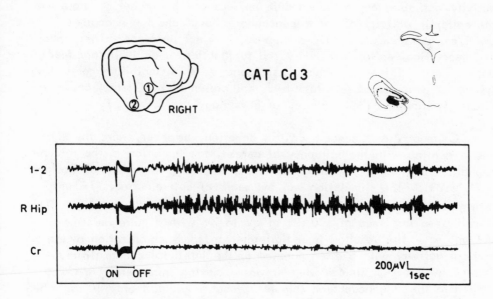

Fig. 18. Cobalt epileptogenic lesion in the right ventral hippocampus. Cat Cd 3, 15 days after cobalt introduction. A caudate train of stimuli (on-off) induces a hippocampal seizure discharge. Stimulation parameters: 13 V, 100/sec, 0.6 msec single-pulse duration. Epilepsia, 10:337-350, 1969.

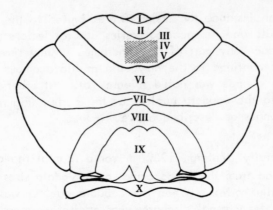

Fig. 19. Scheme of the lobular subdivision of the cerebellar vermis, according to Larsell(14). The paleocerebellar stimulation site is indicated by the dashed area. (Epilepsia, 10:351-362, 1969).

a clonic phase and had already spread to neocortex a 2 per sec spindle activity was observed in the caudate nucleus which was out of phase with the epileptic activity of the rhinencephalic focus and the neocortex (Figure 17E). It seemed to have a suppressive effect upon the rhinencephalic and neocortical epileptic activity and to function as an inhibitory feedback system. This is a rather classic concept of an inhibitory controlling system for generalized seizures which was presented by Gastaut and Fischer-Williams in the Handbook of Physiology in 1959.

Of more direct concern on this occasion, however, were the experiments dealing with the influence of cerebellar stimulation in the rhinencephalic cobalt epilepsy model in the cat (Mutani, Bergamini, & Doriguzzi, 1969). The stimulation was by means of ball electrodes 1-2 mm apart located on the surface of lobules III, IV, and V (Figure 19). The stimuli were for 1 sec at 100/sec at 6V to 7V with a pulse duration of 0.6 ml sec. This resulted in a flattening and desynchronization of the cortical activity with a disappearance of the interictal abnormalities. This might last 1-2 minutes when it was occurring infrequently and was limited to the rhinencephalon (Figure 20) but would last only 10 sec when it was more massive and had spread to neocortical sites. If cerebellar stimulation was given during an ictal phase of amygdala or hippocampal activity it was capable of stopping it regardless of whether it was given during the early tonic or later clonic phase of the ictal discharge so long as it remained confined to the rhinencephalic site (Figures 21 and 22).

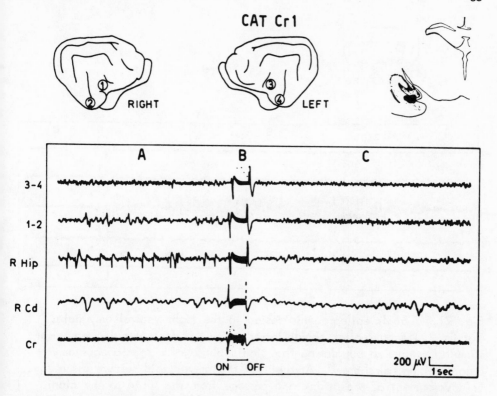

Fig. 20.   Cobalt epileptogenic lesion in the right ventral hippocampus.
Cat Cr 1, 22 days after cobalt introduction.   Effect of paleocerebellar
stimulation on the interictal epileptic activity.   A: hippocampal spikes
rarely propagated to the neocortex.   B: paleocerebellar stimulation (on-
off), parameters 6V, 100/sec, 0.6 msec single-pulse duration.   C: the
interictal epileptic activity has disappeared.   R Hip, right ventral
hippocampus;   R Cd., head of the right caudate nucleus; Cr., paleocerebellar corticogram.   (Epilepsia, 10:351-362, 1969).

If, however, the epileptic discharge had already spread to neocortical
or other subcortical structures cerebellar stimulation was ineffective during the tonic phase but would terminate the seizure if given during the
clonic phase of the neocortical seizure (Figure 23).   The same effect
was obtained if stimulation of the internal capsule was used to activate
the rhinencephalic seizure discharge (Figure 24).

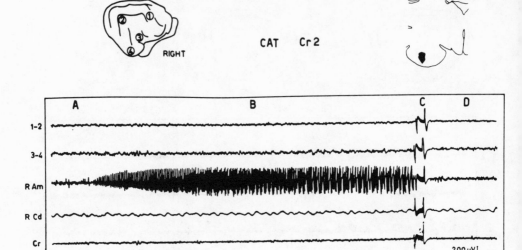

Fig. 21. Cobalt epileptogenic lesion in the right ventral amygdala. Cat Cr 2, 14 days after cobalt introduction. Effect of paleocerebellar stimulation carried out during the clonic phase of a spontaneous amygdaloid seizure discharge. A: onset of the amygdaloid seizure discharge. B: development of the attack and passage from the tonic to the clonic phase. The paleocerebellar stimulation (C) (same parameters as in Fig. 20) arrests the discharge (D). R Am., right ventral amygdala. (Epilepsia, 10:351-362, 1969).

        Adequate precautions were taken to preclude the possibility that these effects were due to spread of current to the reticular formation. Unfortunately no stimulation of the dentate or neocerebellar cortex has been attempted by Mutani as yet. Babb and associates (Babb, Mitchell, & Crandall, 1973) have stimulated both fastigial and dentate systems in hippocampal cobalt epilepsy in cats and they are reporting their results in this symposium. Unlike the caudate system, Mutani did not feel that the paleocerebellar system represented a feedback inhibitory mechanism because he was unable to show that the cerebellum was being constantly "informed" about the activity of the rhinencephalic focus. It should be recalled, however, that in our laboratory when cerebral electrical stimulation was at high voltage and prolonged it was reflected in a change in the unit activity of the cerebellar cortex. Julien and associates

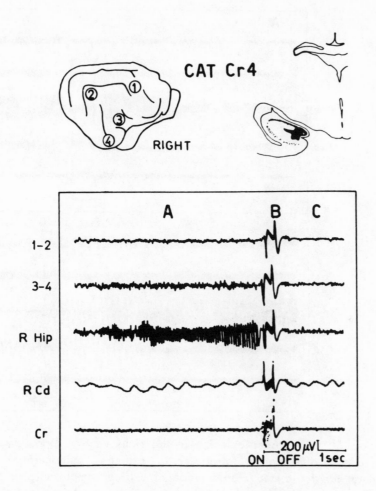

Fig. 22. Cobalt epileptogenic lesion in the right ventral hippocampus. Cat Cr 4, 10 days after cobalt introduction. Effect of paleocerebellar stimulation carried out during the tonic phase of a spontaneous hippo- campal seizure discharge. The paleocerebellar stimulation (B) (paramet- ers: 7V, 100/sec, 0.6 msec single-pulse duration) arrests the discharge. (Epilepsia, 10:351–362, 1969).

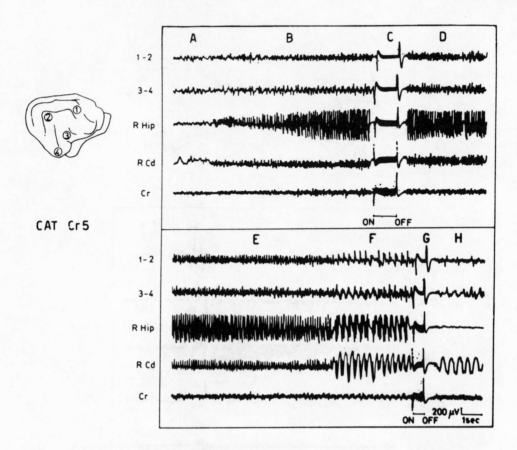

CAT Cr5

Fig. 23. Cobalt epileptogenic lesion in the right ventral hippocampus.
Cat Cr 5, 6 days after cobalt introduction. Effect of paleocerebellar
stimulation on the tonic and clonic phase of a hippocampal seizure discharge with a neocortical involvement: A: pre-ictal biolectric pattern.
B: onset of the discharge which propagates to the neocortex and caudate
nucleus. The paleocerebellar stimulation (C) (parameters: 8V, 100/sec,
0.6 msec single-pulse duration) has no effect on the seizure discharge
which goes on (D, E) developing into the clonic phase (F). The paleocerebellar stimulation (G) (same parameters as during the tonic phase)
stops the attack (H). Note the presence of slow voltage caudate
activity during the clonic phase of the seizure discharge and after its
end. (Epilepsia, 10:351-362, 1969).

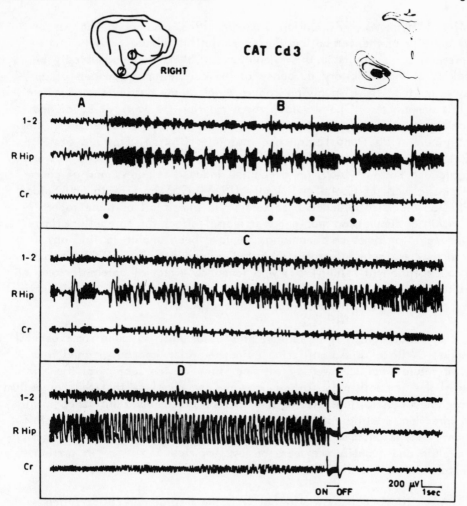

Fig. 24. Cobalt epileptogenic lesion in the right ventral hippocampus. Cat Cd 3, 35 days after cobalt introduction. Effect of the successive stimulation of the internal capsule and paleocerebellum on the activity of the cobalt hippocampal focus. A: Basal activity, B: single capsular shock (dot) (parameters: 13 V, 0.6 msec pulse duration) causes the appearance of a hippocampal spike discharge propagated to the neocortex and cerebellar electrodes. New capsular shocks sustain and enhance the discharge. C: the hippocampal discharge becomes self-sustained, with a tonic and, then, with a clonic pattern (D). Paleocerebellar stimulation (E) (same parameters as in Figure 23) stops the discharge and gives place to a flattened bioelectric pattern (F). The entire hippocampal seizure appears, therefore, to be due to the stimulation of extrarhinencephalic structures: it is produced by capsular stimulation and arrested by paleocerebellar stimulation. (Epilepsia, 10: 351-362, 1969).

(Julien & Halpern, 1972; Julien & Laxer, 1973) also found changes in
unit activity of the cerebellum during penicillin seizure activity and he
is presenting his results in this symposium.   Others will undoubtedly be
speaking of the inhibitory influence of the cerebellum on models of epilepsy other than these involving cobalt which is my particular assignment
in this symposium.   One should perhaps mention the work of Rucci and
associates (Rucci, Giretti, & LaRocca, 1968) on hyperoxic seizures, that
of Kreindler (1962) and Hutton and associates (Hutton, Frost, & Foster,
1972) on penicillin induced seizures in cats, Moruzzi (1941a, b, c) and
Viziola and Postera (1965) on strychnine induced seizures, and of course
the classic work of Cooke and Snider (1953, 1955) and Iwata and Snider
(1957) on electrically induced seizures.   In almost all of these reports
inhibition or suppression was not a universal effect for cerebellar stimulation could at times be enhancing.   I have been unable to find any
instance where cerebellectomy inhibited seizure activity.   Aside from the
single exception of Essig (1967) who found no effect of cerebellectomy on
barbitual withdrawal convulsions in dogs, all other ablation experiments
have resulted in an enhancement of seizure activity.

     In conclusion, I want to take this opportunity to make some general
remarks.   With all the conflicting evidence which can be gleaned from
the literature what can we say with certainty on the subject of the relation of the cerebellum to epilepsy?   One can conclude that the cerebellum
is capable of inhibiting seizures and that its predominant influence is in
this direction.   While species differences exist this is not crucial to this
general conclusion.   Because they do exist, however, further investigation
to explain and quantify the more or less empirical results of its present
clinical application should be performed on the primate brain.

     We still do not know whether it is the medial cerebellar system with
its projection to the reticular formation and hence the cortical activating
system which is responsible for this influence or the lateral cerebellum with
its dento thalamic projection system to the cortex or both.   This is an area
which needs clarification.   A combination of stimulation experiments with
sectioning of outflow pathways will be required to settle this issue.   Certainly from the work of Fadiga and associates (Fadiga, Manzoni, Sapienza,
& Urbano, 1968) it seems clear that the tonic desynchronizing and syn-
chronizing influence on the cerebral cortical rhythmic activity is the exclusive property of the midline cerebellar system rather than hemispherical
outflow.   We do not know if these, however, are identical with the regulation of epileptic activity and the negative results of Grimm and his
associates (Grimm, Frazee, Bell, Kawasaki, & Dow, 1970) in our laboratory would indicate that they are possibly independent.

The work on experimental models of epilepsy do not, in my opinion, clearly indicate whether nuclear or cortical stimulation is the most effective nor can one predict on the basis of present work on models of epilepsy what parameters of stimulation will be most effective. Evidence of electrical stimulation on other types of cerebellar function would indicate, moreover, that a solid prediction can never be made from experiment to experiment or even in single experiment from time to time what effects may be anticipated from cerebellar stimulation. It will, therefore, probably always be necessary in the clinical use of cerebellar stimulation in epileptic patients to rely on a certain amount of trial and error to determine the optimal parameters of stimulation for that particular seizure in that particular electrode placement. Some flexibility will therefore need to be built into the electronic equipment used in our present state of ignorance. Because of these uncertainties it is desirable if for no other reason that this method of treatment be reserved for those cases of epilepsy who fail to respond to more conventional modes of therapy. It would appear, however, not only on the basis of the limited clinical experience thus far but from the results in cobalt experimental epilepsy, that cerebellar stimulation will be less hazardous than cortical excision of epileptogenic foci. It is fortunate that cerebellar stimulation sites are effective for rapid and complete compensation for any inadvertant cerebellar damage is characteristic of a cerebellar lesion. Furthermore, in all its functional attributes it performs a regulatory influence on a nervous mechanism always capable of its own independent activity even when deprived of its cerebellar component. Therefore, the introduction of either stimulation or inadvertant lesion is less apt to produce ill effects than if the system which the cerebellum only regulates were stimulated or lesioned directly.

REFERENCES

ATSEV, E.M., ARUTYUNOV, V., DIMOV, S.P., & CHAVDAROV, D. Dynamics of electrical manifestation of brain activity in cats and rabbits with an experimental epileptogenic focus (Macro- and micro-electrode investigations). In Servit, Z. (Ed.) "Comparative and Cellular Pathophysiology of Epilepsy". New York: Excerpta Medica Foundation, 1966, pp. 221-234.

BABB, T.L., MITCHELL, A.G., & CRANDALL, P.H. Fastigiobulbar and dentatothalamic influences on hippocampal cobalt epilepsy in the cat. 1973 (submitted for publication).

BARTON, G. & DOW, R.S. Effect of cerebellar stimulation on penicillin-induced convulsant activity in the cat. Unpublished data. Laboratory of Neurophysiology, Good Samaritan Hospital & Medical Center, Portland, Oregon, 1965.

CESA-BIANCHI, M.G., MANCIA, M., & MUTANI, R. Experimental epilepsy induced by cobalt powder in lower brain-stem and thalamic structures. Electroenceph. Clin. Neurophysiol. 22:525-536, 1967.

CEREGHINO, J.J. & DOW, R.S. Effect of cobalt applied to the cerebellum on cobalt experimental epilepsy in the cat. Epilepsia, 11:413-421, 1970.

CHAMBERS, W.W. & SPRAGUE, J.M. Functional localization in the cerebellum. I. Organization in longitudinal cortico-nuclear zones and their contribution to the control of posture, both extrapyramidal and pyramidal. J. Comp. Neurol. 103:105-129, 1955a.

CHAMBERS, W.W. & SPRAGUE, J.M. Functional localization in the cerebellum. II. Somatotopic organization in cortex and nuclei. Arch. Neurol. Psychiat. 74:653-680, 1955b.

CHUSID, J.G. & KOPELOFF, L.M. Epileptogenic effects of pure metals implanted in motor cortex of monkeys. J. Appl. Physiol. 17: 697-700, 1962.

CHUSID, J.G. & KOPELOFF, L.M. Epileptogenic effects of metal powder implants in motor cortex of monkeys. Int. J. Neurophysiat. 3:24-28, 1967.

CLARK, S.L. Responses following electrical stimulation of the cerebellar cortex in the normal cat. J. Neurophysiol. 2:19-35, 1939a.

CLARK, S.L. Motor seizures accompanying small cerebellar lesions in cats. J. Comp. Neurol. 71:41-57, 1939b.

CLARK, S.L. & WARD, J.W. The electroencephalogram in cerebellar seizures. Electroenceph. Clin. Neurophysiol. 1:299-304, 1949.

COOKE, P.M. & SNIDER, R.S. Some cerebellar effects on the electrocorticogram. Electroenceph. Clin. Neurophysiol. 5:563-569, 1953.

COOKE, P.M. & SNIDER, R.S. Some cerebellar influences on electrically induced cerebral seizures. Epilepsia, 4:19-28, 1955.

DAWSON, G.D. & HOLMES, O. Cobalt applied to the sensorimotor area of the cortex cerebri of the rat. J. Physiol. 185:455-470, 1966.

DIMOV, S.D. Changes in the cerebral bioelectric activity of rabbits following application of cobalt to the brain cortex (formation and development of epileptogenic focus). In Servit, Z. (Ed.) "Comparative and Cellular Pathophysiology of Epilepsy". New York: Excerpta Medica Foundation, 1966, pp. 235-242.

DOW, R.S. Cerebellar syndromes. In Vinken, P.J. & Bruyn, G.W. (Eds) "Handbook of Clinical Neurology". Amsterdam: North-Holland Publishing Co., 1969, pp. 392-431.

DOW, R.S., FERNANDEZ-GUARDIOLA, A., & MANNI, E. The influence of the cerebellum on experimental epilepsy. Electroenceph.
Clin. Neurophysiol. 14:383-398, 1962a.

DOW, R.S., FERNANDEZ-GUARDIOLA, A., & MANNI, E. The production of cobalt experimental epilepsy in the rat. Electroenceph.
Clin. Neurophysiol. 14:399-407, 1962b.

DOW, R.S. & MORUZZI, G. "The Physiology and Pathology of the
Cerebellum". Minneapolis: The University of Minnesota Press, 1958.

ECCLES, J.C., ITO, M., & SZENTAGOTHAI, J. "The Cerebellum as
a Neuronal Machine". New York: Springer-Verlag, 1967.

ESSIG, C.F. Clinical and experimental aspects of barbituate withdrawal
convulsions. Epilepsia, 8:21-30, 1967.

FADIGA, E., MANZONI, T., SAPIENZA, S., & URBANO, A. Syn-
chronizing and desynchronizing fastigial influences on the electrocortical activity of the cat, in acute experiments. Electroenceph.
Clin. Neurophysiol. 24:330-342, 1968.

FISCHER, J. Elektronemikrokopische befunde bei der epileptogenen
kobalt nekrose im rattengehirn. Experientia, 24:162, 1968.

FISCHER, J. Electron microscope findings on the ganglion cells of an
experimental cobalt-gelatin focus in the rat. Physiol. Bohemsolov.
17:458-459, 1969.

FISCHER, J., HOLUBER, J., & MALIK, V. A new method of producing
chronic epileptogenic cortical foci in rats. Physiol. Bohemoslov.
16:272-277, 1967.

FISCHER, J., HOLUBER, J., & MALIK, V. Neurohistological study of
the development of experimental cortical cobalt-gelatin foci in rats
and their correlation with the onset of epileptic electrical activity.
Acta Neuropath. (Berlin), 11:45-54, 1968.

GASTAUT, H. & FISCHER-WILLIAMS, M. The physiopathology of epileptic seizures. In Field, J. (Ed.) "The Handbook of Physiology,
Vol. I". Baltimore: Williams & Wilkins, 1959, pp. 329-363.

GRIMM, R.J., SAVIC, M., PETERSEN, P.F., & GRIFFITH, J.S.
Halothane anesthesia for squirrel monkeys used in neurophysiology
studies. Laboratory Primate Newsletter, 8:7-16, 1969.

GRIMM, R.J. & FRAZEE, J.G. Suppression of cerebellar evoked responses in cerebral cortex during drowsiness in squirrel monkeys. Int.
J. Neurol. 7 (2,3,4):113-125, 1970a.

GRIMM, R.J., FRAZEE, J.G., BELL, C.C., KAWASAKI, T., & DOW,
R.S. Quantitative studies in cobalt model epilepsy: The effect of
cerebellar stimulation. Int. J. Neurol. 7 (2,3,4): 113-140, 1970.

GRIMM, R.J., FRAZEE, J.G., KAWASAKI, T., & SAVIC, M. Cobalt
epilepsy in the squirrel monkey. Electroenceph. Clin. Neurophysiol.
29:525-528, 1970c.

GRIMM, R.J., FRAZEE, J.G., & OZBAY, S. Afterdischarge bursts in
    cobalt and penicillin foci in primate cortex. Electroenceph. Clin.
    Neurophysiol. 34:281–301, 1973.
HENJYOJI, E.Y. & DOW, R.S. Cobalt induced seizures in the cat.
    Electroenceph. Clin. Neurophysiol. 19:152–161, 1965.
HODSKINS, M.B. & YAKOVLEV, P.I. Anatomico–clinical observations
    on myoclonus in epileptics and on related symptom complexes. Am.
    J. Psychiat. 9:827–848, 1930.
HOLUBAR, J. & FISCHER, J. Electrophysiological properties of the
    epileptogenic cortical foci produced by a new cobalt–gelatine
    method in rats. An attempt to correlate the electrophysiological,
    histological, and histochemical data. Physiol. Bohemoslov. 16:
    278–283, 1967.
HUTTON, J.T., FROST, J.D., & FOSTER, J. The influence of the
    cerebellum in cat penicillin epilepsy. Epilepsia, 13:401–408, 1972.
IWATA, K. & SNIDER, R.S. Some evidences of cerebello–hippocampal
    interrelationships. Anat. Rec. 133:292, 1959.
JULIEN, R.M. & HALPERN, L.M. Effects of diphenylhydantoin and
    other antiepileptic drugs on epileptiform activity and Purkinje cell
    discharge rate. Epilepsia, 13:387–400, 1972.
JULIEN, R.M. & LAXER, H.R. Cerebellar responses to penicillin–induced
    cerebral cortical epileptiform discharge. (Submitted for publication
    in Brain Research) 1973.
KOPELOFF, L.M. Experimental epilepsy in the mouse. Proc. Soc. Exp.
    Biol. Med. 104:500–504, 1960.
KREINDLER, A. Active arrest mechanisms of epileptic seizures. Epilepsia,
    3:329–337, 1962.
MANCIA, M. & LUCIONI, R. EEG and behavioral changes induced by
    subcortical introduction of cobalt powder in chronic rat. Epilepsia,
    7:308–317, 1966.
MANNI, E., HENATSCH, H.D., HENATSCH, E.M., & DOW, R.S.
    Localization of facilitatory and inhibitory sites in and around the
    cerebellar nuclei affecting limb posture, alpha and gamma moto-
    neurons. J. Neurophysiol. 27:210–228, 1964.
MORUZZI, G. Sui rapporti fra cervelletto e corteccia cerebrale.
    I. Azione d'impulsi cerebellari sulle attivita corticali motrici dell'
    animale in narcose cloralosica. Arch. Fisiol. 41:87–139, 1941a.
MORUZZI, G. Sui rapporti fra cervelletto e corteccia cerebrale.
    II. Azione d'impulsi cerebellari sulle attivita motrici provocate
    dalla stimolazione faradica o chimica del giro sigmoideo nel gatto.
    Arch. Fisiol. 41:157–182, 1941b.

MORUZZI, G. Sui rapporti fra cervelletto e corteccia cerebrale.
III. Meccanismi e localizzazione delle azioni inhibitrici e dinamogene del cervelletto. Arch. Fisiol. 41:183-206, 1941c.

MORUZZI, G. Effects at different frequencies of cerebellar stimulation
upon postural tonus and myotatic reflexes. Electroenceph. Clin.
Neurophysiol. 2:463-469, 1950.

MORUZZI, G. & POMPEIANO, O. Inhibitory mechanisms underlying
the collapse of decerebrate rigidity after unilateral fastigial lesions.
J. Comp. Neurol. 107:1-25, 1957a.

MORUZZI, G. & POMPEIANO, O. Effects of vermal stimulation after
fastigial lesions. Arch. ital. de biol. 95:31-55, 1957b.

MUTANI, R. Cobalt experimental amygdaloid epilepsy in the cat.
Epilepsia, 8:73-92, 1967a.

MUTANI, R. Cobalt experimental hippocampal epilepsy in the cat.
Epilepsia, 8:223-240, 1967b.

MUTANI, R. Experimental evidence for the existence of an extrarhinencephalic control of the activity of the cobalt rhinencephalic epileptogenic focus. Part I. The role played by the caudate nucleus.
Epilepsia, 10:337-350, 1969.

MUTANI, R., BERGAMINI, L., & DORIGUZZI, T. Experimental evidence for the existence of an extrarhinencephalic control of the activity of the cobalt rhinencephalic epileptogenic focus. Part 2.
Effects of paleocerebellar stimulation. Epilepsia, 10:351-362, 1969.

NEEDHAM, C.W. & DILA, C.J. Cobalt epilepsy and the reticular
formation. Neurology, 19:310, 1969.

PAYAN, H., LEVINE, S., & STREBEL, R. Inhibition of experimental
epilepsy by chemical stimulation of cerebellum. Neurology, 16:
573-576, 1966.

REIMER, G.R., GRIMM, R.J., & DOW, R.S. Effects of cerebellar
stimulation on cobalt induced epilepsy in the cat. Electroenceph.
Clin. Neurophysiol. 23:456-462, 1967.

RUCCI, F.S., GIRETTI, M.L., & LaROCCA,M. Cerebellum and hyper-
baric oxygen. Electroenceph. Clin. Neurophysiol. 25:359-371,1968.

SPRAGUE, J.M. & CHAMBERS, W.W. Regulation of posture in intact
and decerebrate cat. I. Cerebellum, reticular formation, vestibular
nuclei. J. Neurophysiol. 16:451-463, 1953.

VIZIOLA, R. & PASTENA, L. Azione del cervelletto sulle punte
stricniche del giro sigmoideo del gatto e considerazioni sui rapporti
fra epilessa e cervelletto. Riv. Neurol. 35:259-269, 1965.

ACKNOWLEDGMENTS

This work was made possible through National Institutes of Health Grant
No. 02289.

EXPERIMENTAL EPILEPSY: CEREBRO-CEREBELLAR

INTERACTIONS AND ANTIEPILEPTIC DRUGS

Robert M. Julien

Department of Medical Pharmacology and Therapeutics
University of California at Irvine
Irvine, California

Epilepsy is a term used to describe the repeated occurrence of any of the various clinical forms of convulsive seizures. Convulsive seizures appear to be the normal mode of expression of cerebral cortex and subcortical structures to an excessive, overwhelming discharge originating in a variety of loci. The tonic extensor rigidity and clonic convulsive movements of the clinical grand mal attack result from involvement of motor cortex and the spread of excitation away from the abnormal focal discharge (Adrian, 1936). One fundamental problem in epilepsy involves identification of the mechanism underlying and controlling the "highly explosive" discharges described by Hughlings Jackson (1931) which characterize the cortical epileptic focus (Ward, 1969).

In experimental epilepsy, a variety of topically applied chemical agents produce convulsive episodes which resemble in many respects the behavioral and electrographic characteristics of clinical epilepsy (Ajmone-Marsan, 1969). Of these several epileptogenic agents, penicillin applied topically to cerebral cortex has a rapid onset of interictal spike activity which progresses to spontaneous ictal episodes in about two hours (Julien & Halpern, 1972). These ictal episodes recur frequently and predictably over a period of several hours. In addition, several reports (Prince, 1968, 1969; Matsumoto et al, 1969; Ayala et al, 1970) have characterized the intracellular events in neurons located near the penicillin focus. Most studies have been the intracellular events occurring during the transition from the interictal to the ictal episode. The consensus is that this transition is not a direct action of

the epileptogenic agent, but results from excessive impingement upon
inhibitory neurons such that they may become temporarily inactivated
(Dichter & Spencer, 1968; Kandel & Spencer, 1969). This falling-out
of inhibitory mechanisms would create a favorable situation for development of the ictal episode. To date, however, these inhibitory mechanisms which might exert a restraining action over epileptiform activity
and whose falling-out might predispose to development of the ictal
episode have not been identified.

This failure to clearly identify extra-focal inhibitory mechanisms
which might modulate cerebral cortical excitability has occurred despite
the attempts of numerous investigators to artificially stimulate many areas
of the brain in attempts to limit or terminate abnormal electrographic
activity (Dow, 1965 for review). Of all structures so far investigated,
only two appear when stimulated to significantly reduce or inhibit seizure development. These two structures are the caudate nucleus (La-
Grutta et al, 1971) and the cerebellar cortex. The present investigation
is directed towards a further understanding of the involvement of the
cerebellum both in the modulation of epileptiform activity and in the
action of antiepileptic drugs. Subsequent investigations will examine
more closely the action of the caudate nucleus.

Electrical stimulation of the cerebellar cortex is capable of inhibiting strychnine-induced spinal cord convulsions (Terzuolo, 1954) and
electrically-induced cerebral cortical (Cooke & Snider, 1955) or hippocampal (Iwata & Snider, 1959) seizures. Similarly, cerebellar stimulation during periods of cerebral cortical seizure activity produces a
positive DC-shift in cerebral cortex while simultaneously shortening
seizure duration (Donde & Snider, 1955). In the rat, similar cerebellar
stimulation inhibits cobalt-induced epileptiform activity (Dow et al,
1962). In the cat, penicillin-induced activity is reduced by cerebellar
stimulation (Hutton et al, 1972). Mutani et al (1969) reported that
cerebellar cortical stimulation markedly decreases the excitability of
cobalt-induced epileptic focus in cat amygdalae and hippocampus and
inhibits or stops seizure discharge resulting from activity in either focus.

Since stimulation of the cerebellar cortex tends to limit seizure
activity, one would predict that cooling or destruction of the cerebellar
cortex would exert an opposite action: i.e. augmentation of seizure
discharge. Indeed, it has been demonstrated that such cooling does
tend to intensify seizure activity (Terzuolo, 1954; Dow et al, 1962).
In the human, Cooper and co-workers have reported that electrical
stimulation of cerebellar cortex inhibits epileptiform activity while

ablation of cerebellar nuclei tends to exert a similar effect (Cooper et al, 1973 and elsewhere in this volume).

From these and other studies one would conclude that the cerebellar cortex appears to uniformly demonstrate the ability to limit, terminate, or reduce convulsive activity which may originate in cerebral cortical or subcortical structures. However, cerebellar responses to cerebral cortical epileptiform activity has not been recorded nor has the cerebellum been implicated as a possible site of action of antiepileptic drugs. Both of these important areas will now be discussed.

CEREBELLAR RESPONSES TO EPILEPTIFORM ACTIVITY

In a series of experiments conducted in locally anesthetized, paralyzed cats with penicillin-induced foci in sensory-motor cortex, simultaneous electrode recordings were made in either the cerebellar cortex or the dentate nucleus together with a recording in the anterior sygmoid gyrus (sensory-motor cortex) near the site of penicillin injection (Julien & Halpern, 1972; Julien & Laxer, submitted). Prior to sub pial injection of 5,000 units of penicillin into the anterior sygmoid gyrus, cellular discharge recorded from either Purkinje cells or from cells located in the dentate nucleus are as follows: Purkinje cell (P-cell) discharge is characteristically low and irregular, averaging approximately 10 to 25 Hz. The discharge rate of dentate cells (D-cells) is characteristically higher and much more regular, averaging approximately 35 - 40 Hz. This high discharge rate in the dentate agrees quite closely with the average of 37 Hz reported by Thach (1972).

After a delay of approximately 20 minutes following penicillin injection, P-cells and D-cells both begin to respond to high voltage penicillin-induced epileptiform activity in characteristic manners. In the Purkinje cells, high frequency bursts of cellular discharge commence approximately 20 msec after the initial deflection of the epileptiform "spike" and P-cell discharge persists for approximately 75 - 80 msec (Fig. 1). In the dentate, however, a period of inhibition of discharge is observed during the approximate 100 msec time course of the epileptiform "spike". The D-cell does not discharge until after a delay of approximately 100 msec. Although microelectrode recordings have not been made simultaneously from a P-cell and a D-cell, the time course of these events suggest that the dentate cell does not begin its characteristic discharge burst until after the Purkinje cell burst has ceased. Simultaneous recordings are obviously necessary to further characterize

P - cell

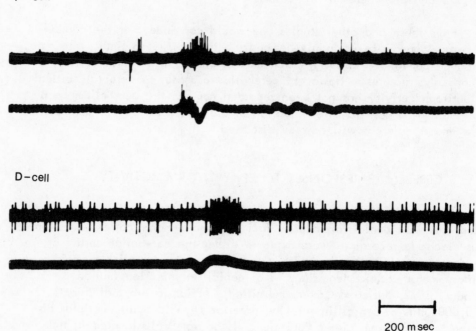

D - cell

200 m sec

Fig. 1. Penicillin-induced bursts of Purkinje cells (upper traces) and dentate cells (lower traces) to activity originating from a focus in anterior sigmoid gyrus. Note that P-cells are evoked after a short (20 msec) latency while D-cells do not burst until approximately 100 msec after the initiation of the focal "spike". Note also the differing rates of spontaneous activity from P-cells and D-cells.

the exact time pattern of these responses. It would be expected, however, that since the Purkinje cell is known to inhibit the discharge of dentate cells (Ito & Yoshida, 1964) such inhibition of D-cell discharge during the P-cell burst would be predicted. In addition, the discharge frequency of the D-cell burst (up to 300 Hz) would also be predicted since rebound facilitation is known to follow P-cell inhibition of the dentate (Eccles et al, 1967). Following this short, high frequency burst of dentate cells, D-cell discharge recovers to normal spontaneous rates after a short delay (Fig. 1).

P-cell responses similar to that shown in Figure 1 have been identified over the entire cerebellar cortex and at sites both ipsilateral and
contralateral to the penicillin focus. Similarly, high frequency dentate
bursts have been recorded from D-cells in both the ipsilateral and contralateral dentate nucleus. Whether these cellular responses in cerebellum
ipsilateral to the focus are a direct result of high voltage discharge or an
indirect involvement as a result of involvement of cortex contralateral to
the focus has not been delineated.

As the penicillin focus continues to develop (and assuming that an
end-tidal CO_2 of 3.0 to 3.2% is maintained and no local anesthetic has
been absorbed from the wound margins), short (2 - 10 sec) bursts of epileptiform activity may be recorded. These short seizure bursts are conducted to the right cerebral hemisphere although they do not develop to maximal voltage or exhibit the characteristic hypersynchrony observed during
the prolonged episodes which develop later (see below). During these
short epileptiform bursts, Purkinje cells throughout all areas of the cerebellum discharge at high frequencies (150 - 200 Hz) for the duration of
the burst and cease discharging following cessation of the episode (Fig. 2).
In the dentate, high frequency discharge bursts of D-cells are similarly
observed during the epileptogenic activity (Fig. 3). Following cessation
of the episode, the D-cells become quiescent and gradually resume spontaneous discharge rates.

As the penicillin focus continues to develop, the short, fast, epileptiform activity described above develops into prolonged ictal episodes
which become maximal, synchronous, and generalized throughout both
cerebral hemispheres. Accompanying development of these prolonged
ictal episodes are distinct alterations in the behavior of cells in the
cerebellum. In the Purkinje cells, cellular discharge abruptly ceases
during this transition from sustained focal discharge to the maximal, synchronous, generalized episode and the Purkinje cells remain quiescent
during the entire convulsive episode (Fig. 4). Following cessation of the
episode, the cells remain quiescent and seldom resume discharging for
20 - 60 seconds. In the dentate, however, a different pattern of cellular activity is observed (Fig. 5). The D-cells continue to behave as
they did during the short episodes in that they continue to discharge in
high frequency bursts and do not cease discharging as did the Purkinje
cells. If anything, D-cell discharge becomes more intense as the episode continues.

From these data, several conclusions may be drawn. First, during
development of the penicillin focus, both the Purkinje cells and dentate

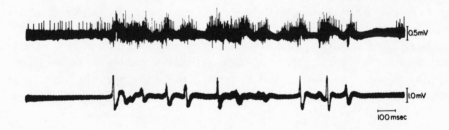

Fig. 2.   Response of a Purkinje cell in contralateral paravermis (upper trace) to epileptiform activity originating in left anterior sigmoid gyrus.

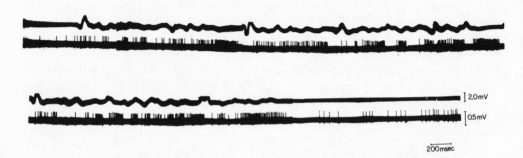

Fig. 3.   Nine second cortical epileptiform burst (upper trace) recorded 45 minutes after penicillin.   Lower trace: discharge of cell located in dentate nucleus.   Upper pair of traces continues with lower pair.   Note the continued discharge of the D-cell during the epileptiform burst and the rapid return to spontaneous discharge rate after termination of the burst.

cells respond to high voltage "spike" activity with characteristic bursts consisting of a Purkinje cell burst commencing 20 msec after the initial phase of the epileptiform spike and persisting for approximately 80 msec. This is followed by a high frequency burst of dentate cells.   Second, there is a "falling-out" of inhibitory discharge (the Purkinje cell) during development of the major, synchronous, prolonged ictal episode.   Third, the observation that Purkinje cells (which have ceased discharging during

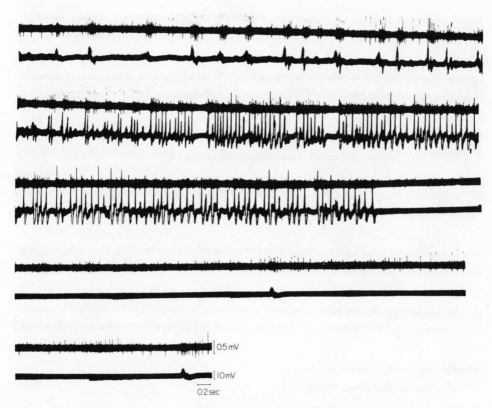

05 mV

10mV

02 sec

Fig. 4.   Discharge of a Purkinje cell in the anterior cerebellar vermis
before, during and after a penicillin-induced epileptiform burst recorded
in sensory-motor cortex.   Note the spontaneous and evoked cellular
discharge (top trace), cessation of cellular discharge during transition
to high voltage seizure activity (left side of 2nd set of traces, and the
return of spontaneous and evoked cellular discharge approx. 10 seconds
following termination of the seizure.   Vertical deflections above the
cerebellar recording during the last half of the seizure are high voltage
spikes from the focus overshooting the cerebellar record.

the ictal episode) do not resume discharging until many seconds following termination of the seizure indicates that the cerebellar cortex is most
likely not involved in the active termination of the epileptiform episode.
The falling-out of inhibition during development of the epileptiform episode, however, implies that loss of cerebellar cortical function may be
involved in development of the episode.   Perhaps other structures such as
the caudate nucleus may be more intimately involved in the active

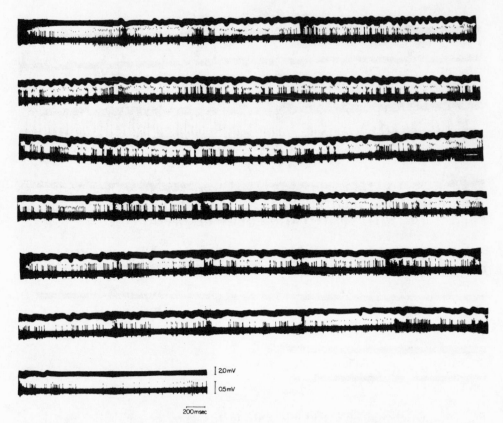

Fig. 5. Thirty second epileptiform burst recorded approximately 1.5 hours after penicillin. Upper trace, recording from focus. Lower trace, discharge of cell located in dentate nucleus. Note continuous high frequency discharge of dentate cell during entire epileptiform episode and rapid return to spontaneous discharge frequency following cessation of the episode (bottom trace).

termination of already initiated convulsive activity. It is important to note that a true cause and effect relationship between the cessation of P-cell discharge and the generalization of seizure activity remains to be elucidated. However, the many experiments of other workers (discussed above) demonstrating the influence of cerebellar cortical stimulation on epileptiform activity indicates that this is likely.

THE CEREBELLUM AND THE ACTION OF ANTIEPILEPTIC DRUGS

The introduction of diphenylhydantoin (DPH, Dilantin) by Merritt and Putnam (1938) signaled the introduction of the first antiepileptic compound which was not a potent depressant of the nervous system. In numerous studies on isolated nerves DPH has been found to exert a "stabilizing effect" (Korey, 1951; Toman, 1952; Toman & Sabelli, 1969) in the absence of depressant effects on conduction velocity or excitability thresholds (Brumlik & Moretti, 1966; Bigger et al, 1968; Julien & Halpern, 1970; Den Hertog, 1972). The only apparent effect of DPH on peripheral nerve is increased "C" fiber excitability following rapid repetitive electrical stimulation (Julien & Halpern, 1970). This reduction of the hypoexcitable period in C fibers following repetitive stimulation is thought to be due to DPH-induced depression of post-tetanic hyperpolaization (Raines & Standaert, 1967; Julien & Halpern, 1970). Such an action of DPH, however, is not depressant in nature as it would tend to increase neuronal responsiveness to single stimuli administered subsequent to repetitive conditioning. It may therefore be concluded that DPH exerts a membrane stabilizing effect protecting the nerve against repetitive activity generated by repetitive stimuli. Normal conduction parameters are unaffected by physiologic doses of DPH.

Similarly, DPH exerts little effect on the parameters of synaptic transmission following single shocks, but does exert a significant depression of the potentiation of synaptic transmission through spinal or ganglionic synapses following repetitive conditioning of either the dorsal root or the preganglionic nerve trunk (Esplin, 1957). Indeed, this block of post-tetanic potentiation by DPH correlates with the drug's ability to modify cortical seizure discharge (Esplin & Zablocka, 1969) and is perhaps the best explanation to date for the anticonvulsant action of the drug. It is not currently known, however, if post-tetanic potentiation is a naturally occurring physiological phenomenon or is an artifact of high frequency electrical stimulation. Similarly, the relation between post-tetanic potentiation and cortical hyperexcitability (or seizure spread) has not been demonstrated.

Aside from these studies of DPH on peripheral nerve and synaptic transmission, there are a few reports on the effects of DPH on discrete cortical circuits which might provide a more adequate explanation for the unique anti-convulsant properties of the compound. Giachetti (1949) first proposed that DPH blocked transmission of convulsive activity from neurons of a primary epileptogenic focus to secondary areas which were themselves normal. Subsequently, other investigators demonstrated that DPH prevents the development and spread of cortical epileptiform activity (Gangloff & Monnier, 1957; Morrell et al, 1959; Strobos and Spudid, 1960; Louis et al, 1968). These reports concluded that the anticonvulsant effect of DPH correlates with limitation of spread rather than with suppression of the primary focus and that the mechanism of action of DPH involves a reinforcement of those systems within the brain which serve to limit seizure propagation rather than a direct action on epileptogenic tissues. Thus, an extra-focal site of action of DPH was suggested but has not been identified.

That this extra-focal site might be cerebellar in origin was indicated by several studies. First, cerebellar ataxia, both reversible and irreversible, has been reported following chronic administration of large doses of DPH (Merritt & Putnam, 1938; Utterback et al, 1958; Roger & Soulayrol, 1959). Selective Purkinje cell degeneration has been reported in patients administered high doses of DPH (DeChamps et al, 1958; Hoffman, 1958; Utterback et al, 1958; Haberland, 1962; Afifi & Van Allen, 1968). Purkinje cell degeneration has also been demonstrated in cat cerebellum (Utterback et al, 1958) while P-cell degeneration has been correlated with DPH blood levels in humans, cats, and rats (Kokenge et al, 1965). Similarly, patients whose seizures were poorly controlled by DPH had P-cell densities significantly lower than those in patients adequately controlled by the drug (Dam, 1970). Finally, DPH appears to be selectively concentrated in the cerebellum (Kokenge et al, 1965).

Thus, since DPH is not a neuronal depressant, since DPH exerts prominent effects on the cerebellum, since Purkinje cells are inhibitory to their projections to cerebellar nuclei (Ito & Yoshida, 1964), and since the net result of stimulation of the cerebellar cortex (Purkinje cells) is limitation of seizure activity, DPH-induced augmentation of Purkinje cell activity would account at least in part for the antiepileptic usefulness of the compound. Thus, experiments were designed to delineate the action of DPH on Purkinje cells and also on representative cells located in a structure to which the Purkinje cells project (the dentate nucleus).

In studies on Purkinje cells, DPH administration is followed by dramatic increases in spontaneous P-cell discharge rate in normal cats and in cats with penicillin-induced epileptogenic foci (Julien & Halpern, 1971, 1972). Purkinje cell discharge rate characteristically increases from a low, random rate of approximately 25 Hz to continuous discharges at greater than 120 Hz (Fig. 6). Increases are usually apparent within 30 minutes after 10 mg/kg doses of DPH and reach maximal discharge frequencies two

hours after DPH administration, then declining slowly over a several
hour period.

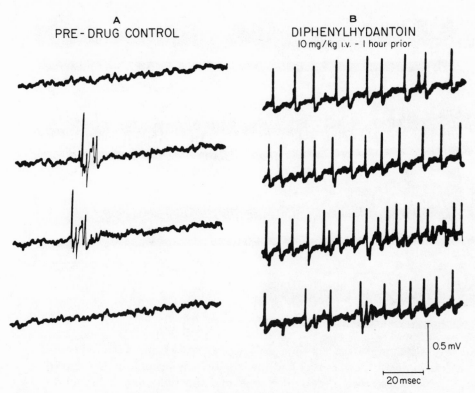

Fig. 6. Spontaneous discharge of a cerebellar Purkinje cell before (A)
and one hour after (B) diphenylhydantoin (10 mg/kg i.v.). Each sweep
is 100 msec in duration.

In cats chronically pretreated with DPH (5 mg/kg i.p. 2 x daily
for 3 days), P-cell discharge rate was sustained at frequencies of approximately 140 Hz in at least 65 cells studied (Halpern & Julien, 1972).
Additional acute doses of DPH(10 mg/kg i.v.) induced no further increases
in P-cell discharge rate in these chronically pretreated animals. In cats
with penicillin-induced epileptiform activity, depression of seizure activity
by DPH was accompanied by sustained Purkinje cell discharge at rates
greater than 120 Hz (Fig. 7). Cerebellectomy subsequent to DPH administration resulted in intensification of epileptiform activity indicating that
the cerebellar cortex is necessary for the drug's antiepileptic action
(Julien & Halpern, 1972).

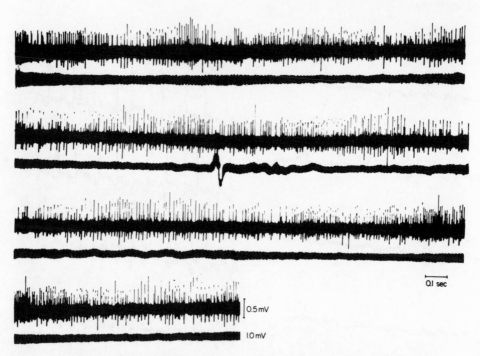

Fig. 7. Discharge of a Purkinje cell (upper trace) and activity near a penicillin focus (lower trace) following diphenylhydantoin (10 mg/kg i.v.). Note sustained P-cell discharge and the reduction in epileptiform activity. The four sets of traces are continuous.

That this augmentation of Purkinje cell discharge subsequent to DPH administration may be the result of a direct action of DPH on the P-cell is indicated by the experiments of Gabreëls (1970). In his doctoral theses, Gabreëls reported that Purkinje cells (either in vivo or in tissue culture) are metabolically more active under the influence of small doses of DPH. Similarly, in studies on Bemegride convulsions in rats, doses of 100 mg/kg DPH produced favorable antiepileptic effects while higher doses (150 - 200 mg/kg) became progressively less and less anticonvulsive. Together with this loss of effectiveness, a cerebellar syndrome emerged and toxic changes became morphologically apparent in Purkinje cells. Finally, in rats with cerebellar cortectomy, DPH had little effect and it was concluded that DPH appears to be antiepileptic only if the cerebellar cortex is intact. These data add further evidence to the present hypothesis that DPH may exert a direct action on cerebellar Purkinje cells and that this action is important in the antiepileptic action of the drug.

If DPH increases the discharge rate of Purkinje cells and if this action is related to the antiepileptic action of the compound, DPH should indirectly decrease the spontaneous discharge rate of cells located in the dentate nucleus. In studies conducted with Dr. K. Laxer in 15 cats, such decreases were observed (Fig. 8). DPH (10 mg/kg i.v.) was found to decrease the spontaneous discharge rate of dentate cells from approximately 37 Hz to rates as low as 5 Hz.

Thus, administration of DPH is followed by significant increases in the discharge rate of Purkinje cells with concomitant slowing of spontaneous activity of cells within the dentate nucleus. In addition, the data concerning the responses of the Purkinje cell during penicillin-induced epileptiform activity together with the reductions of seizure activity which follow cerebellar cortical stimulation leads one to postulate that this augmentation of Purkinje cell discharge may be related to the antiepileptic action of DPH.

Subsequent studies (Julien & Halpern, 1972; Julien, 1972) indicate that phenobarbital and diazepam (Valium) similarly increase the discharge rate of Purkinje cells and such increases occur concomitant with the depression of penicillin-induced epileptiform discharge. Thus, both phenobar-

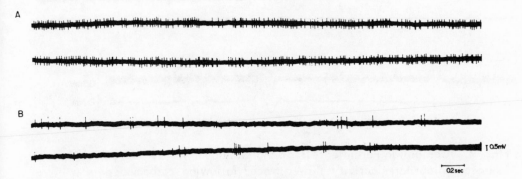

Fig. 8. Spontaneous discharge rate of a cell located in the dentate nucleus before (A) and after (B) diphenylhydantoin (10 mg/kg). Note the drug-induced decrease from 37 Hz to 5 Hz.

bital and diazepam appear to exert their antiepileptic actions at least in
part through a mechanism which is similar to that of DPH.

What appears to be needed is an orally effective, antiepileptic
drug which exerts its seizure-depression action in the absence of Purkinje
cell involvement. Identification of such a drug would provide a compound which might be therapeutically effective in patients unresponsive
to cerebellar-stimulant, antiepileptic compounds such as DPH, phenobarbital or diazepam. From studies on 12 cats with penicillin-induced epileptiform activity, carbamazepine (Tegretol) was found to effectively suppress epileptiform discharge in the absence of augmented Purkinje cell
discharge rates (Fig. 9). Following administration of carbamazepine
(10 - 20 mg/kg i.p) and with the attainment of blood levels in the range
of 4 - 15 ug/ml, carbamazepine effectively suppressed epileptiform activity and Purkinje cell discharge was characteristically low, resembling discharges in non-epileptic animals. However, epileptiform spike activity
was still capable of eliciting high frequency bursts of Purkinje cell discharge. Thus, from these preliminary studies it appears that carbamazepine may be an effective antiepileptic drug which exerts its action through

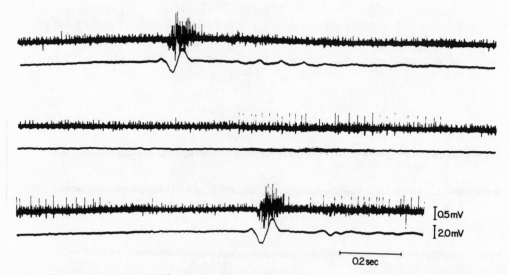

Fig. 9. Cerebellar Purkinje cell discharge (upper trace) and penicillin-
induced epileptiform activity (lower trace) following carbamazepine
(Tegretol*, 20 mg/kg i.p.). Note the low rate of spontaneous P-cell
activity, the reduction in epileptiform discharge, and the P-cell burst
evoked by focal "spike" activity. The three pairs of traces are continuous.

a mechanism which, although yet unidentified, differs from that of other currently available compounds. Carbamazepine, therefore, may be beneficial in those patients unresponsive to other medication. Other studies with carbamazepine (Julien, submitted) indicate that the drug effectively supresses alumina cream-induced electrographic and behavioral seizures in Rhesus monkeys, does not block post-tetanic potentiation in cat spinal cord, and intensifies Premarin-induced 3/sec spike and wave activity in cats. Therefore, the compound would seem to be useful in major seizures with less efficacy in minor seizures such as petit mal. In addition, the lack of effect on Purkinje cells and on post-tetanic potentiation indicates a mode of action different from that of other currently available compounds.

CEREBRO-CEREBELLAR INTERACTIONS IN EXPERIMENTAL EPILEPSY

The well established anatomy of the cortico-Purkinje-dentate-thalamo loop can be displayed in the circuit diagram presented in Figure 10. Epileptiform activity originating in sensory-motor cortex projects via the pyramidal tract to pontine nuclei (PN) and the inferior olive (IO) which in turn project to Purkinje cells and dentate cells (Evarts & Thach, 1969 for review). Activity of the dentate is then projected back through the diffuse nuclei of the thalamus to sensory-motor cortex. In this circuit diagram, the Purkinje cells provide the only known inhibitory control and

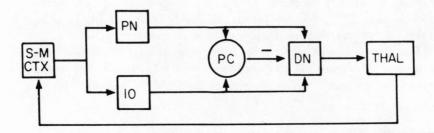

Fig. 10. Block diagram of proposed circuit for cerebrocerebellar interactions in experimental epilepsy. S-M CTx = sensory-motor cortex; PN = pontine nuclei; IO = inferior olive; PC = Purkinje cell; DN = dentate nucleus; Thal = non-specific thalamus. For simplicity the intermediate steps between PN and PC have been omitted. Note that PC is the only inhibitory control.

this control is exerted through projections onto the dentate cells (Eccles et al, 1967; Ito, 1970). Since the only inhibitory control of this circuit is through the P-cell projection to the dentate, Purkinje cell function is essential in order to restrain and modulate activity in the circuit. If as in the major, bilateral, synchronous seizure episode, the Purkinje cell ceases to function (as in Figure 4), there would be no inhibitory influence and the system would be without inhibition and thus be self perpetuating. Similarly, if Purkinje cell activity could be augmented (as by DPH in Figure 6), the circuit would be restrained and epileptiform activity would be inhibited.

Similarly, from Figure 10 one would predict that interruption of the cortico-dentate-thalamo pathway or else increased P-cell activity should decrease seizure activity. On the other hand, stimulation of the circuit or inhibition of the Purkinje cell should increase seizure activity. There is experimental evidence that indeed such predictions may be true. As stated above, electrical stimulation of the cerebellar cortex (P-cells) inhibits or abolishes epileptiform activity. Such stimulation also decreases cellular discharge in the diffuse nuclei of the thalamus and in cerebral cortex (Snider et al, 1970). Also, pharmacologic augmentation of Purkinje cell activity by DPH, phenobarbital, or diazepam correlates with drug-induced depression of seizures. Similarly, ablation of the cerebellar cortex appears to intensify seizure discharge (Dow et al, 1962) and antagonize the antiepileptic action of DPH (Gabreëls, 1970). In the dentate nucleus, electrical stimulation intensifies seizure activity (Mitchell et al, in press; Babb et al, submitted) while, in man, ablation of the dentate inhibits seizures (Cooper, elsewhere in this volume). In diffuse nuclei of the thalamus, electrical or chemical stimulation induces seizure activity (Hunter & Jasper, 1949; Manhke et al, 1971; Mitchell et al, in press) while ablation reduces seizure frequency and duration (Kusske et al, 1972). Thus, experimental evidence is in general agreement with the control diagram of Figure 10 and indicates that this circuit may indeed be important in the modulation of cortical excitability and epileptiform activity.

Obviously, this is not the only circuit within the brain which acts to modulate cortical excitability. This was evidenced by the antiepileptic action of carbamazepine (Fig. 9) which was not exerted through the cerebellum. Indeed, such structures as the caudate nucleus are known to be inhibitory (LaGrutta et al, 1971). The involvement of the caudate, however, in cortical excitability remains to be elucidated.

A final comment appears to be in order. Hobson and McCarley

(1972) demonstrated in cats that the discharge rate of Purkinje cells decreases during transition from waking to synchronized sleep. This observation is of interest to the present discussion since there is much clinical information that seizures frequently occur during this transition from wakefulness to synchronized sleep and synchronized sleep may act as a convulsant, facilitating appearance of generalized bilateral hypersynchrony (Pompeiano, 1969). During the transition from wakefulness to sleep, the EEG becomes synchronous or even hypersynchronous while Purkinje cell discharge is reduced. It is intriguing to speculate that perhaps loss of inhibition (as characterized by loss of Purkinje cell discharge) may be partly responsible for the electrographic hypersynchrony and increased seizure susceptibility which occurs during onset of sleep.

Recently, it was also demonstrated that low frequency dentate stimulation would synchronize activity in non-specific thalamic nuclei (Hayrapetian & Vaghanian, 1970) and it is well known that thalamic stimulation diffusely synchronizes activity throughout cerebral cortex. From Figure 10, loss of Purkinje cell discharge would lead to reverberating synchrony throughout this cortico-dentate-thalamic circuit, facilitating the development of hypersynchrony with increased seizure susceptibility.

The recent report of Cooper et al (1973) that, in humans, electrical stimulation of the cerebellar cortex leads to decreased epileptiform activity indicates once again that the cerebellar cortex via the Purkinje cells exerts a significant restraint over cortical excitability, perhaps through the circuit depicted in Figure 10.

Supported by USPHS grant #NS-09835, National Institute of Neurological Diseases and Stroke, and by a grant from the Rebecca Payne Livingston Foundation.

ACKNOWLEDGMENTS

The author wishes to gratefully acknowledge the technical assistance of Mr. J. Manago and Mr. D. Kunis; the secretarial assistance of Mrs. B. Knudsen; and the participation of Dr. K. Laxer on the dentate experiments.

REFERENCES

ADRIAN, E.D. The spread of activity in the cerebral cortex. J.
    Physiol. 88:127, 1936.
AFIFI, A.K. & VAN ALLEN, M.W. Cerebellar atrophy in epilepsy.
    J. Neurol. Neurosurg. Psychiat. 31:169-174, 1968.
AJMONE-MARSAN, C. Acute effects of topical epileptogenic agents.
    In Jasper, Ward, & Pope (Eds.) "Basic Mechanisms of the
    Epilepsies". Boston: Little, Brown & Co., 1969.
AYALA, G.F., MATSUMOTO, H., & GUMNIT, R.J. Excitability
    changes and inhibitory mechanisms in neocortical neurons during
    seizures. J. Neurophysiol. 33:73-85, 1970.
BABB, T.L., MITCHELL, A.G., & CRANDALL, P.N. (submitted).
    Fastigiobulbar and dentatothalamic influences on hippocampal
    epilepsy in the cat.
BIGGER, J., BASSETT, A., & HOFFMAN, B. Electrophysiological
    effects of diphenylhydantoin on canine Purkinje fibers. Circulation
    Research, 22:221-236, 1968.
BRUMLIK, J. & MORETTI, L. The effects of diphenylhydantoin on nerve
    conduction velocity. Neurology, 16:1217-1218, 1966.
COOKE, P.M. & SNIDER, R.S. Some cerebellar influences on electric-
    ally-induced cerebral seizures. Epilepsia, 4:19-28, 1955.
COOPER, I.S., CRIGHEL, E., & AMIN, I. Clinical and physiological
    effects of stimulation of the paleocerebellum in humans. J. Amer.
    Geriatr. Soc. 21:40-43, 1973.
DAM, M. Number of Purkinje cells in patients with Grand Mal Epilepsy
    treated with diphenylhydantoin. Epilepsia, 11:313-320, 1970.
DeCHAMPS, A., COLLE, G., HOZAY, J., & ROUSSEL, J. Anatomo-
    clinical documents on epilepsy. Acta Neurol. Belg. 58:105-129,
    1958.
DEN HERTOG, A. The effect of diphenylhydantoin on the electrogenic
    component of the sodium pump in mammalian non-myelinated nerve
    fibers. Europ. J. Pharmacol. 19:94-97, 1972.
DICHTER, M.A. & SPENCER, W.A. Hippocampal penicillin "spike"
    discharge: epileptic neuron or epileptic aggregate. Neurology,
    18:282, 1968.
DONDE, M. & SNIDER, R.S. On cerebellar stimulation. Electroenc-
    eph. clin. Neurophysiol. 7:265-272, 1955.
DOW, R.S. Extrinsic regulatory mechanisms of seizure activity.
    Epilepsia, 6:122-140, 1965.
DOW, R.S., FERNÁNDEZ-GUARDIOLA, A., & MANNI, E. The in-
    fluence of the cerebellum on experimental epilepsy. Electroenceph.
    clin. Neurophysiol. 14:383-398, 1962.

ECCLES, J.C., ITO, M., & SZENTAGOTJAI, J. "The Cerebellum as a Neuronal Machine". New York: Springer-Verlag, 1967.

ESPLIN, D.W. Effects of diphenylhydantoin on synaptic transmission in cat spinal cord and stellate ganglion. J. Pharmacol. exp. Ther. 120:301-323, 1957.

ESPLIN, D.W. & ZABLOCKA, B. Effects of tetanization on transmitter dynamics. Epilepsia, 10:193-210, 1969.

EVARTS, E.V. & THACH, W.T. Motor mechanisms of the CNS: cere-brocerebellar interrelations. Ann. Rev. Physiol. 31:451-498, 1969.

GABREËLS, F.J.M. De Invloed van Phenytoine op de Purkinje-cel van de Rat. Doctoral Dissertation, Catholic University of the Nether-lands, 1970. Summarized in Epilepsy Abstracts 5:110, 1972.

GANGLOFF, H. & MONNIER, M. The action of anticonvulsant drugs tested by electrical stimulation of the cortex, diencephalon, and rhinencephalon in the unanesthetized rabbit. Electroenceph. clin. Neurophysiol. 9:43-58, 1957.

GIACHETTI, A. Effect of phenytoin on the transmission of epileptic activity with special reference to Clementi's sensory epilepsy. Arch. Sci. Biol. 33:390-398, 1949.

HABERLAND, C. Cerebellar degeneration with clinical manifestation in chronic epileptic patients. Psychiat. Neurol. 143:29-44, 1962.

HALPERN, L.M. & JULIEN, R.M. Augmentation of cerebellar Purkinje cell discharge rate after diphenylhydantoin. Epilepsia, 13:377-385, 1972.

HOBSON, J.A. & McCARLEY, R.W. Spontaneous discharge rates of cat cerebellar Purkinje cells in sleep and waking. Electroenceph. clin. Neurophysiol. 33:457-469, 1972.

HOFFMAN, W.W. Cerebellar lesions after Dilantin administration. Neurology, 8:210-214, 1958.

HUNTER, J. & JASPER, H.H. Effects of thalamic stimulation in unan-esthetized animals. Electroenceph. clin. Neurophysiol. 1:305-324, 1949.

HUTTON, J.T., FROST, J.D., & FOSTER, J. The influence of the cerebellum in cat penicillin epilepsy. Epilepsia, 13:401-408, 1972.

ITO, M. Neurophysiological aspects of the cerebellar motor control system. Int. J. Neurology, 7:162-176, 1970.

ITO, M. & YOSHIDA, M. The cerebellar-evoked monosynaptic inhib-ition of Deiters neurons. Epxerientia, 20:515-516, 1964.

IWATA, K. & SNIDER, R.S. Cerebello-hippocampal influences on the electroencephalogram. Electroenceph. clin. Neurophysiol. 11: 439-446, 1959.

JACKSON, J.H. "Selected Writings of John Hughlings Jackson",
      Vol. I, on epilepsy and epileptiform convulsions. Ed. by
      J. Taylor, Hodder and Stoughton, London, 1931.

JULIEN, R.M. Cerebellar involvement in the antiepileptic action of
      diazepam. Neuropharmacology, 11:683-691, 1972.

JULIEN, R.M. Carbamazepine (Tegretol): Correlation of blood levels
      with antiepileptic effects in acute and chronic epileptic cats and
      monkeys. (Submitted).

JULIEN, R.M. & HALPERN, L.M. Stabilization of excitable membrane
      by chronic administration of diphenylhydantoin. J. Pharmacol. exp.
      Ther. 175:206-212, 1970.

JULIEN, R.M. & HALPERN, L.M. Diphenylhydantoin: Evidence for a
      central action. Life Sciences, 10:575-582, 1971.

JULIEN, R.M. & HALPERN, L.M. Effects of diphenylhydantoin and
      other antiepileptic drugs on epileptiform activity and Purkinje cell
      discharge rate. Epilepsia, 13:387-400, 1972.

JULIEN, R.M. & LAXER, K.D. Cerebellar responses to penicillin-
      induced cerebral cortical epileptiform discharge. (Submitted).

KANDEL, E. & SPENCER, W.A. Synaptic inhibition in seizures. In
      Jasper, Ward & Pope (Eds.) "Basic Mechanisms of the Epilepsies".
      Boston: Little, Brown & Co., 1969.

KOKENGE, R., KUTT, H., & McDOWELL, F. Neurological sequelae
      following Dilantin overdose in a patient and in experimental
      animals. Neurology, 15:823-829, 1965.

KOREY, S.R. Effect of Dilantin and Mesantoin on the giant axon of
      the squid. Proc. Soc. exp. Biol. Med. 76:297-299, 1951.

KUSSKE, J.A., OJEMANN, G.A., & WARD, A.A.,Jr. Effects of
      lesions in ventral anterior thalamus on experimental focal epilepsy.
      Exp. Neurol. 34:279-290, 1972.

LaGRUTTA, V., AMATO, G., & ZAGAMI, M.T. The importance of
      the caudate nucleus in the control of convulsive activity on the
      amygdaloid complex and the temporal cortex of the cat. Electro-
      enceph. clin. Neurophysiol. 31:57-69, 1971.

LOUIS, S., KUTT, H., & McDOWELL, F. Intravenous diphenylhydan-
      toin in experimental seizures. II. Effect on penicillin-induced
      seizures in the cat. Arch. Neurol. 18:472-477, 1968.

MAHNKE, J.H., BABB, T.L., & VERZEANO, M. The action of chol-
      inergic agents on the electrical activity of the non-specific nuclei
      of the thalamus. Proc. Amer. Assoc. Neurol. Surg., 1971.

MATSUMOTO, H., AYALA, G.F., & GUMNIT, R.J. Neuronal behav-
      ior and triggering mechanisms in cortical epileptic focus. J.
      Neurophysiol. 32:688-703, 1969.

MERRITT, H.H. & PUTNAM, T.J. Sodium diphenylhydantoinate in the treatment of convulsive disorders. J.A.M.A. 111:1068-1073, 1938.

MITCHELL, A.G., BABB, T.L., & CRANDALL, P.H. Influence of a dentate-thalamic pathway on experimental hippocampal epilepsy. Electroenceph. clin. Neurophysiol. (in press)

MORRELL, F., BRADLEY, W., & PTASHNE, M. Effect of drugs on discharge characteristics of chronic epileptiform lesions. Neurology, 9:492-498, 1959.

MUTANI, R., BERGAMINI, L., & DORIGUSSI, T. Experimental evidence for the existence of an extrarhinencephalic control of the activity of the cobalt rhinencephalic epileptogenic focus. Part 2, Effect of paleocerebellar stimulation. Epilepsia, 10:351-362, 1969.

POMPEIANO, O. Sleep Mechanisms. In Jasper, H.H., Ward, A.A. & Pope, A. (Eds.) "Basic Mechanisms of the Epilepsies". Boston: Little, Brown, & Co., 1969.

PRINCE, D.A. Inhibition in "epileptic" neurons. Exptl. Neurol. 21:307-321, 1968.

PRINCE, D.A. Electrophysiology of "epileptic" neurons: Spike generation. Electroenceph. clin. Neurophysiol. 26:476, 1969.

RAINES, A. & STANDAERT, F.G. An effect of diphenylhydantoin on post-tetanic hyperpolarization of intramedullary nerve terminals. J. Pharmacol. exp. Ther. 156:591-597, 1967.

ROGER, J. & SOULAYROL, R. A propos des accidents neurologiques du traitement de l'epilepsie par les hydantoines. Rev. Neurol. 100:783-785, 1959.

SNIDER, R.S., MITRA, D.J., & SUDILOUSKY, A. Cerebellar effects on the cerebrum. Int. J. Neurology, 7:141-151, 1970.

STROBOS, R.J. & SPUDID, E.V. Effect of anticonvulsant drugs on cortical and subcortical seizure discharges in cats. Arch. Neurol. 2:399-406, 1960.

TERZUOLO, C. Influences supraspinales sur le tetanos strychnique de la moelle elineire. Arch. int. Physiol. 62:179-196, 1954.

THACH, W.T. Cerebellar output: Properties, synthesis and uses. Brain Research, 40:89-97, 1972.

TOMAN, J.E.P. Neuropharmacology of peripheral nerve. Pharmacol. Rev. 4:168-218, 1952.

TOMAN, J.E.P. & SABELLI, H.C. Comparative neuronal mechanisms. Epilepsia, 10:179-192, 1969.

UTTERBACK, R.A., OJEMAN, R., & MALEK, J. Parenchymatous cerebellar degeneration with dilantin intoxication. J. Neuropath. exp. Neurol. 17:516-519, 1958.

WARD, A.A.J. The epileptic neuron: Chronic foci in animals and man. In Jasper, Ward, & Pope (Eds.) "Basic Mechanisms of the Epilepsies". Boston: Little, Brown, & Co., 1969.

THE EFFECT OF CHRONIC STIMULATION OF CEREBELLAR

CORTEX ON EPILEPSY IN MAN

I. S. Cooper, I. Amin, S. Gilman and J. M. Waltz

Departments of Neurosurgery and Neurology
St. Barnabas Hospital
Bronx, New York

The purpose of this report is to summarize our observations of the effects of chronic stimulation of the cerebellar cortex in 7 patients with intractable epilepsy and one patient totally incapacitated by generalized intention myoclonus. These 8 patients represent part of a series of 28 cases in whom we have attempted to utilize the inhibitory function of cerebellar cortex to achieve a therapeutic modification of motor behavior. The remaining 20 patients were incapacitated by various types of spasticity and/or rigidity. Preliminary results in this latter group have been reported separately (Cooper, Crighel, & Amin, 1973).

This therapeutic approach was conceived on the basis of abundant anatomic and electrophysiologic evidence that cerebellar cortex modifies sensory information and motor behavior both via descending cerebello-nucleofugal reticulo spinal pathways and via ascending nucleofugal-thalamo-cortical connections (Cooper, 1973; Cooper, Crighel, & Amin, 1973). A brief review of some of the principal contributions is germane to this communication.

The powerful inhibitory activity of cerebellar cortex was demonstrated in the last century when Lowenthal and Horsley (1897) and Sherrington (1897) independently reported the relaxation of decerebrate rigidity by stimulation of anterior lobe at cerebellum. Twenty-five years ago Fulton (1948) stated that the importance of inhibitory action of anterior cerebellum could not be too greatly stressed.

Moruzzi (1950) reported the remarkable observation that stimulation

119

of anterior lobe (paleocerebellum) could produce either a decrease or an increase of decerebrate rigidity from the same point, depending upon the frequency of stimulation. He found that with frequencies of 10 cycles/sec. increase of decerebrate rigidity might be achieved while frequencies of 100 to 300 cycles/second invariably produced a decrease. Moruzzi held that temporal summation was responsible for reversal from inhibition to fac- ilitation. Furthermore, he noted that the decrease of frequency of stimu- lation could be compensated for by increasing the duration of each stimu- lus, but that a train of repetitive stimuli was always necessary in order to produce an inhibitory or facilitatory effect.

Moruzzi concluded, therefore, that there is a temporal summation within cerebellar cortex, as well as in the deep nuclei or reticular cen- ters. A reticulo-spinal pathway to internuncial neurons which then brought about inhibition of spinal motoneurons has been held to account for the powerful inhibition achieved by paleocerebellar stimulation. Fur- thermore, Moruzzi suggested that high frequency paleocerebellar stimula- tion can overcome synaptic resistances in contralateral bulbo-reticular centers, irradiating from the ipsilateral center, to produce bilateral motor influence.

In addition to its profound effect on spinal motoneurone activity, cerebellar cortex has been demonstrated to have important modulating effects via both thalamic and brain stem relays upon cerebral cortex, as well as interactions with afferents to widespread areas of cortex and ef- ferents from it. Soriano and Fulton (1947) found that spasticity is much stronger in monkeys if extirpation of areas 4 and 6 is associated with ab- lation of anterior lobe of cerebellum. Walker (1938) had earlier shown that electrical stimulation of Crus I and II of neocerebellum led to marked alteration of spontaneous electrical activity of the cerebral motor area, and to a lesser extent in parietal and temporal regions. Henneman, Cooke, and Snider (1952) later showed a much more extensive widespread cerebellar projection to cerebral cortex.

Snider (1967) has conclusively demonstrated cerebellar influences on sensory systems at the cerebral level, via projections through many thal- amic nuclei, as well as diencephalic tegmentum. Both anatomic and electrophysiologic evidence supports the presence of cerebro-cerebellar loops which not only interact at brain stem levels, but by means of which the cerebrum feeds back information to cerebellum and, in turn, has its activities modulated by cerebellum. In a review paper, Snider (1950) offered some speculations on the possible functional significance of cere- bro-cerebellar loops. He later developed the thesis that cerebellum helps to regulate levels of responsiveness in sensory systems as a temporal

modulator to "switch or gate" ascending activity depending on the "neurologic need" of the organism.

It would seem apparent that this abundant evidence of the ability
of cerebellum to inhibit peripheral manifestations of motor hyperactivity
at the sponal motoneurone level, its ability to modify sensory information
in the brain stem and in cerebro-cerebellar loops, as well as its direct
connections via VL to motor cortex, should lead to speculation concerning
the relationship of cerebellar function to epilepsy.

Moruzzi (1950) postulated that cortical convulsive discharges tend
to evoke the activity of paleocerebellar suppressor mechanisms. Cooke
and Snider (1955) investigated the possibility of cerebellar mechanisms
involved in cerebral seizure activity. They showed that cerebellar stimulation could alter electrical patterns of the seizure discharges in cerebrum,
and that stimulation voltages as low as 7V in cat cerebellar cortex could
completely stop a seizure discharge which was induced by 60V applied to
cerebrum. One explanation which these authors suggested was that cerebellar excitation of the reticular activating system may have been responsible for the breakdown of the synchronized seizure discharges.

Dow et al (Dow, Fernández-Guardiola, & Manni, 1962) studied the
influence of cerebellum on chronic epileptic activity in unrestrained unanesthetized rats. Epilepsy was induced in these animals by application of
cobalt powder to the right frontal lobe. In a series of varied experimental conditions these investigators found the cerebellar influence on chronic
epilepsy to be essentially inhibitory. In some cases of generalized cobalt
induced seizure, augmented by parenteral administration of an additional
convulsive agent, megimide, cerebellar stimulation was not effective.
Dow and his associates attributed this to depression and increased threshold
of cerebellum to electrical stimulation caused by megimide.

Generally, however, electrical stimulation of anterior cerebellum
inhibited seizures in Dow's studies. Furthermore, the inhibitory effect on
the seizure activity of cerebral cortex was generalized and not localized
to the contralateral hemisphere. This led Dow et al to suggest that cere-
bello-reticular connections play a role in this inhibitory effect, a conclusion harmonious with Moruzzi's view that paleocerebellar stimulation affects both ipsilateral and contralateral brain stem reticular formation.

The most recent physiologic finding which contributed to the concept
of chronic cerebellar cortical stimulation was the demonstration by Ito and
Yoshida (1964) that the synaptic effect of Purkinje cell discharge

is uniformly inhibitory. Conversely, the major aspect of the second cerebellar efferent stage, the nucleofugal impulses of dentatus, fastigium and
interpositus, is purely excitatory (Eccles, Ito, & Szentágothai, 1967). A
steady tonic discharge of these deep cerebellar nuclei, and of Dieters
nucleus, give rise to depolarization in the membrane of nuclei in the
brain stem, reticular formation, various thalamic nuclei, including VL
and the red nucleus. Stimulation of cerebellar cortex induced inhibitory
Purkinje cell discharge, which goes either down the spinal cord to moto-
neurones, to participate in control of motor movement, or is directed to
cerebral cortex via brain stem, reticular formation, thalamus, and diencephalon, modulating motor and other behavioral activity of these higher
levels.

Thus the cerebellar cortex can be thought of as a potential store-
house of inhibition designed to react to a complex inflow of information,
which the Purkinje cell inhibitory outflow can modify at various nervous
system levels of information processing mechanisms. The concept of chronic cerebellar stimulation is based upon the thesis that this Purkinje cell
inhibition can be prosthetically induced to modify neurologic activity
which is abnormally and undesirably heightened by pathologic facilitation
or disinhibition (Cooper, 1973; Cooper, Amin, & Gilman, 1973; Cooper
& Gilman, 1973).

It would appear, on the basis of these consistent experimental data
from Sherrington, Lowenthal and Horsely, Fulton, Moruzzi, Snider, Dow
et al, Ito and Yoshida, and Eccles et al, as well as many others, that
the enormous expanse of cerebellar cortex and its potential of Purkinje
cell inhibitory discharge offers the possibility of modulating motor behavior
and tone as the pedals of a mighty organ modulate the output of its chimes.

This investigation represents an initial effort to study the various combinations of pathologic substrata, physiologic conditions, electrode placements, and combinations of stimulation parameters which may prove to be
therapeutically fruitful. The data resultant from this therapeutic effort are
of a preliminary nature but will, we hope, lead to improved therapy of
presently intractable neurologic disorders and also contribute to our understanding of the complex function of the human brain.

Both Snider (1973) and Dow (1973) have suggested to us that for
descriptive purposes of the human cerebellum we refer to anterior and
posterior cerebellum rather than paleo and neocerebellum. For the purpose of this communication, therefore, we shall use this nomenclature.

SURGICAL TECHNIQUE

For electrode placement on anterior cerebellum, that is cerebellar cortex anterior to the posterior superior fissure, the cerebellum is approached from the superior surface of the tentorium cerebelli. A small occipital craniectomy with gentle retraction of the occipital lobe of cerebrum allows exposure of the tentorium. A small flap is incised in the tentorium medial to the lateral sinus. This approach was perfected in human cadaver disections prior to its use in patients.

A plate of silicon coated mesh with four pairs of platinum disc electrodes, affixed similar to those previously employed on the surface of human spinal cord for dorsal column stimulation, is applied beneath the tentorium to the cortex of anterior lobe of cerebellum (Fig. 1). This approach also exposes part of Crus I of posterior cerebellum, which may also be affected by the most laterally placed pair of the four pairs of surface electrodes. The cortex of posterior cerebellum, principally Crus I and II of the posterior lobe, is approached by a routine suboccipital craniectomy (Fig. 2). Bipolar stimulation between four or more pairs of electrodes is produced simultaneously. In some cases electrode bearing plates have been placed on both anterior and posterior cerebellar cortex. It is now our practice to apply electrodes to both anterior and posterior lobe cortex in all cases. Various protocols of simultaneous or alternating stimulation have been assessed. The electrode plate location is confirmed by x-ray (Fig. 3). The electrodes are stimulated through an antenna fixed subcutaneously on the chest, by means of a trans-epidermal inductive coupling (Fig. 4). Rectangular pulses, of one millisecond width, with a rate of 7 - 200 c/s and an intensity of 0.5-14 volts were used for stimulation.

The 8 patients to be reported have been followed for 7 to 11 months since electrode implantation. Periodically, clinical examination, motion pictures, electromyograms, EEG recordings, detailed psychological examinations, and ancillary electrophysiologic tests have been performed.

The parameters of stimulation have varied from case to case, and have been changed, depending upon effects noted in individual cases. The most commonly employed frequency in the epileptic patients has been 7 - 15 cycles per second. This was instituted because during empirical trial in our first case an aura and seizure was elicited by stimulation at 200 c/s and interrupted by stimulation at 10 c/s. The voltage generally varies from 5 to 14 V, although some electrophysiologic testing has been performed at 0.5 to 1.0 volt.

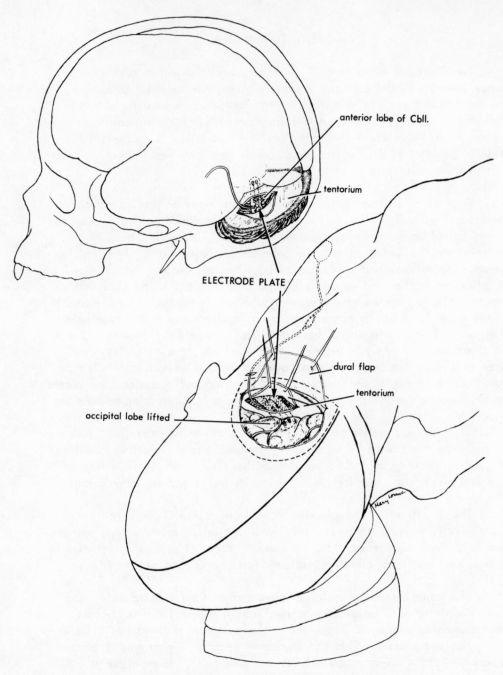

Fig. 1. Surgical approach through the tentorium, after retraction of occipital lobe, which is employed for placement of electrode plate on anterior cerebellum.

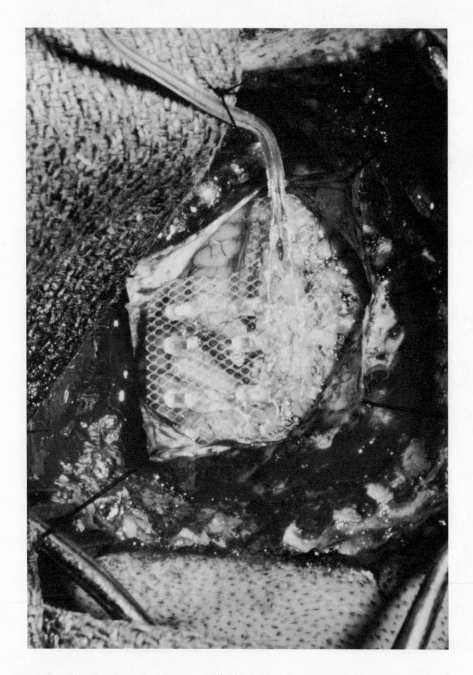

Fig. 2. Placement of silicon mesh bearing 8 pairs of bipolar electrodes on posterior cerebellum.

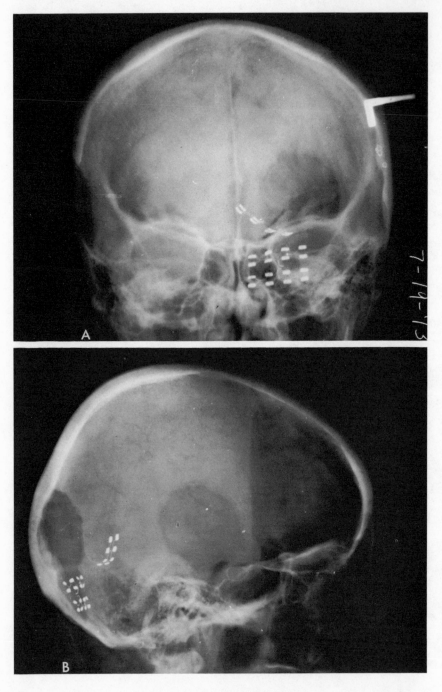

Fig. 3A and B. Anterior and lateral roentgenograms demonstrating electrode arrays on anterior and posterior cerebellum.

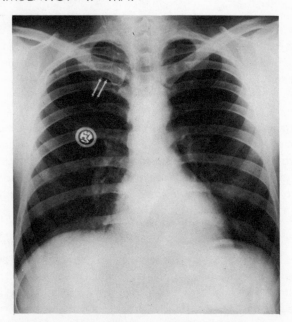

4A. Chest roentgenogram demonstrating position of subcutaneous receiver which is attached to the intracranial electrodes.

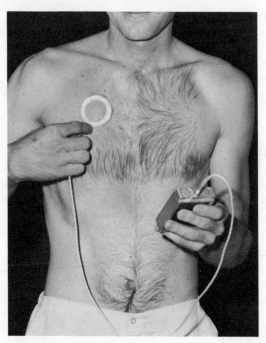

4B. Demonstration of placement of antenna from power pack over the sight of the subcutaneous receiver.

Originally stimulation was applied when the patient felt an aura, in order to attempt to abort the usually succeeding seizure.   However, the technique was modified to provide chronic automatic stimulation throughout the day in an attempt to prevent both auras and seizures.   For this purpose an automatic timed power pack stimulator was developed.

The stimulator is designed to deliver predetermined electrical impulses to two separate areas of the cerebellum.   The energy requirements of this system necessitate an external power source which transmits signals across the skin by means of radio waves to two implanted receiver-electrode assemblies.   A totally implantable device is desirable and being investigated with several engineering and biophysical colleagues.

The external signal generator consists of a radio transmitter which feeds two separate loop transmitting antennas.   The implanted portion of the system contains two miniaturized passive radio receivers with connectors, and two bipolar electrode arrays.   One array contains eight small platinum electrode buttons on a silicone rubber-coated dacron mesh pad, while the other contains sixteen electrode buttons (Fig. 5).   Other arrays are contemplated.

After the electrode arrays are implanted on the cerebellum, they are connected by tunnelling to the two radio receivers which are placed in pockets about half an inch beneath the skin just below each clavicle. When stimulation is to commence, the two transmitting antennas are taped directly over each receiver and are then plugged into the two antenna sockets on the transmitter (Fig. 6).

When the system is turned on, the transmitter begins generating a pulse-modified radio signal at a carrier frequency of 2.1 MHz. A special timing mechanism within the transmitter causes this signal first to feed one antenna for a number of minutes, and then the other for the same period. Consequently, the cerebellum is stimulated continuously, but in two separate areas alternately.   One or the other of the leads may be used to stimulate only anterior or posterior cerebellum, with a silent period of non-stimulation if that is deemed desirable.

The pulse rate is variable within its range by the "RATE" control knob.   There are also two controls labelled "VOLTS" which vary the output to each antenna between .1 and 14 volts.   A fourth control on the transmitter is a red button called the "JAM" button.   Should the patient sense the prodromal symptoms of a seizure he can push this button, thereby stimulating both electrode arrays simultaneously rather than alternately. This has been found successful in aborting an attack in some instances.

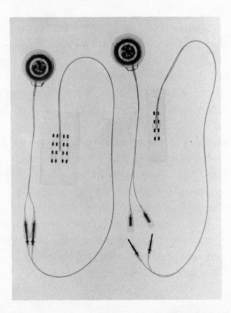

Fig. 5. Photograph of the 2 electrode arrays currently in use. On the left is an 8-pair array, connected to a receiver. On the right is a 4-pair array, demonstrating the male-female plug arrangement which is used to connect the electrodes to the receiver during surgery.

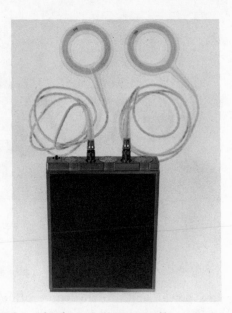

Fig. 6. Power pack, which is automatically timed to stimulate, alternately, 2 antennas, which are also demonstrated.

The primary power supply for the transmitter is an internal isolated battery pack containing six replaceable Mallory RN-12 1.5 volt primary cells. Each system is also supplied with an auxilliary plug-in power unit which plugs into any 110 volt AC outlet. This is designed for use during the sleeping hours or other periods of inactivity to conserve the battery pack in the portable transmitter (Fig. 7).

On the basis of our experience thus far it appears that stimulus frequency in the range of 10 - 20 is the effective range in aborting or preventing seizures, while high frequency stimulation of approximately 200 cycles per second is effective in reducing spasticity. However, these rates should not yet be considered conclusively as the optimal rate of stimulation. Further clinical experience is necessary to define the parameters of stimulation in various circumstances. This automatic timed stimulator, which we have elected to refer to as a brain pacemaker, was developed in collaboration with Avery Laboratories.

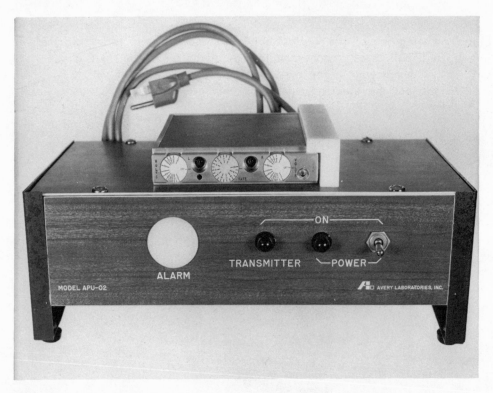

Fig. 7. Auxiliary plug and power unit which can be attached to any 110-volt AC outlet. This is used during the sleeping hours or any periods of inactivity to conserve the battery pack in the portable transmitter.

RADIOGRAPHIC PLOTTING OF ELECTRODE IMPLANTATION
ON CEREBELLAR MAP

The x-rays which are used for these measurements are taken at 12 feet and therefore eliminate any coefficient of enlargement. Two x-ray projections are necessary, an absolute AP and lateral projection. The mid points of the bipolar platinum disc electrodes are used in the plotting.

Anterior Cerebellar Electrode Position

The anterior cerebellar electrode bank position is determined by means of three measurements, A, E, and F. In the lateral x-ray, the direction of the electrode bank is determined by direct observation, the most superior pair is towards the midline and the most inferior pair will lie laterally and their direction from the medial pair determines an anterior or posterior direction. (In the example Fig. 8 the electrode bank is directed posteriorly).

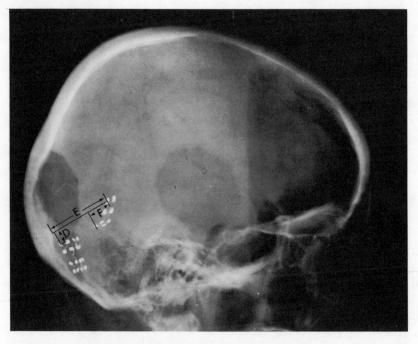

Fig. 8. Lateral x-ray, demonstrating measurements E, D, and F, described in the text, which are used for plotting positions of the electrodes on the cerebellar surface.

The internal occipital protuberance is the main point of reference and distance E is then determined from the lateral x-ray, measuring from the internal occipital protuberance to the midpoint of the superior electrode (to the posterior one, if the bank is directed posteriorly or to the anterior electrode if the bank is directed anteriorly). This electrode is also the most medial and its distance from the midline is determined in the AP x-ray as distance A.

The line from internal occipital protuberance to the most medial electrode is distance E and becomes a baseline from which a line is then dropped at right angles to it, passing through the midpoint of the most lateral electrode (posterior or anterior, as the case may be depending on the bank's direction). The distance between these two electrode midpoints becomes distance F and establishes the angle of the electrode bank from the midline when viewed from the superior surface of the cerebellum. These measurements are than transferred to the cerebellar (map, Fig. 9). The electrode points are then determined by means of a template that has been made corresponding to the midpoints of the electrode banks of 8 and 16 contacts.

On the cerebellar map, point 3 is determined first by its distance E along the midline from the internal occipital protuberance and its distance from the midline (distance A). Using the template point 3 is marked and the template is then rotated until point 4 is located. Point 4 is the lateral point of a right angled triangle whose altitude is distance F. The hypotenuse is predetermined by the template. The remaining electrode points are then plotted through the template.

Posterior Cerebellar Electrode Position

The posterior cerebellar electrode bank's position is determined by three measurements also, B, C, and D.

In Figure 10, the AP x-ray projection distance B is the distance of the midpoint of the superior medial electrode from the midline and C the distance from the midline of the inferior medial electrode midpoint. In the lateral x-ray, the distance D is determined by the distance of the superior medial electrode below the internal occipital protuberance perpendicular to line E.

The electrode bank's position is mapped on the cerebellar map again (Fig. 11), using a template where point 1 is located by the distance

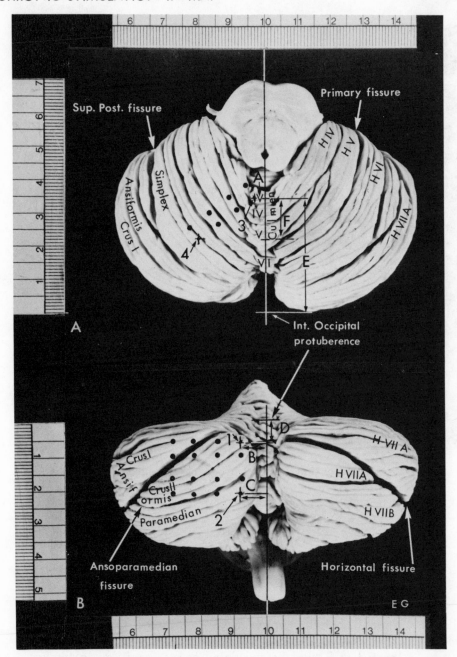

Fig. 9A. Superior, or subtentorial view of the cerebellum, demonstrating mapping of the electrodes on this surface.
Fig. 9B. Posterior view of the cerebellum demonstrating mapping of 8 pairs of bipolar electrodes on Crus I and Crus II.

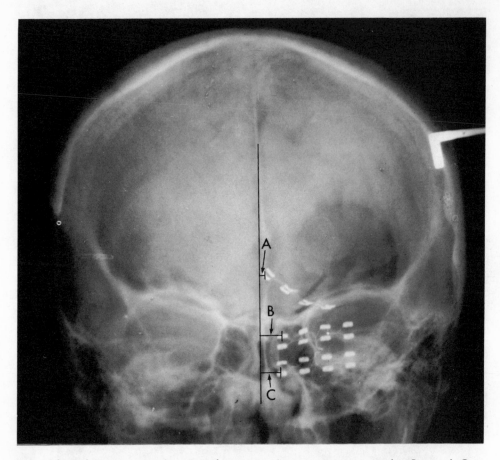

Fig. 10. AP x-ray projection demonstrating measurements A, B, and C, described in text.

D below the internal occipital protuberance and distance B lateral from the midline. The template is applied and point 2, the inferior medial electrode, is located and then the remaining points are filled in through the template using either an 8 or 16 electrode template.

The cerebellar map was obtained by careful dissection of a normal cerebellum and by observations at operation and autopsy (Fig. 12).

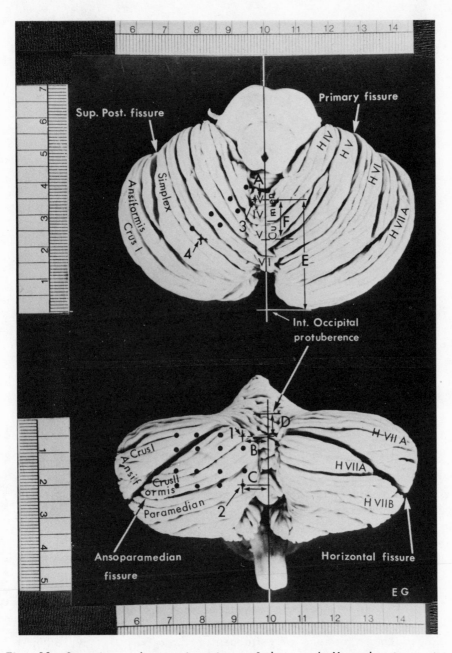

Fig. 11. Superior and posterior views of the cerebellum showing points 1, 2, 3, and 4 which determine application of the template.

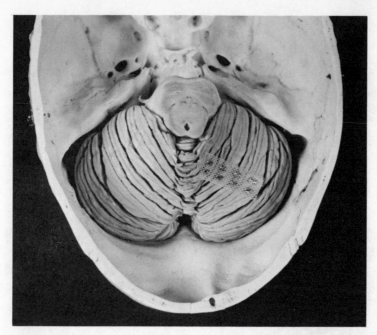

Fig. 12. A view of the anterior cerebellum, with electrode array in place. This photograph was made in an anatomical specimen, following removal of the tentorium, permitting a view of the subtentorial anatomy of the cerebellum.

CLINICAL OBSERVATIONS

Seven patients with intractable epilepsy and one with intractable generalized myoclonus have undergone chronic cerebellar stimulation. Each patient was incapacitated by seizures despite long term, competently managed medical treatment. Follow-up period at the time of this report is 4 to 11 months.

The preliminary clinical observations will be briefly summarized and certain physiologic studies under way will be referred to.

Three of the seven patients suffered psychomotor epilepsy. In each there was also occasionally grand mal, and in two of the three uncontrollable violent temper tantrums were frequent. These patients have all had marked evidence of seizure control, although one of three appears to have regressed after six months. Two of these three cases have also had control

of the behavior disorder since onset of cerebellar stimulation.   Brief
reports of these three cases follow:

Case No. 1 (W.A.) - The patient is a 24-year old male admitted
to hospital on October 30, 1972 with a chief complaint of uncontrolled
epileptic attacks.   He was well until age 16 when he was struck in the
right temple by a baseball.   He felt dazed, but did not lose consciousness.   At age 17 he fell and struck his occipital region while playing
basketball.   At age 20 the patient developed the first of a series of epileptic attacks all of which have been similar in nature.   Each begins with
a feeling in the abdomen which he describes as "stage fright" or "nervousness".   He would lose consciousness but continue to perform complex motor
activities such as walking and talking.   However, his speech was inappropriate to the situation.   At times he simply sat and stared straight ahead.
After 30-45 seconds he regained consciousness and seemed well except for
a feeling of being slightly "dazed".   Often he would have only an aura
of nausea and nervousness which frequently occurred as often as 20 times
a day.

His convulsive attacks varied in frequency from 1 - 5 per day.   He
also tended to have clusters of attacks up to 30 or 40 per day, for one
week out of each month during the year prior to admission (Fig. 13).
He has taken a number of medications but none has reduced the seizure
frequency.

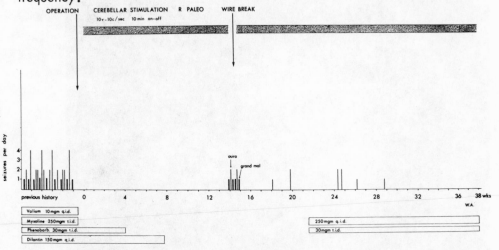

Fig. 13. A graph demonstrating the seizure pattern in Case 1 (W.A.)
prior to and following onset of anterior cerebellar stimulation.   During
the 2 months subsequent to the preparation of this graph the patient has
improved further, so that he is taking mysoline 250 mg b.i.d., without
any other medication.   He has had no additional seizures.

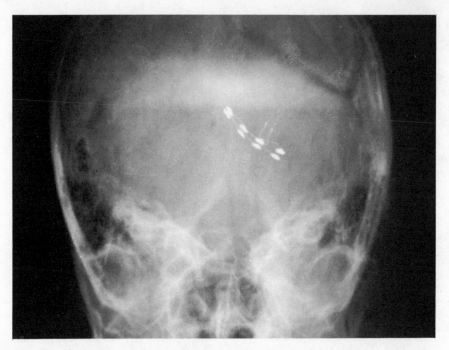

Fig. 14A. Roentgenogram demonstrating position of electrodes on the surface of anterior cerebellum in Case 1.

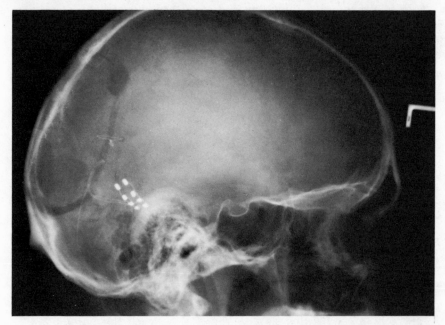

Fig. 14B. Lateral roentgenogram demonstrating position of electrodes on anterior cerebellum in Case 1.

One year prior to admission he had bilateral carotid arteriograms and
a pneumoencephalogram which showed no abnormality. At one time he
developed a seizure while driving an automobile and had an accident,
which caused him to lose his license. He attended college for 1-1/2 years
but because of the frequency of his attacks he could not pursue his career
further and, at the time of admission to hospital, was working on his father's farm. However, both his lethargy due to drug intoxication and his
frequent seizures limited his activities on the farm to minor activities of
little practical value. Neurological examination revealed no abnormalities.
EEG showed a diffuse abnormality compatible with an epileptic disorder.
On two occasions an electroencephalogram with pharyngeal leads demonstrated bilateral spiking in the temporal lobe regions. At the time of admission the patient was receiving dilantin 100 mg 3 times daily, mysoline
250 mg 3 times daily, and phenobarbital 32 mg 3 times daily.

On November 7, 1972 the patient was subjected to a sub-occipital
craniotomy with implantation of an electrode over the right anterior cerebellum (Fig. 14). Initially he turned on the stimulator himself using 10
volts and 10 cps every time he perceived an aura. This aborted the seizures which ordinarily would have followed. However, while being interviewed by us one day he was observed to have a seizure, and it was obvious that he was incapable of responding sufficiently rapidly to abort the
seizure by turning on the stimulation unit himself. Accordingly, he was
placed on a schedule of regular stimulation of 10 volts at 10 cps for 5
minutes every hour throughout the day. Subsequently this was increased to
10 volts for 10 minutes every hour, and finally to 10 minutes on and 10
minutes off, through 24 hours each day.

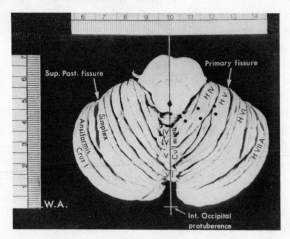

Fig. 14C. Estimated position of the 4 electrode pairs, indicated by black
dots, over the right anterior cerebellum in Case 1. Note the proximity
to the midline of the most medial electrodes and the fact that both H-IV
and H-V are covered by the electrodes.

Initially during his hospitalization his seizure frequency was noted to drop when he was placed on a program of regular stimulation. His medications were progressively reduced and then completely eliminated by December 18, 1972.

He was discharged from hospital on January 24, 1973. He developed 3 attacks at home and the patient discovered that the wire lead from his power pack was broken. Accordingly he was advised to resume a small dose of medication, namely, mysoline 250 mg tid, and to return to New York for correction of the power pack defect.

At present he is virtually seizure free. Momentary staring spells have been observed but these occur no more frequently than once per week. He continues to take approximately 20% of the medications he took preoperatively, and all signs of drug intoxication such as lethargy, gingival hypertrophy and anorexia have disappeared. He is alert, has gained 25 pounds, and is gainfully employed.

No adverse signs of 10 months of chronic stimulation unilaterally, of anterior lobe of cerebellar cortex have been observed.

Case No. 2 (M.C.) – This 16-year old male was admitted to hospital January 9, 1973 complaining of seizures and behavioral disorders. The patient was thought to have been normal until age 4 when he developed clumsiness in walking and complained of having "dizzy spells". He seemed slower in intellectual and manual skills than other children, a finding which was confirmed by detailed examinations by physicians when the patient was 6 years old. He was sent to a special school where he did well in sports, particularly baseball and football, but was slow intellectually. He continued to have episodes in which he complained of "dizziness" and at age 6 years he developed a series of behavioral abnormalities which have persisted to the present.

Retrospectively the parents believe that the patient's dizzy spells and frequent temper tantrums at age 4 may have represented seizure disorders. At age 6 he developed a series of attacks which have varied in character but usually consisted of an aura that something is about to fall on his head. He then developed a pain in the sub-occipital region. Next he developed clonic blinking of his eyes accompanied by closing and opening movements of his mouth. These usually terminated with generalized weakness and gradual recovery of consciousness. Frequently, however, the patient continued to have blinking movements of the eyes and movements of the mouth accompanied by violent flailing movements of all his limbs, with frothing at the mouth. At times these violent flailing movements appeared to be purposeful and were destructive. At times he has physically attacked other individuals and destroyed furniture. Once he punched a window with his fist and developed a large laceration of the forearm. Seizure frequency became much worse in the year prior to admission during which time the patient had been having daily episodes with major attacks lasting up to 1 hour 4 times daily. The family history was significant in that a maternal aunt had suffered grand mal seizures during adult life.

At the time of admission the patient was receiving mysoline 250 mg 3 times daily, phenobarbital 32 mg 3 times daily, and valium 5 mg 3 times daily. A pneumoencephalogram performed elsewhere in October 1972 was said to reveal left cerebral atrophy. Neurological examination revealed no abnormalities apart from a dull normal intellect. EEG consisted of a diffusely abnormal high voltage record. H.V. produced a mild build-up and spike like activity bilaterally. It was thought that this EEG was consistent with the patient's seizure disorder.

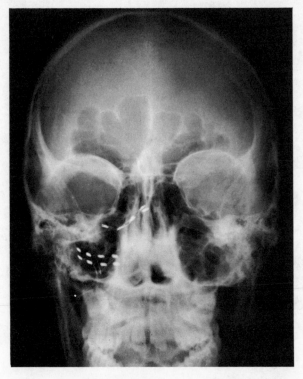

Fig. 15A. Anteroposterior roentgenogram demonstrating position of electrodes on anterior and posterior cerebellum in Case 2 (M.C.).

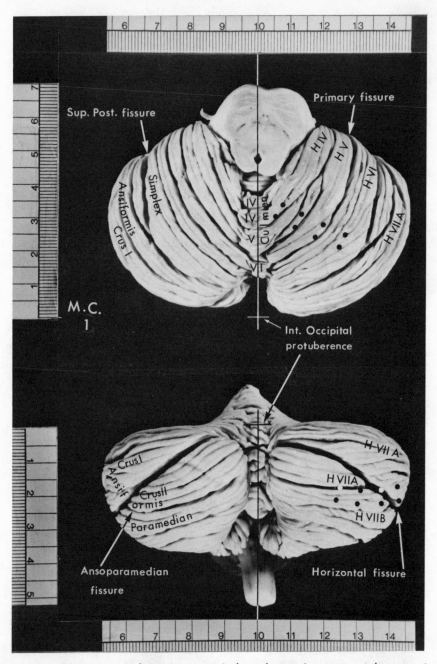

Fig. 15B. Plotting of the position of the electrodes over right anterior and right posterior cerebellum.

On January 16, 1973 the patient was subjected to a sub-occipital craniectomy in which a right anterior and posterior cerebellar electrode was placed (Fig. 15). The patient was stimulated with 10 volts at 10 cps 10 minutes out of every hour initially. Subsequently this was increased to 10 cps with a regimen of 10 minutes on and 10 minutes off, alternating right anterior and posterior cerebellar cortical stimulation. There was marked decrease in seizure frequency following insertion of these electrodes (Fig. 16) and the patient was discharged from hospital.

During this period there was a marked change in the patient behavior. Although he had been sullen, hostile and unresponsive preoperatively, he became open, pleasant, responsive and sociable with the medical staff and with other patients. His spells of aggressive behavior, believed to be epileptic equivalents, disappeared.

His family reported a month after onset of stimulation that, for the first time in his life, the patient responded to painful stimuli. They related as an example that previously he would often put his finger in the flame of a candle at the church altar without complaining of pain. The appreciation of pain, however, became evident, and apparently within normal range within one month after onset of stimulation. This observation

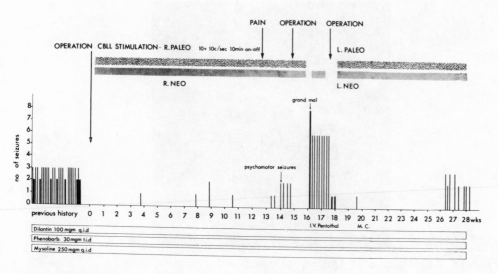

Fig. 16. Chart of patient's seizure pattern before and after onset of chronic cerebellar stimulation. A detailed explanation appears within the test of this case report (Case 2, M.C.).

of the parents, confirmed by the patient, is difficult to intrepret at present. Additionally, the family reported that prior to this procedure the patient had never shown emotional response that seemed to be relevant to a particular situation. His general attitude was sullen, hostile, and withdrawn. During the months following onset of stimulation this behavior was modified. He became properly responsive to cheerful or sad stimuli. On one appropriate occasion, within the family setting at home "he cried real tears for the first time", according to his father.

In May of 1973, however, the patient noted a sensation of pain and paresthesias in the right side of his neck when the power pack discharged to the electrodes on the right anterior cerebellum. Within a few days his psychomotor type seizures, i.e., eye blinking and lip smacking, returned readmission to hospital.

Recordings with a probe inserted into his neck at the site of the pain and paresthesias revealed a leak in the lead to the right anterior electrode plate. The lead in the neck was exposed surgically and a small blood clot was observed within the insulation of the wire (Fig. 17, 18). Despite an attempt to repair this lead, however, the electrodes on the right anterior cerebellum continued to be non-functional, as revealed by failure to produce a stimulus artifact in EEG recordings when the power stimulus was applied.

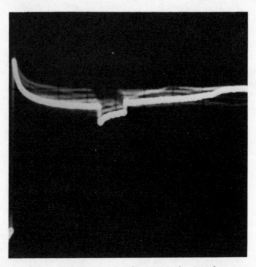

Fig. 17. Oscilloscopic tracing of electrical discharge in the subcutaneous tissues in the neck in Case 2, due to defect in the insulation of the wire leading from the intracranial electrodes to the subcutaneous receiver.

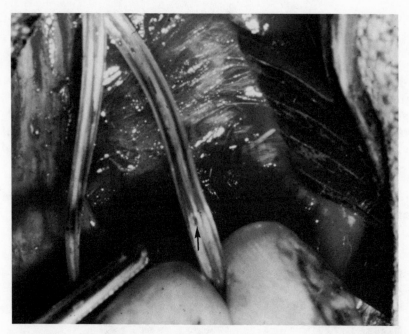

Fig. 18. The lead wire is exposed in the neck, demonstrating seepage of blood through the insulation, as described in the text.

Accordingly, on June 20, 1973 electrodes were placed on left anterior and posterior cerebellar cortex (Fig. 19). These have been stimulated alternately at 10 cps and 10 volts since that time. However, the patient's seizure frequency has returned approximately to its preoperative status. The present seizures differ from those observed previously in that the patient does not lose consciousness during the episodes; he retains the ability to speak and respond appropriately to questions. Moreover, if his extremities become involved in jerky movements the left upper extremity remains uninvolved, the extremity movements when present are adductor in type, and quite different from the violent clonic movements observed prior to surgery. Additionally, the patient often asks repetitively "Why isn't the first electrode working?"

It appears that at the time of leakage in the delivery of current to the right anterior cerebellar electrodes, the patient escaped from control of the prosthetically induced cerebellar inhibition of his seizures. Furthermore, installation of contralateral electrodes has not re-established this control. It is of interest to note that the right anterior cerebellar

electrodes, which apparently were effective when functioning, covered
lobules IV, V, and VI, while the left anterior electrodes lie virtually
entirely within lobule IV.

At present it is our plan to discontinue stimulation for a period and
then reinstate it in various sections of cerebellar cortex, trying various
parameters of stimulation. For the time being, this case must be considered as having demonstrated dramatic response to stimulation, with partial
recurrence, either due to instrumentation failure or escape from effects of
inhibition, or both. The difference in location of the right anterior
cerebellar electrode, which was effective, and that of the left anterior
cerebellar electrode, which thus far has not been effective, is also worthy
of consideration and further study.

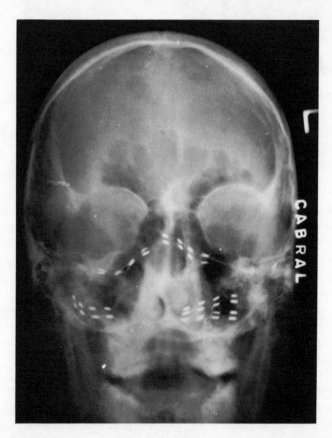

Fig. 19A. AP roentgenogram showing additional placements surface
electrodes on the left anterior and posterior cerebellum in Case 2.

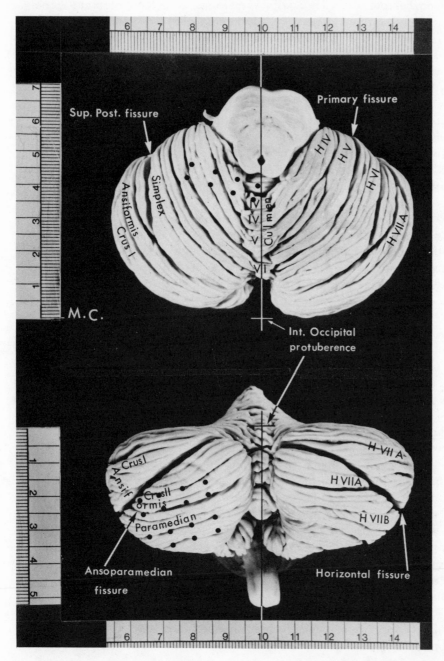

Fig. 19B. Estimated positions of electrodes on the left cerebellum in this case.

Case No. 3 (S.H.) - This 18-year old white male was admitted to
hospital on February 22, 1973 with complaints of psychomotor and generalized seizures, marked aggressive murderous behavior, and severe depression. The patient was the product of a normal gestation and birth. At
6 months of age he had a generalized seizure in association with a fever.
Subsequently he had repeated generalized convulsions until the age of 2
years. He then developed frequent staring spells, each lasting 1-5 seconds, without loss of postural tone. They occurred daily or on alternate
days and often he would have multiple attacks in a single day. These
spells disappeared at age 10, but were replaced by grand mal attacks and
sudden bursts of behavior inappropriate to the situation for which he was
amnesic, as well as intermittent unprovoked episodes of aggressive destructive behavior, which have continued to time of admission.

A typical grand mal attack began with an aura of spinning of the
environment or a sensation of light-headedness. The patient emitted a
cry, fell to the floor, and developed tonic-clonic convulsive movements.
The convulsion lasted between 2 and 8 minutes and was succeeded by
somnolence which persisted for several minutes to several hours. The seizures occurred with a frequency of approximately 15 to 30 times per month.

In addition to his seizure disorder the patient has had a number of
abnormal perceptual experiences. He has had feelings of deja vu, sensations of light-headedness, or spinning of the environment without subsequent epileptic attacks. He has also had feelings of severe anger,
hostility, and depression.

His depression had become so severe that he had attempted suicide
on several occasions. The first was in December of 1972 when he shot
himself in the chest with a rifle. A thoractomy was required for removal
of the bullet. In January of 1973 he took an overdose of barbiturates
but informed his parents he had done so and was treated promptly. On
several occasions subsequently he had slashed his wrists in attempts to
commit suicide. For many years he has had severe behavioral problems,
becoming easily angered and frequently violent, getting into fights with
his fellow students when in school, smashing furniture and often striking
his mother. He quit school in the tenth grade and worked intermittently
as a baker's assistant. His medication on admission included phenobarbital
15 mg 4 times daily and dilantin 100 mg 4 times daily. The past history
and family history were unremarkable. Neurological examination revealed
no abnormalities.

On February 28, 1973 the patient was subjected to a sub-occipital

craniectomy with implantation of electrodes over the right anterior cerebellum and posterior cerebellum (Fig. 20). Subsequently the patient was

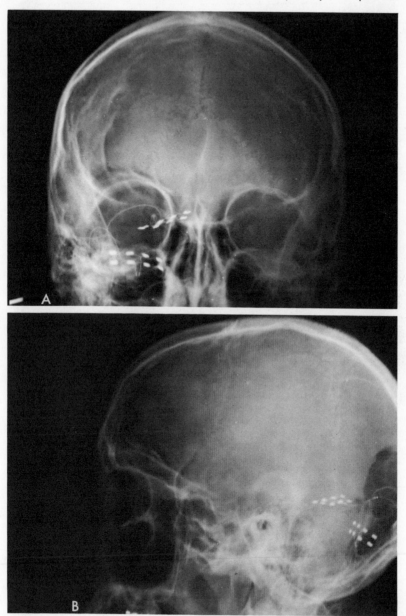

Fig. 20A and B. AP and lateral roentgenograms demonstrating position
of electrodes placed on the right anterior and posterior cerebellum in
Case 3 (S.H).

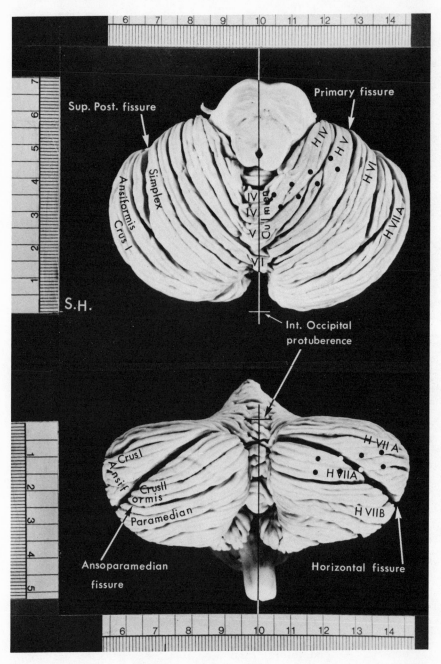

Fig. 20C. Estimated position of electrodes in the same case plotted on the anterior and posterior cerebellum.

stimulated trans-epidermally with 10 volts at 10 cps with a schedule of 10 minutes on and 10 minutes off alternately. From the time of onset of stimulation the patient had no grand mal or psychomotor seizures whatsoever. It is worthy of note that following placement of the electrodes stimulation was not started for 24 hours, during which time several seizures occurred. He was discharged from hospital on April 11, 1973 and continued to have no seizures until May 13, 1973. On that day 13 tonic-clonic seizures occurred in a single day. It was found that a wire in his stimulator had become broken during a night of alcoholic intoxication. The wire was repaired the following day and he has subsequently had no seizures over a period of observation of 2-1/2 months.

In addition to the decrease in seizure frequency the patient has developed a remarkable change in personality. Previously sullen and uncommunicative, he has become considerably more out-going, interested in his environment, and obviously less depressed. He is now gainfully employed as an apprentice in a machine shop. Thus, the patient's seizure disorder appears to have responded well to chronic stimulation, alternating between cerebellar cortex of anterior (H IV and H V) and posterior lobes (H VIIA) of the right side. The fact that placement of electrodes without stimulation failed to produce seizure arrest, plus the recurrence of seizures during one day when the power pack wire was broken provide some element of serendiptitious controlled study.

This patient's psychomotor and grand mal convulsions plus his aggressive behavioral epileptic equivalents of his entire 18 year lifetime appeared to have been favorably modified by chronic cerebellar stimulation during the 5 month period of its utilization.

One patient (Case No. 4) suffered from both grand mal and petit mal seizures for 47 years. Her clinical history is summarized in the following case report.

Case No. 4 (M.B.) - This 56-year old widowed housewife entered hospital on February 22, 1973 with complaints of poorly controlled seizures. The patient was well until age 7 years when she developed petit mal attacks which occurred initially 2 - 3 times per day. In the 5 - 10 years prior to admission the attacks had increased in frequency to 10 - 12 per day. Each episode consisted of a momentary loss of consciousness accompanied by an upward rolling of her eyes but no loss of postural tone. Each attack lasted only a few seconds. At the age of 13, accompanying the onset of her menses, she developed grand mal attacks characterized by sudden loss of consciousness without warning. She would fall with all limbs tonically flexed, then develop clonic movement of the limbs, often with bladder incontinence and tongue biting.

Initially occurring 2 - 3 times per year, the seizures had increased to 2 - 3 times per month in the two years prior to admission to hospital. She has never had an aura except for an occasional feeling of "nervousness". She began taking phenobarbital at age 13 and increased the dose to 32 mg 5 times daily just prior to admission. At age 40 she started taking dilantin and gradually increased the dosage to 400 mg daily. At age 54 she developed dilantin toxicity, consisting of severe ataxia, and consequently reduced the dilantin dosage to 100 mg per day. At age 54 she began taking valium 5 mg per day.

The family history was significant in that the patient has a 19-year old son who developed petit mal at age 5 and is currently well controlled with zarontin. He has had one grand mal attack. The past history was negative, except for a fractured dorsal vertebra at age 31 following a seizure. Physical and neurological examination revealed no abnormality except for marked dorsal kyphosis and scoliosis. The EEG was diffusely abnormal, revealing intermittent slow waves and occasional spikes bilaterally.

On February 26, 1973 a sub-occipital craniectomy was performed and a set of platinum stimulating electrodes was placed over the right anterior (H IV, V, VI) and posterior (H VII A) cerebellum (Fig. 21). From that time stimulation was carried out trans-epidermally with settings of 10 volts at 10 cps alternately 10 minutes on and 10 minutes off. During an observation period of 5 months after stimulation the patient developed no grand mal seizures at all. She developed one grand mal seizure following surgery, but prior to stimulation. The incidence of her petit mal attacks progressively decreased as shown in Figure 22. She was discharged May 24, 1973 receiving dilantin 100 mg twice a day and phenobarbital 32 mg three times daily. Her only complaint was of having occasional brief jerking movements of all of the extremities which she had previously. These lasted a fraction of a second and were apparent only to the patient.

This patient represents a case of grand mal and petit mal epilepsy of 47 years' duration. She received medication to the point of marked toxicity symptoms without seizure control. She has responded, during the 5-month period of cerebellar stimulation, by abolition of grand mal convulsions and virtual, but more gradual, control of her petit mal attacks.

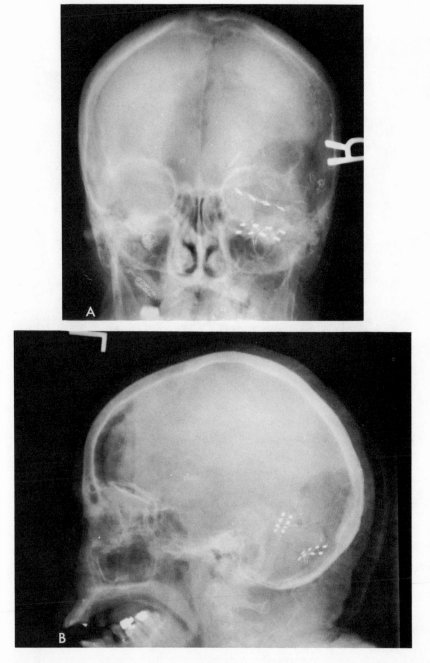

Fig. 21A and B. AP and lateral roentgenograms demonstrating position of electrodes placed on the right anterior and posterior cerebellum of Case 4 (M.B.).

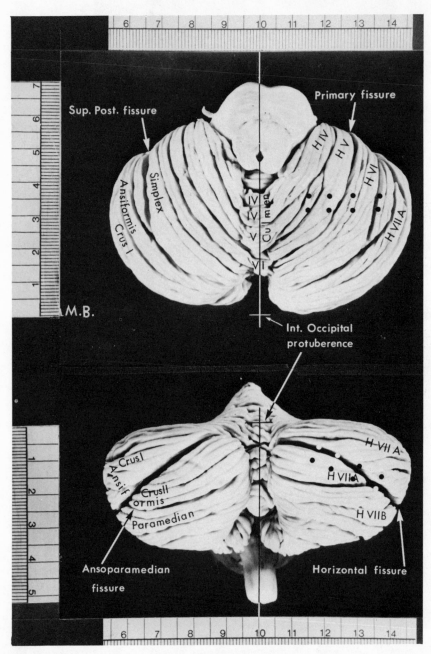

21C. Estimated position of the electrodes on the anterior and posterior
cerebellum in this case.

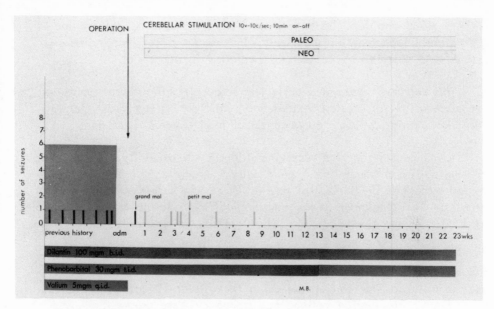

Fig. 22. A graph illustrating the seizure pattern of Case 4 (M.B.) before and after onset of chronic cerebellar stimulation. As indicated in the text grand mal was eliminated from the time of cerebellar stimulation onset. Petit mal gradually decreased and disappeared by the end of the 12th week.

One of the patients in this series was incapacitated by left-sided focal or Jacksonian seizures. This case is reported as follows:

Case No. 5 (W.B.) - This 23-year old male was admitted to hospital on December 18, 1972 with complaints of total incapacitation due to uncontrollable seizures. The patient was well until age 7 when he was struck in the left temple by a ball which did not cause him to lose consciousness. At age 10 he began having seizures which within the next 2 years were of such severity and frequency as to render the patient incapacitated. By the time of admission to our service they occurred daily, often 3 to 6 times in a 24-hour period. The seizures began with an aura of a burning sensation in the left hand, a "good" feeling in his abdomen, and unpleasant taste or odor, or a feeling of anxiety. Next he developed clonic movements of the left hand and then the left leg. Rarely he would fall to the floor and lose consciousness, at times also developing shaking movements of the right limbs.

In 1965 and 1967 he underwent a right temporal lobectomy and right frontal lobectomy, respectively, in another center, having been studied and operated by competent specialists in this field.

His seizures occurred slightly less frequently after these operations, but subsequently progressed in frequency until during the year prior to admission, during which they occurred at least several times daily.

On admission he was receiving dilantin 400 mg daily, phenobarbital 120 mg daily, and mysoline 1 gram daily. Neurological examination revealed nystagmus on horizontal gaze. There was a left upper quandrant anopsia. The remainder of the neurological examination was unremarkable. An EEG revealed slow and sharp wave activity in the left temporal region.

On December 19, 1972 a sub-occipital craniectomy was performed and electrodes were implanted over the right anterior cerebellum (H IV, V). Stimulation was carried out using 10 volts at 10 cps for 5 minutes every hour. Stimulating voltage and frequency were progressively increased until he received 14 volts for 30 minutes every hour. Moreover, it was found that stimulation applied when the patient felt an aura in his left hand could abort a seizure. Furthermore, on one occasion he developed an aura followed by a left focal seizure, involving arm and leg, during electroencephalography. Cerebellar stimulation promptly stopped the clinical convulsion and markedly changed the electrical seizure discharge (Fig. 23).

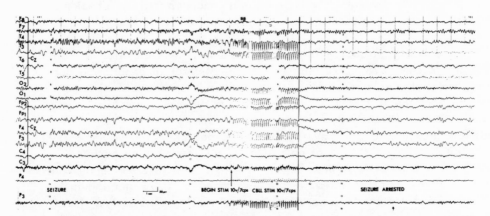

Fig. 23. Electroencephalogram in Case 5 (W.B.) demonstrating abnormal electrical discharge and seizure arrest by cerebellar stimulation, as described in the text.

His seizure frequency diminished by approximately 50%. However, he continued to have a sufficient number of seizures that it was considered necessary to implant a second set of electrodes. Accordingly, on January 18, 1973 electrodes were placed over the cortex of the left anterior (H VI) and posterior cerebellum (H VIIA). Postoperatively he did well but on January 25 he developed a sudden decrease of his level of consciousness. Exploration of the operative site revealed an epidural hematoma which was evacuated. The hematoma was found to have compressed the cerebellum slightly. Following evacuation of the hematoma he complained of difficulty with his vision and on testing had a visual acuity of 20/200 o.u. There was no field defect other than that observed preoperatively and it was concluded that he suffered from amaurosis secondary to ischemia of the occipital lobes.

Slowly he has regained visual function. Alternate stimulation of anterior cerebellum and posterior cerebellum have decreased his seizure frequency significantly, so that he is virtually seizure free at present. At the patient's request a trial period without constant stimulation was carried out, during which the patient turned on the power pack whenever he felt an aura in order to abort his attacks. This, according to the patient's report, was successful, but gradually the number of auras which occurred daily increased. Consequently, chronic stimulation of left anterior and posterior cerebellum reinstated, with subsequent reduction of spontaneous auras and with continued seizure control.

Evaluation of this case is made particularly difficult by the right temporal and frontal lobectomies which were performed prior to his eventual admission to our service. It is further complicated by the surgical sequela of a posterior fossa epidural hematoma, which made his postoperative recovery lengthy, and produced visual difficulty which took two months to clear. Nevertheless, there is clear cut evidence that cerebellar cortical stimulation could abort his focal seizures, if applied promptly at the onset of an aura. Furthermore, when anterior and posterior cerebellar stimulation was carried out throughout the 24 hour period a marked alleviation of auras ensued. These recurred when chronic stimulation was interrupted, and decreased with the reinstitution of chronic automatic stimulation.

Two cases (cases 6 and 7) of grand mal seizures, unpreceded by any aura, have been subjected to unilateral anterior lobe stimulation in one case, and to unilateral anterior and posterior cerebellar stimulation in the other.

In both cases the number of seizures during the post stimulatory
period has been approximately 50% of that during the pre-stimulatory
period. Both cases reside at a great distance from our hospital, and
since they were operated early in the series do not yet have the automa-
ted power pack stimulators which were subsequently developed. Consequently, day-time stimulation has been irregular and nocturnal stimulation
lacking.

A definite but incomplete inhibition of seizures appears to have resulted in these cases. Specific case reports will be presented when further studies and data are available.

An additional case has been included in this series because it illustrates the powerful inhibitory effect of cerebellar cortical stimulation;
because it demonstrates effectively the bilateral effect of unilateral anterior cerebellum stimulation, and because the patient was totally incapacitated by intractable generalized myoclonus, a symptom observed in certain epileptics which has been particularly intractable to treatment.

Case No. 8 (D.C.) – This 39-year old woman was admitted to
hospital November 13, 1972 complaining of involuntary movements of all
limbs. The patient has undergone an operation for an inguinal hernia in
1970. During surgery she suffered a cardiac arrest from which she was
resuscitated but it was not ascertained with certainty how long she suffered complete cessation of all cardiac activity. In the early postoperative days, as she gradually recovered consciousness she noted involuntary
myoclonic movements afflicting all four limbs. The movements interfered
with all purposeful use of her limbs and with her capacity to ambulate.
The movements occurred constantly, even during sleep if she moved, and
prevented her from feeding or dressing herself. She was totally bedridden
and tried to lie absolutely still to avoid the myoclonic-seizure-like activity that was induced by any motion.

She also complained of strange nocturnal "seizures" which she described as follows: "I would have terrible nightmares if I fell asleep,
which awoke me. At those times my arms would be folded tightly
against my chest and my legs held out stiffly. I could not move for
several moments. These occurred once or twice every night."

She had apparently suffered no loss of intellectual competence as a
result of her cardiac arrest. On admission to hospital from a chronic
nursing facility she was receiving valium 15 mg 3 times daily and dilantin
100 mg 3 times daily. Neurological examination revealed a patient with

constant myoclonic jerking movements of all limbs. She was unable to
sit unassisted or to walk, even with assistance. Any attempt to move the
head, neck, or limbs produced an exacerbation of her myoclonic movements.

On January 5, 1973 a sub-occipital craniectomy was performed and
electrodes were inserted over the anterior cerebellum (H IV, V, VI) on
the right side (Fig. 24). Stimulation was applied initially 10 volts 10
cps 5 minutes per hour, subsequently 10 minutes per hour, and then 10
minutes every 1/2 hour. The rate was then increased to 200 cps. There
was no apparent improvement for the first few weeks, but progressively
the movements diminished to the point that she was able to sit without
any involuntary movements whatsoever. The flapping violent movements
of her upper extremities have ceased and she can feed herself, drink from
a glass without difficulty, and carry on all activities of daily living,
except walking, unaided (Fig. 25). She continued to have great difficulty in standing, however, owing to a severe ataxia of the trunk. Accordingly, left posterior cerebellar electrodes (H VIIA, VIIB) were implanted
on June 20, 1973 (Fig. 26). Since the time of the second implantation
there has been essentially no further objective change in her status, although the patient reports a subjective feeling of improvement, particularly a feeling of less tenseness in the mornings. Nocturnal stimulation
has been started only since July 1973. She states that the nightmares
and nocturnal "seizures" have ceased. The patient illustrates several
facts worthy of attention and further study. So far as our investigation
of the literature can determine she is the first case of generalized intention myoclonus following cardiac arrest to respond favorably to any therapeutic procedure. In addition, it is important to note that improvement
was gradual and progressive; a fact noted also in several of our spastic
patients. The bilaterality of response to unilateral stimulation; the lack
of any adverse sensory, motor or intellectual function following 10 months
of such stimulation; and the reversal of totally incapacitating generalized
intention myoclonus of 3 years' duration are all worthy of note.

Dow has pointed out, after examining this patient and the chart of
her cerebellar electrode placements, that the anterior lobe electrodes
cover the lobules thought to "represent" the upper limbs, but not the
anteriormost lobules representing the lower limbs. This is one possible
explanation for the dramatic complete abolition of myoclonus from head,
neck, upper limbs and trunk, with a lesser alleviation in the lower
extremities.

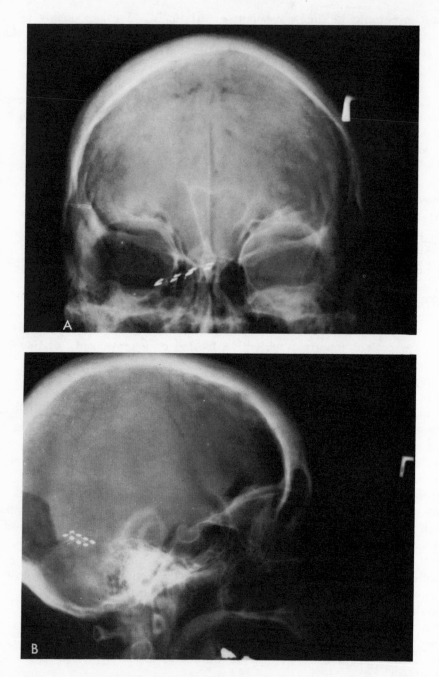

Fig. 24A and B. AP and lateral roentgenograms demonstrating position of electrodes on the right anterior cerebellum in Case 8 (D.C.).

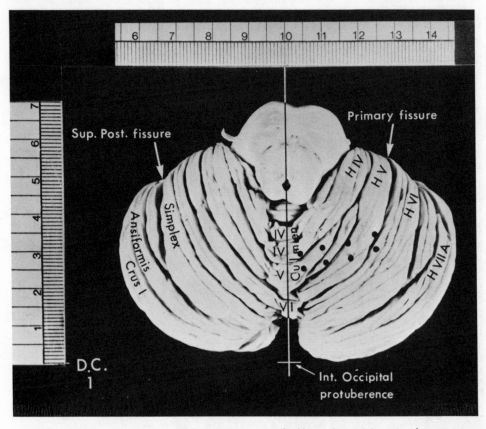

24C. Estimated position of anterior cerebellar electrodes in this case.

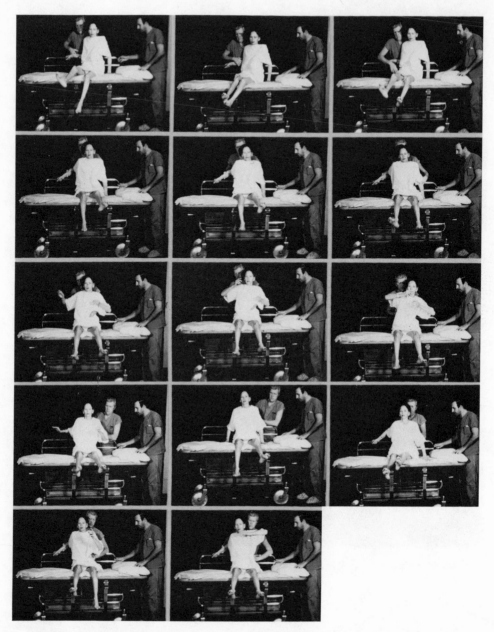

Fig. 25A. Movie frames demonstrating the intractable myoclonic jerks suffered by D.C., Case 8. Any attempt at movement of any part of the body resulted in violent spasms and myoclonic jerks of the head, neck, trunk, and all 4 limbs, resulting in total incapacitation.

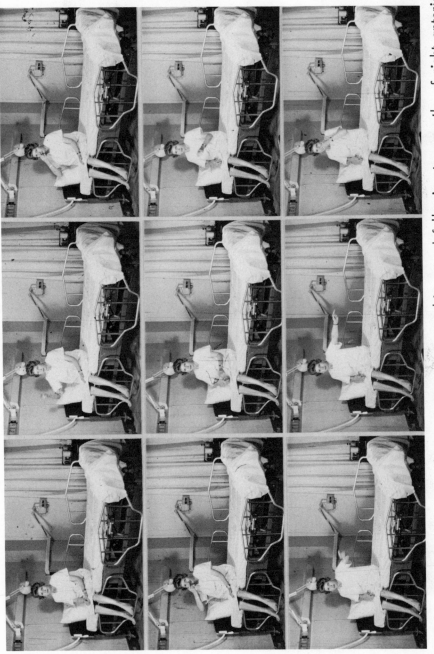

Fig. 25B. Individual frames from a cinematogram graphic record following two months of right anterior cerebellar stimulation. There is total abolition of myoclonic jerks of the head, neck, upper trunk and both upper extremities.

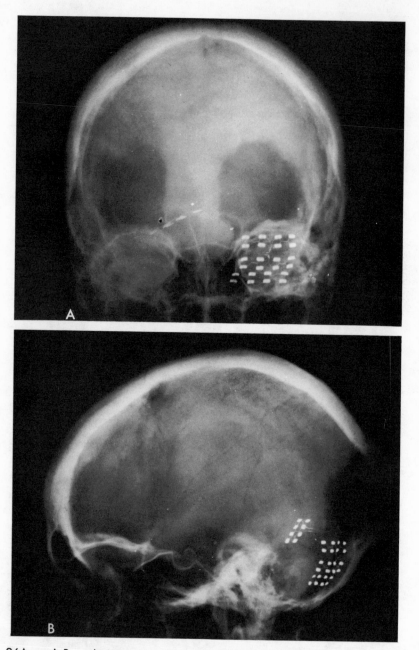

Fig. 26A and B. Anteroposterior and lateral roentgenograms demonstrating the position of 4 pairs of bipolar electrodes over the right anterior cerebellum and 12 pairs of bipolar electrodes over the left posterior cerebellum in Case 8 (D.C.).

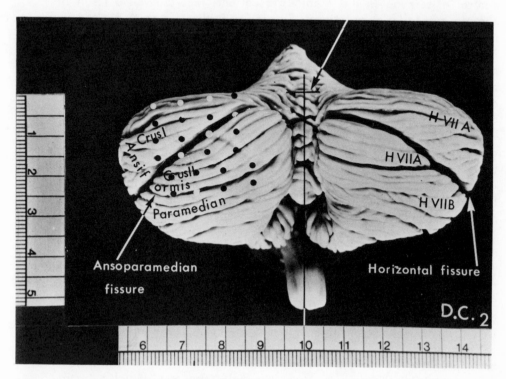

26C. Estimated position of the 12 pairs of bipolar electrodes over the left posterior cerebellum in this case.

NOTE:–Cases number 1, 3, and 8 were available for personal demonstration to all those attending the symposia, as were 2 of the patients under treatment for previously intractable spasticity.

DISCUSSION AND CONCLUSIONS

It appears justified to conclude that the dramatic amelioration or control of seizures in the 7 epileptic patients reported was a result of chronic cerebellar stimulation. The series is thus far quite limited in number. Moreover, a controlled double blind study is not morally justified in such an investigation of clinical results. However, the fact that these patients were intractable to previous therapy, including medication to the point of intoxication; the fact that seizures occurred following craniotomy, but prior to onset of cerebellar stimulation in several cases; and the fact that seizures, which had previously been controlled, recurred when there was a mechanical failure in the stimulating apparatus would all seem to mitigate against the likelihood of coincidence or a placebo effect producing the seizure arrest or control which has been demonstrated in these cases. Obviously, a larger series of cases and longer period of follow-up is necessary in order to assess the long term efficacy of this procedure.

It is notable that the inter-ictal electroencephalogram in these cases was not appreciably changed even though clinical seizures were controlled. However, this is not surprising since medical therapy which successfully controls seizures often fails to produce EEG changes. Recently, Sherwin et al (Sherwin, Eisen, & Sokolowski, 1973) reported that although there is a correlation between plasma levels and brain levels of phenobarbital and diphenylhydantoin, they could not demonstrate a relationship between brain phenobarbital levels and spike discharges in both humans and cat. They do not infer, however, that phenobarbital is not of value in the control of seizures, but merely that spike activity may continue despite substantial concentrations of drug in plasma and brain.

The fact that cerebellar stimulation did arrest both the clinical seizure and the concomitant ictal EEG discharge on 2 occasions in Case 5 (W.B.), see Figure 24, is particularly noteworthy. This finding suggests a possible cerebellar interference with electrical seizure discharge as demonstrated in cat (Cooke & Snider, 1955), rat (Dow, Fernandez-Guardiola, & Manni, 1962), and monkey (Snider, 1973), but not upon background or inter-ictal EEG.

Such a finding is in keeping with other observations of cerebellar function. For example, anterior cerebellar stimulation does not appear clinically to affect muscular tone in normal limbs, either in animals or human, but does lessen tone in spastic extremities. These observations are in keeping with Snider's hypothesis, previously referred to, that the cerebellum is a modulator which arises to the needs of the organism.

The case of intractable generalized myoclonus, remarkably controlled by anterior cerebellar stimulation, Case 8, was included in this report for several reasons. First, the same type of myoclonic phenomena is seen in certain cases of epilepsy. Secondly, its control by chronic cerebellar stimulation, visibly demonstrable by the pre- and post stimulation cinematograph, lends credence to the clinical observations in the epileptic patients. Third, and of particular significance, is the fact that there was a gradual, increasing, cumulative beneficial effect for several months; a finding also observed in our series of spastic cases treated by this method.

This cumulative effect leads us to speculate that chronic cerebellar stimulation leads to a build up of chemical changes in neurotransmitter systems. If this is so, an eventual reconditioning or normalization of some abnormal brain functions, mediated by chemical systems, may take place during chronic stimulation of cerebellar cortex.

The confirmation of cerebellar inhibition of myoclonus in cat (Bickford et al., 1973, this volume), which did not endure, since acute rather than chronic stimulation was employed, points up the potential value of a cumulative effect of chronic cerebellar stimulation.

One can only speculate at this time concerning the principal sites of cerebellar cortical inhibition which might prevent or arrest convulsions and also change the ictal EEG without affecting the inter-ictal electro-encephalographic record. It is our hypothesis that the bulbar reticular substance, affected directly or via fastigioreticular pathways is principally involved in this process. Both downstream (cortico-fugal) and upstream (corticopetal) data are modulated by cerebellum at the reticular level. However, cerebellar effects are so widespread and complex, that even if this hypothesis is correct, it is undoubtedly incomplete. Neurophysiologic and neurochemical laboratory studies are currently in progress to investigate this aspect of the problem.

Thus far, several patients in our overall series of patients receiving chronic cerebellar stimulation have been stimulated for more than one year. There has been no sign that over that period of time such stimulation produces any undesirable motor, sensory, intellectual or emotional changes.

Favorable emotional changes, that is, amelioration of unprovoked dangerous aggressive behavior in 2 patients with psychomotor epilepsy, were not accompanied by any sign of intellectual dullness or other aberration. On the contrary, these patients became more "normal" intellectually and socially. This aspect of our study is reviewed in detail by Riklan et al in this monograph.

It seems worthy of note that in one of the two patients in whom aggressive behavior was controlled, a normalization of response to painful stimuli occurred. This is only a single observation, but additionally supports the view that the cerebellum, which sometimes may appear to act capriciously from case to case, actually does encompass a flexibility which allows it to modulate data according to the needs of the organism.

Several cases illustrate the fact that cerebellum, particularly anterior cerebellum, exerts a profound contralateral as well as ipsilateral effect. This is particularly well demonstrated by the control of bilateral myoclonus by chronic stimulation of the right anterior cerebellum. This bilateral effect has also been notable in our series of patients undergoing stimulation for spasticity.

There are several technical questions still unanswered at this time. One cannot say what elements of cerebellar cortex are being preferentially stimulated. It is our assumption that all cellular and nerve fiber components of the cerebellar cortex are stimulated. However, the obvious inhibitory effect of stimulation (Figures 24, 27, 28) allows us to presume that the ultimate effect of cerebellar cortical stimulation is a rather massive inhibitory Purkinje cell discharge.

Whether the present parameters of stimulation are optimal is not yet known. Questions have been raised which indicate that the current achieved at 10 Hz and 10 volts may be insufficient. Others, however, have raised the possibility of eventual vascular or neuronal coagulation by these same parameters. We are conducting parallel long term laboratory studies in support of our clinical investigation to help answer these as yet unanswered questions. In the meantime, we are encouraged by the fact that the method we are employing has resulted in seemingly unequivocal improvement not only in epilepsy, but also in intractable myoclonus and spasticity of diverse etiology. Furthermore, there is no evidence of any deleterious effect. Consequently, we conclude that chronic stimulation of cerebellar cortex merits judicious, meticulous clinical trial and evaluation in selected cases of epilepsy and generalized myoclonus which have not responded to medical therapy and are not candidates for more conventional surgical techniques of focal cerebral extirpation.

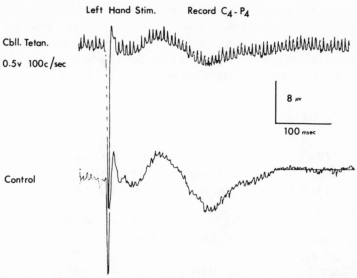

Left Hand Stim.   Record C₄ - P₄

Cbll. Tetan.

0.5v 100c/sec

8 µv

100 msec

Control

Fig. 27. Demonstration of reduction of sensory evoked response by simultaneous stimulation of anterior cerebellum. Both the control and electroencephalographic records represent 25 averaged responses. The sensory
response was evoked by stimulation of the left medial nerve; the response
was recorded over the left parietal lobe; and cerebellar stimulation was
carried out 100 cycles per second and 0.5 volts.

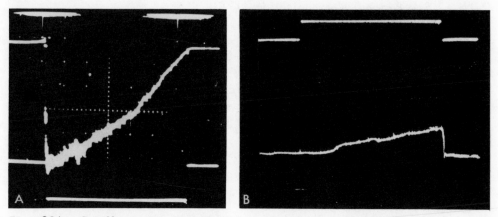

Fig. 28A. Oscilloscopic recording of monosynaptic reflex in man, induced by vibration of the Achilles tendon 100 cycles per second. This
represents a normal response.
Fig. 28B. The same monosynaptic reflex response, in the same patient,
after 5 consecutive minutes of anterior cerebellar stimulation at 10 cycles
per second at 10 volts. Anterior cerebellar stimulation has repeatedly
resulted in marked diminution of this reflex response.

It would seem desirable that specialized centers employing the technique develop a common clinical protocol, employ a universally accepted method of cerebellar mapping of electrode sites, and pool their clinical data in order to further evaluate the clinical and scientific results of chronic cerebellar stimulation.

REFERENCES

COOKE, P. & SNIDER, R.S.   Some cerebellar influences on electrically induced cerebral seizures.   Epilepsia (Anest.) 4:19–28, 1955.

COOPER, I.S.   Chronic stimulation of paleocerebellar cortex in man. Lancet, 1:206, 1973.

COOPER, I.S., AMIN, I., & GILMAN, S.   The effect of chronic cerebellar stimulation upon epilepsy in man.   Tr. Am. Neur. Assn. 98: (in press) 1973.

COOPER, I.S., CRIGHEL, E., & AMIN, I.   Clinical and physiological effects of stimulation of the paleocerebellum in humans.   J. Amer. Geriatr. Soc. 21:40–43, 1973.

COOPER, I.S. & GILMAN, S.   Chronic stimulation of the cerebellar cortex in the therapy of epilepsy in the human.   In Field, W.S. (Ed.) "Neural Organization and its Relevance to Proesthetics". New York: Intercontinental Book Corp., 1973, pp. 371–375.

DOW, R.S.   Personal Communication, 1973.

DOW, R.S., FERNÁNDEZ-GUARDIOLA, A., & MANNI, E.   The influence of the cerebellum on experimental epilepsy.   Electroenceph. Clin. Neurophysiol. 14:383–398, 1962.

ECCLES, J.C., ITO, M., & SZENTAGOTHAI, J.   "The Cerebellum as a Neuronal Machine".   New York: Springer-Verlag, 1967.

FULTON, J.F.   The cerebellum reconsidered.   Chapt. IV in "Functional Localization in Relation to Frontal Lobotomy".   New York: Oxford University Press, 1949.

HENNEMAN, E., COOKE, P.M., & SNIDER, R.S.   Cerebellar projections to the cerebral cortex.   Res. Publ. Ass. Nerv. Ment. Dis. 30:317–333, 1952.

ITO, M. & YOSHIDA, M.   The cerebellar-evoked monosynaptic inhibition of Dieters neurons.   Experientia, 20:515–516, 1964.

LOWENTHAL, M. & HORSLEY, V.   On the relations between the cerebellar and other centers.   Proc. Roy. Soc. London, 61:20–25, 1897.

MORUZZI, G.   "Problems in Cerebellar Physiology".   Springfield: Charles C. Thomas, 1950.

SORIANO, V. & FULTON, J.F.   Interrelation between anterior lobe of
     the cerebellum and the motor area.   Fed. Proc. 6:207-208, 1947.
SHERRINGTON, C.S.   Double (antidrome) conduction in the central
     nervous system.   Proc. Roy. Soc. London 61:243-246, 1897.
SHERWIN, A.L., EISEN, A.A., & SOKOLOWSKI, C.D.   Anticonvul-
     sant drugs in human epileptogenic brain.   Arch. Neurol. 29:73-
     77, 1973.
SNIDER, R.S.   Recent contributions to the anatomy and physiology of
     the cerebellum.   Arch. Neurol. Psychiat. 64:196-219, 1950.
SNIDER, R.S.   Functional alterations of cerebral sensory areas by the
     cerebellum.   In Fox, C.A. & Snider, R.S. (Eds.) "The
     Cerebellum".   Amsterdam: Elsevier Publishing Co., 1967, pp. 322-
     333.
SNIDER, R.S.   Personal Communication, 1973.
WALKER, A.E.   An oscillographic study of the cerebro-cerebellar
     relationships.   J. Neurophysiol. 1:16-23, 1938.

PARAMETERS OF MOTION AND EMG ACTIVITIES DURING SOME SIMPLE MOTOR TASKS IN NORMAL SUBJECTS AND CEREBELLAR PATIENTS

C. A. Terzuolo and P. Viviani

Laboratory of Neurophysiology
University of Minnesota Medical School
Minneapolis, Minnesota

Although the analysis of the connections and properties of the elements of the cerebellar cortex and nuclei has added much to our knowledge (Eccles, Ito, & Szentagothai, 1964; Llinas, 1969), the problem of defining the roles exerted by the cerebellum on motor activities remains widely open. One way of approaching part of this problem is to ask questions concerning the utilization of sensory input data in the control of ongoing movements and how this utilization is affected by cerebellar lesions. Indeed, anatomical and physiological data indicate that several sensory inputs are used in the tasks performed by the cerebellum. When movements of the limbs are considered, a prominent role in their control should be assigned to those input signals generated by motion, that is, by the event which the cerebellum is contributing to control. Therefore, an analysis of the input–output relations between parameters of the motion and motor outputs to agonist and antagonist, both under normal conditions and following cerebellar lesions, becomes a logical necessity. By this approach one can hope to find clues as to the logic by which different types of movements are controlled by the system which comprises the cerebellum. If so, one can eventually envision specific operations, at different sites within the system, adequate to implement this logic. Consequently, single unit recordings in trained animals may eventually be used to test specific hypothesis. Note also that for the outlined program of work to be useful, it should include an analysis of the time dependent characteristics of the input–output relations to be examined. Therefore, the motor tasks to be used should be appropriately chosen and the dynamic characteristics of the afferents data, as well as those of the relation between motor output and motion, should be sufficiently understood to be accountable for when examining (and eventually modeling) the data. All these requirements are met by motor tasks involving the human forearm since: 1) the dynamic characteristics of the stretch reflex have been investigated (Berthoz, Roberts, & Rosenthal, 1971; Poppele & Terzuolo, 1968; Roberts, Rosenthal, & Terzuolo, 1971; Rosenthal, McKean, Roberts, & Terzuolo, 1970) and the dynamic properties of the main receptors involved are sufficiently known (Lennerstrand & Thoden, 1968; Matthews & Stein, 1969; Poppele & Bowman, 1970; Poppele & Terzuolo, 1968; Rosenthal, McKean, Roberts, & Terzuolo, 1970), including the fact that human muscle spindles have the same properties as the cat's spindles (Kennedy & Poppele, 1973); 2) the transfer characteristics between EMG activities and muscle tension for the human biceps and triceps muscles are known (cf Soechting & Roberts, 1973), and the influence of the mechanical properties of the system on the relation between EMG and torque have been studied (Vivien, Soechting, & Terzuolo, 1973).

Note that the choice of human subjects is dictated by the necessity of defining the contribution by intentional motor commands in the performance of the chosen motor tasks. Using these data one can then hope to be able to define conditions under which trained animals can be used as adequate models for the studies mentioned above. Accordingly, the first paper of this series will consider the data on human subjects (both normal and cerebellar patients), while the one which follows will be centered on the comparison between the data obtained in normal human subjects and in trained squirrel monkeys, under comparable experimental conditions (Terzuolo, Soechting, & Palminteri, 1973).

METHODS

Members of the Laboratory volunteered as normal subjects. The 3 cerebellar patients we examined (2 male and 1 female) were selected because of their case histories. All underwent surgery at the Department of Neurosurgery, University of Minnesota Hospitals. An abstract of the case history of each of them is given at the end of this section.

Figure 1 illustrates the apparatus used. Notice that some of the parts of the set-up were adjustable to insure a comfortable accomodation and the proper experimental conditions for all subjects. The pivot point of the lever (P) was made to lay in the axis of rotation of the elbow joint. Under this condition, and with the handle of the lever adjusted to lay in the palm of the hand, the lever duplicates quite precisely, and without appreciable resistance due to friction and mechanical constraints, the movements of the forearm.

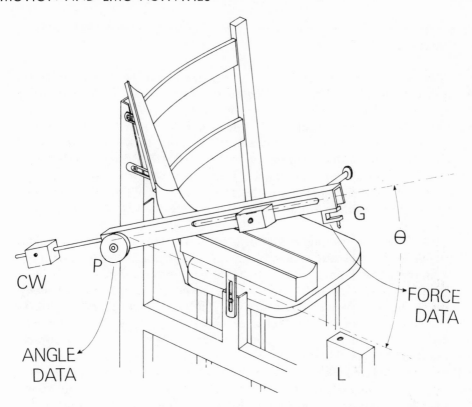

Fig. 1. Experimental set-up - The linear potentiometer (P), located at the pivot point which lay in the axis of rotation of the elbow joint, measures the angle Θ. The lever is locked in the horizontal position by the mechanical system L which releases the lever when a given tension (measured by strain gauge G) is exceeded. A counterweight (CW) balances the downward torque due to the forearm-lever complex.

To exclude that movements of the wrist contributed to the perform-ance two sets of data were compared. One of these sets was obtained with the forearm and hand enclosed in a cast of plaster which was fixed rigidly to the handle of the lever. These data were superimposeable to those obtained without the cast. when the handle was gripped by the hand in supine position. Therefore, the latter procedure was routinely used.

The inertia of the lever could be varied continuously by shifting a mass along the lever. The downward torque introduced by this mass and by the mass of the forearm-lever complex was eliminated by using a

counterweight placed at a suitable distance on the opposite site of the
pivot point (CW in Fig. 1).

The lever could be locked in the horizontal position by a mechanical system (L in Fig. 1) which released the lever when a given tension
was exceeded. The resistive force to be overcome to initiate the movement could be varied continuously between a few hundred grams and 35
kgs. A strain gauge tension transducer (G in Fig. 1) was mounted on
the lever which permitted to measure in each trial the force exerted by
the subject and its decay with time. This decay was not instantaneous,
for mechanical reasons inherent to the set-up. From 20 to 40 msec were
required for the force to fall to zero after the lever was unlocked.

The change in the angle of the lever with respect to the horizontal
position (Θ in Fig. 1) was measured by using a linear potentiometer
placed at the pivot point. The output voltage, after suitable amplific-
ation, was sampled (150 points in 800 msec) and the data were punched
on cards. The electromyographic activity (EMG) was recorded simultaneously with the movement (in most experiments) both from biceps and triceps muscles by means of Teflon coated wires (.0045" in diameter) which
were inserted through the skin using a 23-gauge needle. The needle was
then retracted leaving only the small wire electrode. In a few experiments several of such electrodes were inserted to assure a sampling from
different muscle capita. Since no significant differences were observed
by recording from different regions a single wire electrode for each muscle was used in subsequent experiments. The EMG data were sampled
(1500 points for each of the two channels during the 800 msec sampling
time) and stored in digital form. Synchronization between displacement
and EMG data was insured by using a trigger for the beginning of the
sampling, this trigger pulse being generated by the release of the locked
lever. Data were processed off-line and displayed graphically by using
a digital x-y plotter. The figures shown are reproductions of these plots.

Summary of Case Histories of Cerebellar Patients

M. Y. (female, age 48). Preoperative neurological signs: broad
gate, positive Romberg. A very large meningioma, attached to the lower
surface of the tentorium and extending in front of the left cerebellar hemisphere, was present which compressed very markedly the cerebellum.
Substantial trauma was suffered by the cortex of the left cerebellar hemisphere during surgical procedures. Subsequent to surgery the following
neurological signs were present: Romberg, ataxia, adiadochokinesia,

tremor, dysmetria, rebound, ipotonia and nystagmus. These signs were
still present, although attenuated, 2 and 5 months after surgery, except
for the nystagmus and Romberg. At the time at which this paper is written (20 months after the surgery) the clinical symptoms are very markedly
reduced.

S. S. (male, age 43). Operated on in October 1969 for a very
large acoustic neurinoma, the removal of which necessitated the amputation of the lateral 1/3 of the right cerebellar hemisphere. After surgery the following cerebellar signs were present: adiadochokinesia, dysmetria, ataxia. At the time of our study (2 years after surgery) adiadochokinesia and rebound were still obvious.

E. H. (age 48). This patient was first operated on in 1949 and
1960 for angioblastoma localized to the right cerebellar hemisphere. In
1971 a new and rather extensive amputation of this cerebellar hemisphere
was required. Cerebellar signs present before and after surgery in 1971:
nystagmus, ataxic gate, dysmetric, adiadochokinesia, rebound, tendency
to fall toward the side of the cerebellar lesion. These symptoms were
still present at the time of our examination (1 year after surgery).

RESULTS

The motor tasks used were designed principally to evidentiate the
alterations in motor performance known as dyssynergia, i.e. the disruption
of the smooth control of movements. This sign is already recognized to
result from inappropriate timing and amount of motor command (Altenburger,
1930; Hoffman, 1934). The following two prominent aspects of dyssynergia
will be considered: a) the so-called "rebound phenomenon"; and b) adia-
dokokinesia. The first of these two signs is due to a failure to slow down
or to arrest fast movements automatically, that is, without the participation of intentional commands. The second consists of the inability by
cerebellar patients to perform rapidly alternating intentional movements
(cf Altenburger, 1930; Holmes, 1932). The movements initiated by overcoming a resistive force which quickly decays to zero (see Methods) will
be termed throughout this paper as "ballistically initiated movements".

Unintentional Deceleration of a Ballistically
Initiated Movement in Normal Subjects

The first question we asked is the following: What are the characteristics of the unintentional control of a ballistically initiated movement,
the absence of which produces the rebound phenomenon in cerebellar
patients?   To answer this question normal subjects and cerebellar patients
were instructed to initiate a flexion movement of the forearm by applying
to the locked lever a force sufficient to obtain its release.   The resistive
force was adjusted for each subject to approximate the maximum tension
that he was capable of exerting in our testing situation, in which the
initial angle between the arm and forearm is approximately 135°.   Therefore, the acceleration of the forearm, once the lever was unlocked, was
nearly the maximal that could be achieved by each subject.   This controlled condition is similar to that which is used clinically in testing for
the rebound phenomenon.   The instruction was also given that the movement, once initiated, shall be continued "as fast as possible" until the
forearm had completed the largest flexion anatomically permissible.   This
instruction was added to insure that a braking action on the ongoing movement would not be intentionally applied by the subject.

In 5 out of 7 normal subjects the displacement curves, under the
above stated conditions, showed a marked inflexion in 35% to 60% of the
trials (and in one subject in all trials), indicating a decrease in the rate
of change of the displacement (velocity) soon after the onset of the movement.   Moreover, in 65% of the trials in which the visual inspection of
the time course of the displacement (acceleration) revealed that the movement did not decelerate at a constant rate.

The data shown in A and B of Fig. 2 and in Fig. 3 were obtained
from 3 normal subjects.   They encompass all the features we observed in
our control group.   The upper and lower sets of curves in Fig. 2A and B
describe the time course of the displacement and of the acceleration,
respectively, of two subjects.   The latter data (as well as the velocity
data) were obtained numerically from the smoothed displacement data
(double-sided smoothing by exponential interpolation with cut-off frequency
at 30 Hz).   Since a delay in the sampling ($\simeq$ 40 msec) was introduced
by the trigger and the computer routines, the beginning of the acceleration was made to coincide with its actual time origin by appropriately
delaying the displacement before computing its derivatives.   The introduction of this delay influences the computed value of the acceleration
for the first 4 or 5 data points.   However, since we shall not use these
data in a strictly quantitative way we shall simply remark on the influence

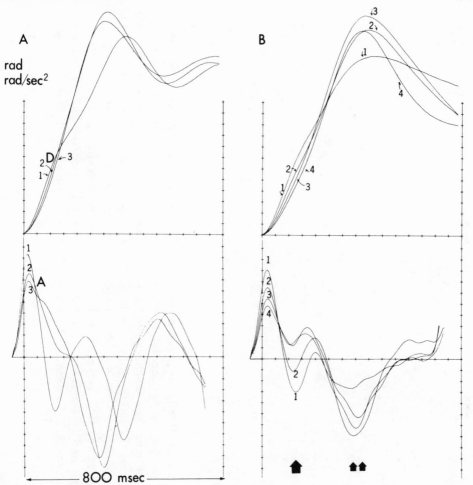

Fig. 2.   Displacement and acceleration data obtained from normal subjects when the instruction is given to proceed with the flexion movement
of the forearm "as fast as possible" after the lever is unlocked - The two
sets A and B are from 2 normal subjects.   The sub-set labeled D contains
the displacement curves and that labeled A the corresponding acceleration
curves.   The numbers permit to identify the same trial in each sub-set.
The trials were chosen among those available in the two subjects to
encompass all the features present, for this type of motor task, in all
normal subjects we studied.   The value of the resistive torque was
slightly reduced in successive trials, following trial No. 1.   The single
arrow in B identifies the notch of the inertial torque introduced by the
automatic control system and termed "unintentional deceleration".   The
double arrow marks the deceleration due to mechanical constraints by
anatomical factors.   Ordinates: 0:12 rad and 12 rad/sec^2 per division.

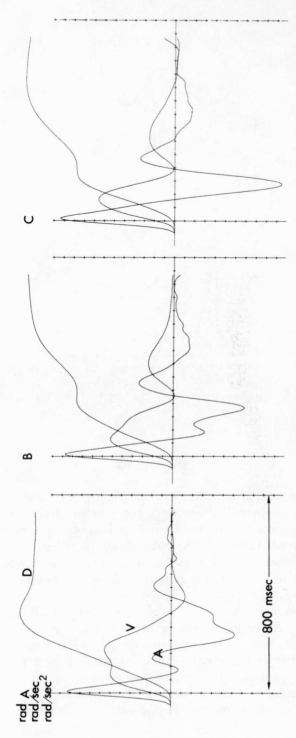

Fig. 3. Unintentional arrest of the ballistically initiated movement – The curves illustrate the parameters of the motion (D, displacement; V, velocity; A, acceleration) in three representative trials of a normal subject. The "unintentional deceleration" (see text) has only a modest influence on the time evolution of the displacement in trial A. In B and C, instead, the movement is temporarily arrested, in spite of the intention by the subject to accelerate the movement initiated by overcoming a near maximum resistive force. The EMG tracings for these three trials are fully considered in Fig. 6. The specific features of the movement parameters are fully considered in the text. Ordinates: 0.12 rad, 1.2 rad/sec and 12 rad/sec² per division in this and subsequent figures. Abscissa: 800 msec total sampling time in all figures (unless otherwise stated).

of data processing by pointing out their effects, as displayed in some of the records to be shown. One last point. Since the acceleration curve also describes the time course of the inertial torque we shall refer to these two parameters interchangeably, although for the latter the appropriate units would have to be used by taking into account the moment of inertia (cf Viviani & Terzuolo, 1973).

By examining Fig. 2A and B it will be noted that a more or less obvious notch is present in the acceleration curves at the time indicated in B by the single arrow. The amplitude of this notch differs in different trials, being larger when the value of the first peak of the acceleration is greater. This fact is particularly obvious in the subject whose data are shown in B. Note that when the negative value of the inertial torque is substantial at the time indicated by the single arrow (as in curve A1 and B1) an inflection in the corresponding displacement curves becomes obvious. This feature is very prominent in 2 of the trials illustrated in Fig. 3, to be considered shortly. Since this behavior takes place in spite of and in opposition to the intent by the subject to proceed with the movement "as fast as possible" it will be referred to as "unintentional deceleration". It will be shown below to be an event which depends on the timing and amount of the motor commands to both agonist and antagonist. When of sufficient magnitude it leads to the arrest of the ongoing movement and its absence can be construed to be responsible for the rebound phenomenon in cerebellar patients. Attention shall not be paid to the values of the inertial torque at the time marked by a double arrow since anatomical factors, which normally limit the forearm flexion, no longer permit an unrestricted motion.

Figure 3 shows other examples of the unintentional deceleration of the ballistically initiated movement in a third normal subject. The velocity data have been added in this figure to provide a full description of parameters of the movement. The effect in the displacement curve introduced during data processing by both smoothing and delay procedures is shown, the time for the beginning of the sampling being situated, as in the previous figure and all subsequent ones, at the origin of the time axis. These displacement curves should be compared with those shown in Fig. 6 where the same data are plotted without delay and smoothing. It can be appreciated that no visually noticeable effect is introduced by both procedures except for the data points near to the time origin of the displacement.

In the trials illustrated in A and B of Fig. 3 two negative peaks of the inertial torque are clearly identifiable before the mechanical factors

mentioned above intervene to distort the data. The influence on the velocity of the movement by these unintentional decelerations is readily apparent. As for the trial illustrated in C, the examination of the EMG
data (Fig. 6) will show that the two decelerations present in B become
fused in C.

At this time, and on the basis of the movement's parameters only,
the following conclusions can already be reached:

1) The time of occurrence of the earlier deceleration is quite constant in the same subject and varies little among different subjects (see
Fig. 2). In all subjects the value of the inertial torque becomes negative 60 to 95 msec after the beginning of sampling, when the unintentional deceleration is sufficiently large. By taking into account the delays introduced by the trigger and sampling routines the time lag from the
onset of the acceleration is of about 100 to 135 msec.

2) The unintentional deceleration is not an all-or-none event and
its magnitude is positively correlated with the value of the acceleration
parameter at its first positive peak. This last point will be considered
further below.

Absence of Unintentional Deceleration in Cerebellar Patients

We will now present the data obtained in cerebellar patients ipsilaterally to the lesion. The data shown in Fig. 4A and B are representative of the behavior exhibited by one of these patients (M.Y.) 20 days
after surgery, while the data shown in C and D were obtained from the
same subject approximately 5 months after surgery. Notice that the maximal resistive torque that this subject was capable to overcome was rather
modest (4 kgw.m at 5 months after surgery). This fact largely accounts
for the small acceleration. A second factor which contributes to this
behavior resides in the fact that cerebellar patients are apparently incapable of producing a maximal contraction of the agonist without simultaneously engaging to a substantial extent also the antagonist (see below).

No obvious unintentional deceleration is present in the records of
Fig. 4, nor in any other measurement made in this patient at three different times (20 days, 2 and 5 months after surgery). The inertial torque
never became negative before 200 msec from the beginning of sampling.
However, the time at which the acceleration reaches its first positive
peak is not different, 5 months after surgery, from that of normal subjects,

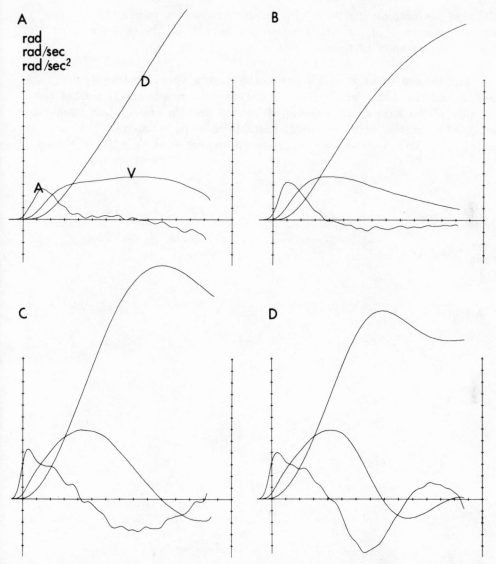

Fig. 4. Performance of the same motor task as in Figs. 2 and 3 by a cerebellar patient (M.Y.) - A and B are representative of the performance of the motor task at 20 days after surgery. C and D were instead obtained at 5 months after surgery. The movement parameters in this figure and subsequent ones are labeled as in Fig. 3. Note: a) the absence of a negative going peak in the acceleration; b) the lower velocity (the peak value being attained at a much later time than in normal subjects, even 5 months after surgery); c) the bumpy appearance of the inertial torque curves (tremor).

although the absolute value of this parameter remains rather small. The
bumpy appearance of the acceleration curves will be shown later to be
due to the presence of tremor.

As for the other 2 cerebellar patients, the data consistently indicate
that no unintentional deceleration of the ongoing movement is present on
the side of the cerebellar lesion. However, only in one subject were the
peak values of the acceleration comparable to those measured in normal
subjects. Figure 5 shows two representative samples of the data obtained

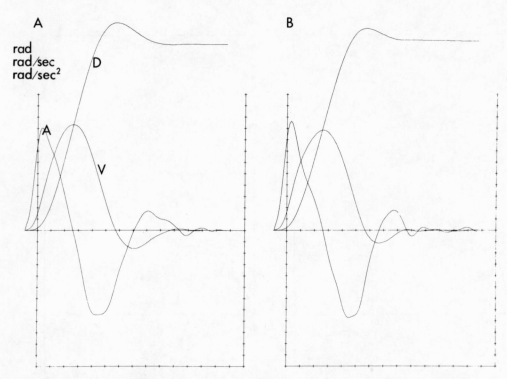

Fig. 5. Absence of "unintentional deceleration" in cerebellar patients –
In this patient (S.S.), although the value of the first positive peak of the
acceleration is comparable to that of normal subjects, there is little evidence in any of the trials (the two shown in A and B being representative
examples) of the "unintentional deceleration" illustrated in Figs. 2 and 3.
Note, in fact, that the inertial torque changes signs at a much later time
than in the three records of Fig. 3, when the position attained (angle Θ)
is such to imply already an impediment to the motion by mechanical
factors, (as pointed out in Fig. 2B).

in this patient (S.S.) who had been operated upon more than two years prior to our testing. In no trials did the inertial torque become negative before 140 msec from the beginning of sampling. Therefore, adaptive properties of the central nervous system cannot overcome completely the deficit resulting from cerebellar lesions. Confirmation of this point was obtained by determining the pattern of motor activities which in normal subjects accounts for the unintentional deceleration of a ballistically initiated movement, and by showing that this pattern is absent in the cerebellar patients we examined.

Pattern of Motor Activities Associated, in Normal Subjects, with a Ballistically Initiated Movement

Figure 6 illustrates the EMG data obtained in the same 3 trials shown in Fig. 3. The displacement curve and that describing the acceleration have been included for the purpose of illustrating their time relationships with the motor output. In this and subsequent figures the EMG of the biceps is shown by the trace labeled B, while that of the triceps is labeled T. Notice that in Fig. 6 no delay was introduced in the data processing before differentiation. Consequently, the values of the acceleration at its first positive peak are larger than those shown in Fig. 3. The reason for not using the delay in this figure is twofold: a) to illustrate the influence upon the value of the acceleration by the delay introduced during data processing; b) to demonstrate that the time of the peak for this quantity is indeed that shown in previous figures, in which a delay was used.

Some features of the electromyographic activity are common to all trials in Fig. 6; they are also found to varying degrees in all normal subjects from all recording sites within both the agonist and antagonist. These features are:

1) the presence of a silent period in the EMG of the agonist, which begins shortly after the lever is unlocked (35 to 50 msec, when taking into account the delay of the trigger and that of the sampling routine);

2) a burst of activity in the antagonist, during the above described silent period of the agonist;

3) a burst of activity in the agonist which ends its initial silent period. The duration of this burst can vary greatly from trial to trial. No activity is ever present in the antagonist during this time.

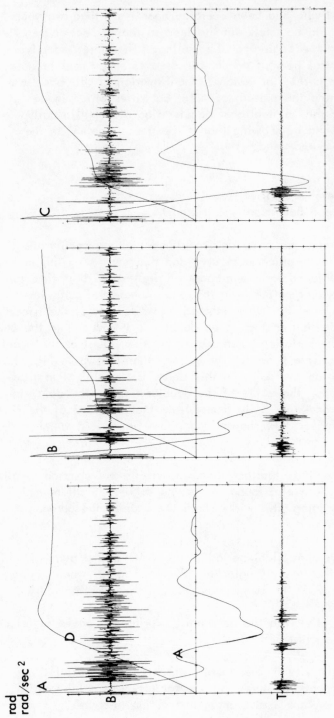

Fig. 6. Relations between the EMG of agonist and antagonist and movement's parameters during the "unintentional deceleration" – The three trials illustrated are the same as in Fig. 3. Reference to this figure shall be made for the velocity parameter. The EMG activities of the biceps (tracing labeled B) and triceps (tracing labeled T) were sampled simultaneously with the displacement data (see Methods). The EMG data were differentiated before plotting.

4) a second silent period of the agonist during which activity is constantly observed in the antagonist (cf B and C of Fig. 6). In trials evolving as in A of Fig. 6 the activity of the agonist is reduced but not totally suppressed;

5) a resumption of activity in the agonist. The characteristics of this activity vary greatly from trial to trial.

In summary, a highly structured pattern of motor activity is present in the agonistic and antagonistic muscles of normal subjects following the ballistic onset of the movement. The general structure of this pattern is invariant and consists of reciprocally alternating periods of activity and inactivity in the agonist and antagonist which begin, soon after the onset of the movement, with a silent period of the agonist. Characteristically the number of these cycles depends on whether or not the movement is successfully arrested by the unintentional deceleration.

The data just presented confirm and extend the findings of other authors who performed similar experiments in normal subjects. In particular, Alston et al (1967) noted that in their experimental conditions (maximum resistive force 6.70 kg. w) there can be several – 3 or more – "distinct silent periods" in the EMG of the agonist. These authors recorded the electromyographic activity by means of large surface electrodes. Therefore, there can be no doubt that the discrete sampling obtained by recording with a wire electrode (as in our experiments) is representative of the behavior of the majority of motor units involved. The behavior of the antagonist was not examined by these authors, but Angel et al (1965) reported the presence of the burst of activity in the antagonist during the first silent period of the agonist under the same conditions. It can therefore be contended that the motor pattern we have here described is a normal concomitant of ballistically initiated movements, even when the resistive force is less than the maximum which the subject can overcome. However, when the resistive force is negligible the first burst of the triceps may be absent.

The effect of this highly structured pattern of activity in the agonist and antagonist is rather obvious when one compares the curves describing the inertial torque and the simultaneously recorded EMG. Only a few points need to be stressed.

1) When the intentional command resulting from the instruction to proceed with the movement "as fast as possible" is overriding (as in the trial illustrated in Fig. 6A), the activity of the agonist which follows the

first silent period is quite substantial.

2) The duration of the first burst of agonist together with the timing of the second burst of the triceps determine whether or not the movement is carried on in a seemingly smooth fashion from the viewpoint of displacement (as in trial A of Fig. 6) or the movement is arrested as in records B and C.

3) Only when the unintentional deceleration is modest (as in trial A of Fig. 6) are there several bursts of activity in the antagonist (3 to 5), which may last until the steady position of the forearm is attained. Instead, of the unintentional braking action has succeeded in arresting the movement (as in B and C of Fig. 6) no new cyclic pattern of agonist-antagonist activity is reinstated.

4) The intentional action to proceeding with the movement "as fast as possible" (that is, to accelerate the ongoing movement) has no access to the effector muscle until the first cycle of reciprocal activity in the agonist and antagonist (silent period of the agonist with concomitant activity in the antagonist) is completed. This motor output need not be sustained, being not infrequently fractioned into bursts.

As a comment to points 1) and 4) above we can note that when the ongoing movement is effectively arrested by the unintentional deceleration, it is because the intentional commands have failed to intervene by prolonging the first burst of the biceps. In this case the effectuation of the intentional action takes place after the end of the second pause of the agonist. It would therefore seem as if the intentional commands operate essentially by modifying the characteristics of the pattern ignited by the ballistically initiated movement without altering its general structure. More data on this subject will be presented later.

Coming now to comment on point 2) above, some features of the activity of the antagonist deserve to be considered in relation to the parameters of the movement.

The magnitude of the first burst of the triceps varies from trial to trial although statistically it is found to be larger in those trials in which the acceleration is greater (Terzuolo, Soechting, & Viviani, 1973). This fact accounts for and supports the statement made earlier, when Fig. 2 was presented, that the magnitude of the initial and small unintentional decelerations, which barely affect the rate of displacement, is related to the value of the acceleration at its first positive peak. Moreover, this triceps activity occurs in close time relation to the peak of the acceleration. Therefore, if it is supported by input data generated by the movement, derivatives higher than velocity are involved. Instead, the timing of the second burst of the triceps apparently depends on whether or not the intentional action to accelerate the ballistically initiated movement succeeds in prolonging the first burst of biceps. By inspecting Figs. 3 and 6 one can see that in trial C, in which the unintentional deceleration is the most effective (the absolute value of the deceleration being the highest), the second burst of the triceps occurs at the peak of velocity. Instead in trial A, where the unintentional deceleration is the least effective, no activity is present in the triceps at the peak of the velocity resulting from the ballistic onset. However, the increase in acceleration caused in this trial by the intentional action to accelerate the motion (prolongation of the first burst of the biceps) brings about a burst of activity in the triceps which occurs, as in trial C, at the peak of the velocity attained as a result of the biceps activity. Although in intermediate cases, such as in trial B of Fig. 6, the time relation between the second burst of the triceps and the velocity parameter is less clear, we have little doubt in asserting that also in these cases this burst occurs in close coincidence with the peak velocity caused by the first burst of the biceps.

The timing of the subsequent burst of the antagonist will be considered in the Discussion.

Cerebellar Participation in the Generation of the Patterning of Motor Output Associated with a Ballistically Initiated Movement

Since a braking action is absent in cerebellar patients, the question shall be posed whether the motor pattern identified above as being responsible for the unintentional deceleration is absent in cerebellar patients. If so, such pattern could be construed as being generated with the participation of cerebellar activities.

Figure 7 shows the EMG data obtained in the same trials illustrated in Fig. 4C and D in Fig. 5. It is quite obvious by inspecting these records that the highly structured pattern of activity in both agonist and antagonist, described above, is absent in these patients. These records are representative of all trials in the 3 cerebellar patients we examined.

Their main features can be summarized as follows:

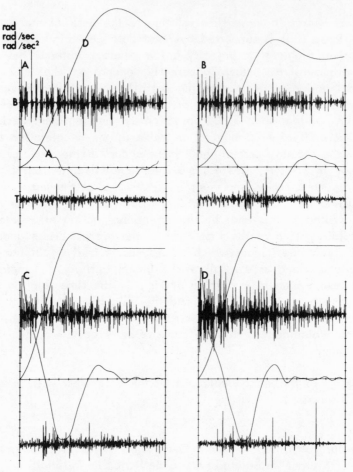

Fig. 7. Absence of a structured and reciprocally organized motor output in cerebellar patients – The 4 trials are representative of the data obtained in 3 cerebellar patients. A and B are from patient M.Y. at 5 months after surgery; C and D are from patient S.S. at 2 years after surgery. The EMG data are to be compared to those of Fig. 6. This comparison permits to identify the main features of the motor output which depends from the functioning of the automatic control system. Note: a) the absence of a silent period in the agonist soon after the onset of the movement; b) the absence of the structured and reciprocally organized activity responsible, in normal subjects, for the "unintentional deceleration"; c) the grouping (particularly in A and B) of the activity of the agonist in short bursts, which clearly influence the inertial torque being responsible for the so-called "intentional tremor" (the amount of smoothing used while processing the displacement data before proceeding to the numeral differentiation being the same as that used in Fig. 6); d) the coactivation of agonist and antagonist(trial C). The details are considered in the text.

1) The activity of the agonist continues almost unperturbed after the lever has been unlocked. When the EMG activity is fragmented, as in records A and B of Fig. 7 (tremor, see below), it is not possible to ascertain whether or not a total pause in the activity of the biceps is present some time after the initiation of the movement. In general, it can be safely stated that the motor activity of the biceps declines gradually, when the velocity of the movement is low (as in A and B of Fig. 7), or remains almost unchanged until after the maximal displacement anatomically possible is attained (D of Fig. 7). When the velocity is high (as in record C and D), some decline in the activity of the agonist may be present in some trial (as in C and D, 2 years after surgery).

2) Some instructured activity is observed in the antagonist, both before the onset of the movement and during the movement which ceases only after the steady-state position is attained (D of Fig. 7). Constantly lacking is the first burst of the triceps, which occurs at or near the peak of the acceleration.

3) There is a lack of agonist-antagonist reciprocity. The activity of the antagonist (as in C of Fig. 7) almost invariantly occurs in unison with activity in the agonist. This overlap in the timing of the activity of agonist and antagonist will be further emphasized when examining the performance during tracking movements.

4) When tremor is present, the EMG of the agonist is fractioned in short bursts which are largely responsible for the bumpy appearance of the curve of the inertial torque (A and B of Fig. 7). Notice that the tremor is only present in the agonist (a point which will be reinforced by other data to be presented later) and that there is no silence in the background activity of the antagonist during these bursts of activity of the agonist, stressing again the lack of reciprocity between agonist and antagonist.

The conclusions to be drawn from the data just presented are as follows: The shortening of the biceps following the onset of the movement has little effect on the excitability level of the biceps alpha motoneuron population in the 3 cerebellar patients we examined. Moreover, the activity of the triceps seems to be largely independent from the parameters of the motion. Therefore, it would seem that segmental reflex mechanisms alone are inadequate to account, in normal subjects, for the presence and general structure of the motor pattern which is ignited by a ballistically initiated movement and for the reciprocity between agonist and antagonist. Cerebellar activities would seem to be involved. Finally, it can be stated that the absence of silent period in the agonist together with the lack of activity in the antagonist are responsible for the absence of unintentional deceleration in cerebellar patients, and therefore for the "rebound" phenomenon.

The observations on the cerebellar tremor (summarized at point 4), will be considered under a separate heading later on.

Intentional Arrest of a Ballistically Initiated Movement by Normal Subjects and Cerebellar Patients

In the experiments to be now described the subjects were instructed to arrest intentionally the ongoing movement "as soon as possible" after its onset, and to maintain the position attained. The movement itself was initiated ballistically in the way described previously.

The first general question we asked from this experiment was the following: Is a pattern of reciprocal activity in agonist and antagonist also involved in the intentional arrest of the ongoing movement by normal subjects? The answer to this question is affirmative. Moreover, the activity responsible for the intentional arrest is injected constantly at the time at which the unintentional one is operating.

In Fig. 8A two sets of curves are shown which were obtained from the same normal subject. The behavior illustrated by set U for (unintentional) is that described under a preceding heading, while that of set I (for intentional) is the one to be here considered. The time origin of the curves of this last set was arbitrarily delayed in plotting the data to permit the independent examination of each set. This examination should leave no doubt that the intentional command is preventing the continuation of the flexion movement at the same time at which the curves in set U indicate that the rate of displacement begins to change as a result of the unintentional deceleration. This point can actually be decided unequivocally by examining the acceleration curves shown in Fig. 8B. The value of these parameters becomes negative between 60 to 95 msecs after the beginning of sampling. This range is the same as that reported above for the unintentional deceleration.

The EMG data presented in Fig. 9 also show that the general structure of the motor pattern in agonist and antagonist which is responsible for the intentional arrest of the movement is similar, in its general features, to that which was previously shown (Fig. 6) to be responsible for the unintentional deceleration. By comparing the EMG data under these two

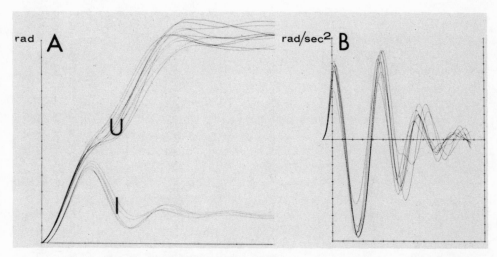

Fig. 8. Comparison between the time of occurrence of the "unintentional deceleration" and of the intentional arrest – The two sets of displacement curves shown in A illustrate, for the same normal subject, the performance during the two motor tasks considered, that is, when the instruction is given to proceed with the ballistically initiated movement "as fast as possible" (set U) and when the instruction is given to "stop the movement as soon as possible" (set I). The time origin of the latter set was delayed in plotting the data to permit the independent visualization of each set. Note that the rate of rise is the same in the two sets, the resistive force being the same. The intentional commands to arrest the movement clearly arrest the flexion at the same time that the "unintentional deceleration" is operating during the first type of motor task. This point is further illustrated in B, in which it is shown that the inertial torque during the intentional arrest assumes a negative value in the same range of times encountered (see Figs. 2 and 3) for the "unintentional deceleration". For A only: abscissa 106 msec per division.

experimental conditions the following main points can be made:

1) The time at which the first silent period begins in the biceps, following the onset of the movement, and that of the first burst of activity in the triceps fluctuate within the same limits in both experimental conditions.

2) The activity of the triceps is greatly accentuated by the inten-

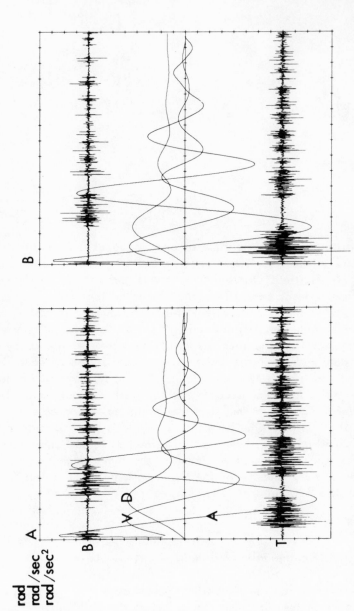

Fig. 9. Motor output to the agonist and antagonist accompanying the intentional arrest of the ballistically initiated movement – The 2 trials shown are from the same subject whose data were also presented in Fig. 6. Note that the oscillatory behavior is sustained by a reciprocally organized motor output to the agonist and antagonist. The time relationships between these motor outputs and the parameters of the motion are fully considered in the text.

tional action to arrest the movement, much in the same way as the first burst of activity of the biceps was previously shown to be affected by the opposite intentional command (Fig. 6A).

A few other features of the records shown in Fig. 9 deserve comment. It will be recognized by inspecting these data that the arrest of the movement is accomplished with the participation of the reciprocally organized activity in antagonist and agonist. This patterning is obviously contributing to the oscillatory behavior of the inertial torque, which in turn determines the damped oscillations of the displacement curve. Since the command to arrest the movement is not intentionally formulated in terms of reciprocally alternating activity in the antagonist and the agonist, this feature of the motor pattern should therefore be generated independently. Indeed, it can be seen in the records that, as the oscillatory behavior decreases, a condition prevails in which both agonist and antagonist are simultaneously active. This condition is ultimately responsible, as to be expected, for the immobilization of the joint at the angle attained as a result of the damped oscillation.

The pattern of reciprocal organized motor output we have just described was found to be absent in cerebellar patients.

The records of Fig. 10A and B are from the same patient as in Fig. 4, while those shown in C and D of the same figure are from the same patient as in Fig. 5. Both sets are representative of the behavior exhibited in all trials by each patient. Some features are common to both of them, as well as to the other patient we examined. There is an extreme paucity of damped oscillation (compare the oscillations of the inertial torque with those shown in Fig. 9 for a normal subject). Accordingly, the position at which the forearm is finally arrested is closer to the maximum displacement initially attained than in normal subjects. In spite of this behavior, which is examined quantitatively in another paper (Viviani & Terzuolo, 1973), the movement is rather effectively arrested by one of the patients (records C and D), while in the other patient the intentional command is much less effective (compare the displacement curves in Fig. 10A and B to those in Fig. 4, in which the subject was not requested to arrest the movement). The reason for this difference has to be found in the timing at which activity begins in the triceps (compare, in Fig. 10, A and B to C and D). This difference in behavior between these two cerebellar patients remains unexplained. We can note, however, that dysmetria was only present in the patient (M.Y.) in which the intentional activation of the antagonist was delayed. We shall come back to this point soon.

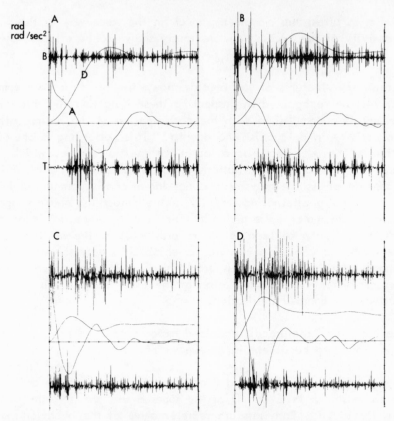

Fig. 10.   Absence in cerebellar patients of a structured motor output and
of an oscillatory behavior during the intentional arrest of an ongoing
movement – The data are from the same patients as in Fig. 7 (M.Y.:
trials A and B; S.S.: trials C and D).   Dysmetria was very marked in
one of them (M.Y.) but not in the other.   These EMG data have to
be compared to those of Fig. 9.   The absence of oscillations is characteristic of cerebellar patients.   Accordingly, the angle Θ at the end
of the sampling is larger than in normal subjects.   This fact is particularly obvious in A and B, since the motor commands to the triceps are
substantially delayed in this patient with marked dysmetria.   Note also
the absence of a reciprocal behavior in agonist and antagonist, although
in C and D some reciprocal behavior appears to be present.   These two
trials were selected since this behavior is more obvious than in the other
trials available.   Even so, co-activation of agonist and antagonist is
present, especially at the beginning of the tracing.   Note that the frag-
mentation of the motor output into bursts is more marked in the patient
with a very obvious tremor (trials A and B) and that this feature predom-
inates in the muscle activated by intentional commands (first the biceps
and then the triceps).

As for the activity of the agonist, it does not cease during the intentional activation of the triceps. Even when a reduction in this activity is present (as in trials A and D of Fig. 7) the peak negative value of the inertial torque is smaller than that attained at the first positive peak. This is the opposite of what occurs in normal subjects where the activity of the triceps does not overlap that of the biceps, the peak negative value of the inertial torque being in these subjects consistently larger than that of the first positive peak (Viviani & Terzuolo, 1973).

In conclusion, no reciprocally organized activity in the agonist and antagonist contributes, in cerebellar patients, to the intentional arrest of the ongoing movement. Activation of both agonist and antagonist appears to be the way in which these subjects successfully arrest the ongoing movement.

The delayed activity of the triceps, illustrated in A and B of Fig. 10, could be suggested to be at the basis of dysmetria. This symptom was indeed quite marked in this patient. It can also be suggested, from the data so far presented, that the inability to execute rapidly alternating movements (adiadochokinesia) may result from the impossibility to activate independently agonist and antagonist (cf Holmes, 1932). This behavior, however, might not be an exclusive characteristic of subjects with cerebellar lesions, since the coordination required to bring about rapidly alternating intentional movements is not infrequently rather poor in the non-dominant side of normal subjects. This was observed in two of our normal subjects. Moreover, Soechting et al (Soechting, Stuart, Hawley, Paslay, & Duffy, 1971) have reported the coactivation of agonist and antagonist, in normal subjects, during a motor task similar to the one we are considering. We can only state that in our data the peak negative value of the inertial torque was constantly larger than that of the preceding positive peak (cf Viviani & Terzuolo, 1973). This behavior can only result if the activity of the triceps is segregated in time, and does not overlap that of the biceps.

Relationship Between the Characteristics of the EMG Pattern
and the Parameters of the Movement

Having demonstrated that the general structure of the motor pattern described under the preceding heading depends on the presence of the cerebellum, it remains to be seen if the specific characteristics of this output bear a relation with sensory input data. To this end one can change the inertial load, therefore affecting the time evolution of the motion.

It will be noted in Fig. 9 that the activity of both biceps and triceps occurs mostly while each muscle is being stretched, this activity
being greater at the peak of velocity. This temporal relation is particularly obvious for the first burst of the biceps and the second burst of
the triceps, since the EMG activity clearly precedes in time the displacement and ceases before the peak stretch is attained. This temporal
relation between velocity of stretch and motor output already suggests the
involvement of primary spindle afferents (stretch reflex), the output of
these receptors being in phase with velocity when stretched sinusoidally
at a frequency equal to that of the oscillations initiated, in the records
of Fig. 9, by the intentional arrest of the movement (cf Poppele & Bowman, 1970; Poppele & Terzuolo, 1968; Rosenthal, McKean, Roberts, &
Terzuolo, 1970).

The data shown in Fig. 11 further stress the dependency of the
motor output on sensory input data. They were obtained by imposing an
inertial mass in the way described under Methods. Records shown in A
and B of Fig. 11 have to be compared with those of Fig. 9, having been
obtained from the same normal subject, while the data shown in C and
D of Fig. 11 are from the same cerebellar patient whose data without
inertial mass are shown in C and D of Fig. 10.

In all normal subjects the frequency of the oscillation was decreased
by the addition of the inertial mass. This expected result is considered
in detail in another paper (Viviani & Terzuolo, 1973). Relevant in the
present context are the corresponding changes in the characteristics of
the motor outputs. These changes strongly favor the hypothesis that the
oscillatory behavior is supported by reflex activities since the increase
in the period of the oscillations and the spacing between bursts, in both
biceps and triceps muscles, proceed pari passu. Note also that an overlap is still present between the EMG activities of the agonist and antagonist and the velocity at which these muscles are being stretched particularly in the case of the second burst of the triceps. However, one
gains the qualitative impression that the motor outputs may begin to overlap partially the displacement. A quantitative analysis of these data is
provided elsewhere (Soechting, 1973) with the conclusion that in normal
subjects the causal relation between parameters of the motion and motor
output is supported by sensory data since the phase relation between the
motion and the impulse density is almost unaffected by the addition of
an inertial mass. A dependency of the motor output from sensory input
data is not found, instead, in the cerebellar patient. This point is

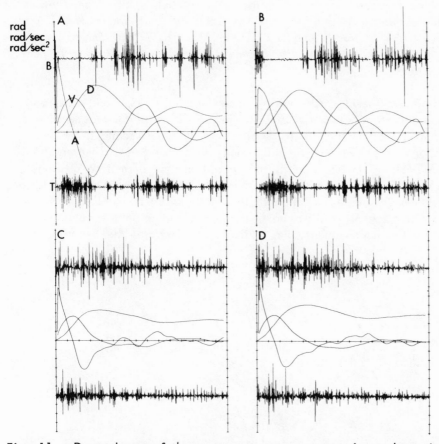

Fig. 11.   Dependency of the motor output on sensory input data, in
normal subjects - Trials A and B are from the same normal subject as in
Fig. 9.   Trials C and D are from the same cerebellar patient as in Fig.
10C and D.   The data from the normal subject illustrate the fact that
the specific characteristic of the motor output are related to the time
evolution of the moment.   They were obtained by increasing the inertial
load with respect to the trials presented in Fig. 9.   The EMG activity
which supports the oscillatory behavior maintains with respect to the
parameter of motion approximately the same phase relation even though
the period of the oscillation is increased by increasing the moment of
inertia.   In C and D oscillations are absent, no reciprocal behavior of
agonist and antagonist is present and the arrest of the movement is
obviously due to the simultaneous activation of both muscle groups.

examined quantitatively elsewhere (Soechting, 1973). Here it suffices to note that no obvious differences in the motor output is introduced, in cerebellar patients, by changing the inertial load (compare records C and D of Fig. 10 to records C and D of Fig. 11). These last records emphasize again the lack of reciprocity between agonist and antagonist in cerebellar patients.

Adiadochokinesia. Alternating movements of flexion and extension which approximate a sinusoidal motion can easily be performed, with a minimal amount of training (2 to 3 trials lasting some seconds), by tracking an appropriate acoustic stimulus. This motor task, described in detail elsewhere (Vallbo, 1971), reveals that the frequency of motion attainable is much higher in the normal side than on the one of the cerebellar lesion. Account, however, must be taken of the fact that in normal subjects the maximum frequency attainable can be somewhat higher in the dominant side than in the nondominant one. Figure 12 illustrates the behavior in

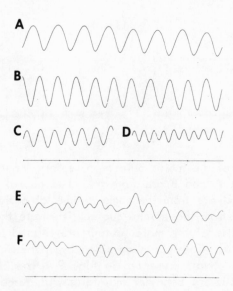

Fig. 12. Adiadochokinesia – This figure provides a comparison of the performance in the normal side (A, B, C and D) and in the cerebellar side (E and F) when the patient is asked to impart a sinusoidal movement to the lever by tracking a sinusoidally modulated acoustic input. Only the displacement curve is shown. In A, B, C and D the frequencies to be tracked were 1, 2, 3 and 4 respectively. In E and F the patient was attempting to track a frequency of 1.5 Hz.

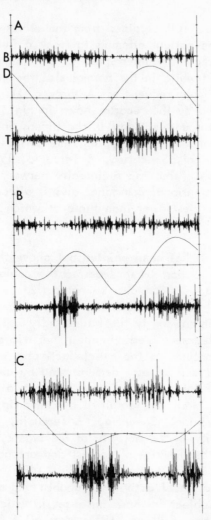

Fig. 13. Behavior of a pair of antagonistic muscles during an intentionally controlled movement in cerebellar patients – The motor task was the
same as that described in the legend of Fig. 12. The frequency to be
tracked in A was 1 Hz. Although up to this frequency the cerebellar
patients usually do not have difficulty in performing adequately the task,
as shown by the displacement trace, the EMG data clearly shows that
the activity of biceps and triceps are not confined to not overlapping
times, as it is the case in normal subjects (see Fig. 1 of Ref). When
the subject is asked to track a higher frequency (1.5 Hz or above) the
performance becomes erratic (B and C), this behavior being due to the
fact that agonist and antagonist are frequently coactivated, during the
task, leading to the distortions and frequency arrests of the movement.

one cerebellar patient, the result obtained from the others being similar. It will be noted that as the patient attempts to track a frequency of 1.5 cycles/sec the motion is frequently interrupted in the side of the cerebellar lesion (records E and F) while in the normal side the motion is still sinusoidal even at much higher frequencies (A through D). The reason for this behavior is provided by the records shown in Fig. 13. It can there be seen that the motor unit activity in the biceps and triceps is not confined into discrete and non-overlapping time periods, as in normal subjects (cf. Fig. 1 of Viviani, Soechting, & Terzuolo, 1973), but these activities frequently overlap. Thus the reciprocity between agonist and antagonist resulting from intentional commands also is affected by cerebellar lesions, even at frequencies lower than those at which adiadochokinesia becomes obvious.

Cerebellar Tremor. It has been pointed out above that the grouping of the motor unit activity in short bursts leads to the cerebellar tremor. By examining Fig. 10B and C it can also be noted that as the emphasis of the intentional action shifts from the biceps to the triceps, the patient being instructed to arrest intentionally the ballistically initiated movement, the bursting activity also becomes predominant in the triceps. Therefore, the tremor is essentially confined to the muscle activated by the intentional command. This fact can be best demonstrated by auto-correlating the activity of agonist and antagonist. Figure 14 shows a typical example. The auto-correlation (Fig. 14A), was obtained by converting the EMG data into impulse density (cf. Viviani, Soechting, & Terzuolo, 1973). It shows the presence of a periodicity in the activity of the biceps, while the cross-correlation between the activity of agonist and antagonist indicates the absence of reciprocity in the two muscles (Fig. 14B). Such reciprocity, and indeed the alternation of activity in agonist and antagonist, is instead present in normal subject in those instances in which physiological tremor (cf. Lippold, Redfearn, & Vuco, 1957; Marshall & Walsh, 1956) occurs during a prolonged attempt to overcome a very large resistive force. An example of this behavior is illustrated in Fig. 15A. In B the activity of the agonist and antagonist was cross-correlated to demonstrate the appearance of the cross-correlogram when reciprocity is present. This cross-correlogram should be compared to that of Fig. 14B.

DISCUSSION

In our view the following points have been adequately substantiated by the data presented above to warrant their acceptance:

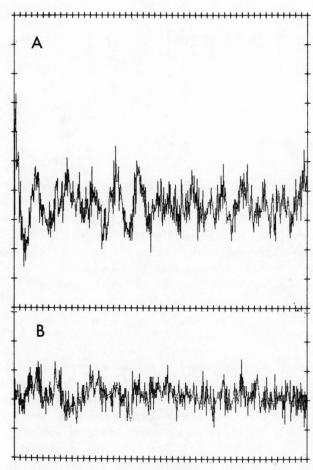

Fig. 14. Cerebellar tremor in the agonist muscle – A. Autocorrelogram
of the EMG activity of the biceps for the trial illustrated in Fig. 7A.
To obtain this autocorrelogram the EMG was first converted into impulse
density (each impulse being made equal in length to the sampling interval), and the autocorrelation was subsequently made utilizing each successive interval. Ordinates in arbitrary units. In B the cross-correlation
between agonist and antagonist is shown from the same trial (compare to
Fig. 15B).

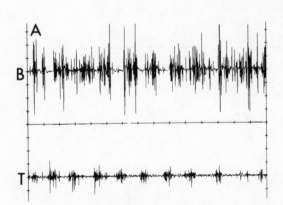
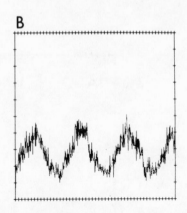

Fig. 15. Tremor in a normal subject during sustained effort – A illustrates the tremor present in some of the trials, from a normal subject,
when the resistive force was too large and the lever could not be released
from the locking device (triggering of the sampling was done manually).
This record is shown since the cross-correlogram between biceps and triceps
activity presented in B was obtained from this trial. This cross-correlogram demonstrates the reciprocal behavior of agonist and antagonist and
should be compared to that of Fig. 14B.

1) A motor pattern is generated in normal subjects, by a ballistically initiated movement which is characterized by alternating periods of
activity and inactivity in both agonist and antagonist. This pattern begins
with a silent period in the EMG of the agonist while the antagonist becomes active, the activity in the two muscles being reciprocally organized.

2) The above pattern was not found to be present in 3 patients with
surgical cerebellar lesions.

3) Specific characteristics of this pattern, which depend on the
absolute value of the initial acceleration, are responsible for a deceleration of the ballistically initiated movement which occurs in spite of the
instruction to proceed with the movement "as. fast as possible". This deceleration can be so powerful to effectively arrest the movement. The
EMG activities responsible for this deceleration are absent in cerebellar
patients, leading to the rebound phenomenon.

4) When the instruction is given to arrest the ballistically initiated movement "as soon as possible", the intentional commands in normal subjects gain access to the triceps within the same range of times in which activity is injected into this muscle as part of the pattern responsible for the unintentional deceleration (point 3 above). In both cases the acceleration becomes negative within the same range of times from the onset of the movement. The instruction to proceed with the ballistically initiated movement "as fast as possible" (that is, to accelerate the movement once this is initiated) is translated into action in concomitance with the first or second bursts of the biceps. Therefore, the intentional actions either to arrest or to accelerate the ongoing movement apparently gain access to the effector muscles at times in which activity is programmed to be present in these muscles as a part of the motor pattern generated by the ballistic onset of the movement.

5) The intentional action to arrest the ballistically initiated movement is accomplished, in normal subjects, by means of reciprocally organized activity in the antagonist and agonist. Such behavior is not present in subjects with cerebellar lesions. Therefore, the intentional commands most likely do engage the system which comprises the cerebellum. The specific characteristics of the resulting activity are largely dependent on sensory input data.

6) The reciprocal behavior of agonist and antagonist is either absent or greatly reduced as a consequence of cerebellar lesions, whether this reciprocal behavior is supported by sensory input data (point 5 above) or it depends on intentional commands (sinusoidal motion).

Input Data Which Contribute to the EMG Pattern Present
During a Ballistically Initiated Movement

A discussion of the origin and mechanisms of each of the components of the motor pattern described at point 1) is in order. We may begin this task by considering the silence in the motor output of the biceps which is instated soon after the onset of the ballistically initiated flexion movement. This silent period, described by Hansen and Hoffman (1922) and termed by these authors "unloading reflex", has been investigated extensively in human subjects, also by means of electrical stimulations applied to the muscle nerve while the subject is contracting intentionally the muscle (Hansen & Rech, 1925; Higgins & Lieberman, 1968; Hoffman, 1934; Merton, 1951; Schwerin, 1936; Sommer, 1939). Merton (1951) compared the characteristics of the muscle twitch with the pause in alpha motoneurons' activity and concluded that the pause in spindle primary afferents

during the twitch could adequately account for the silent period of the
alpha motoneurons.   He felt no need for advocating the participation of
an active inhibitory event mediated by afferent activity from Golgi tendon
organs.   The same point of view was expressed by Jansen and Rudjord
(1963).   Moreover, Angel et al. (Angel, Eppler, & Iannone, 1965) and
Alston et al. (Alston, Angel, Fink, & Hoffman, 1967) demonstrated that
displacement of the forearm, and therefore shortening of the agonist, is
essential for determining the presence of the silent period, in agreement
with the conclusions of Struppler et al. (Struppler, Landau, & Mehls, 1964).
Finally Struppler and Schenck (1958), Chaion, Chermitte and Scherrer
(1961) and Arrigo (1963) reported that the silent period is reduced or absent in cerebellar patients, although data by other authors (cf. Lieberman
& Higgins, 1968) contradict these findings.   Our results confirm the absence
of the silent period in cerebellar patients for the case of ballistically initiated movements and establish that, in normal subjects, intentional commands
directed to accelerate this movement do not override the mechanisms responsible for this abrupt cessation of the motor output to the agonist. These
two facts are here interpreted to mean that this silent period normally requires the participation of the cerebellar activities.   In particular, segmental reflex mechanisms alone would appear to be inadequate to produce this
silent period, as well as the simultaneous activation of the antagonist,
since both features are absent in cerebellar patients.   However, afferent
data are obviously involved in triggering and/or regulating this reciprocal
behavior in agonist and antagonist.   To discuss this point we shall first
consider the reciprocal actions upon agonist and antagonistic alpha motoneurons by the afferent activity from the primary endings of muscle
spindles.

Among the observations made when the instruction was given to proceed with the ballistically initiated movement "as fast as possible", the
following ones tend to deny a quantitative and, therefore, direct relationship between the activity from primary afferents of the agonist and antagonist and the reciprocally organized motor output: 1) the silent period of
the agonist frequently begins significantly earlier than the time at which
activity is present in the antagonist; 2) the pause in activity of the agonist
varies modestly from trial to trial (irrespectively from the value of the resistive torque and, therefore, the initial acceleration) while the presence
and amount of the first burst of the triceps varies as a function of the resistive torque, being absent in many of the trials in which the initial acceleration is modest; 3) there is a significant time delay between the end
of the first burst of the agonist and the second burst of the antagonist.

Therefore, we do not feel compelled to assign an overriding role, as far as the reciprocity between agonist and antagonist is concerned, to the segmental reflex mechanisms subserved by primary afferents, without advocating the intervention of a supraspinal control. The absence of such reciprocity in cerebellar patients further supports this viewpoint.

Coming now to consider more closely the possible effect of changes in primary spindle afferents upon the silent period of the agonist, it hardly needs to be mentioned that experimental data became available in recent years strongly indicate that alpha and gamma motoneurons are co-activated during intentional movements (for a review cf. Granit, 1970). Moreover, the data of Vallbo (1971) obtained in man during isometric intentional contractions clearly indicate the presence of a strong gamma componet, since the primary endings are activated during intentional twitches. It could therefore be contended that in our experimental conditions the unloading of the muscle spindles of the biceps, consequent to this shortening during the forearm flexors might be inadequate to produce a pause in the firing of the primary endings. However, we feel that the activity in the primary ending most likely ceases during the ballistic onset of the movement, even if a high background of gamma fusostatic activity is present (Chen & Poppele, 1973; Soechting, 1973), because of the high rate sensitivity of these receptors (Lennerstrand & Thoden, 1968; Matthews & Stein, 1969; Rosenthal, McKean, Roberts, & Terzuolo, 1970).

The fact reported by Alston et al. (Alston, Angel, Fink, & Hoffman, 1967) that the duration of the silent period is related to the amount of displacement is in keeping with this viewpoint. More importantly the silent period begins at or near the peak of the acceleration. Therefore, an input signal in phase with this parameter should be involved. The dynamic characteristics of joint receptors (McCall & Williams, 1971) and primary endings of muscle spindles (Henatsch, 1972; Poppele & Bowman, 1970; Poppele & Terzuolo, 1968; Rosenthal, McKean, & Roberts, 1970) are known to approximate this requirement when the motion is sufficiently fast. Even so, the drop in excitatory drive to the biceps alpha motoneurons by the suppression of primary spindle afferents would seem to be inadequate per se, to account for the first silent period of this muscle under our experimental conditions. Indeed, one would have to postulate that the excitatory drive to the alpha motoneurons by the intentional commands would be inadequate per se to induce impulse activity. This possibility would accentuate the role of the gamma loop in supporting motor outputs (cf. Granit, 1970). However, data by Vallbo (1971) indicate that, in man, alpha motoneurons can be activated by intentional commands before the gamma loop is brought into action. Therefore, we conclude that under our experimental conditions either the intentional commands are suppressed or the

alpha motoneurons are submitted to an inhibitory action. The first subject has been considered in a separate paper (Terzuolo, Soechting, &
Viviani, 1973) dealing with the possible role of cerebellar activities in
the formation of intentional motor commands. Here we shall instead focus
upon the possible contribution to the silent period of the agonist by sensory input data.

First of all, the possible participation in producing the silent period
by Golgi tendon organ afferents shall be mentioned. This subject has been
treated extensively by Granit (1970). It suffices here to say that this inhibition is "facultative" in the words of Granit, and it is regulated, at
least in the cat, by supraspinal centers which receive inputs from the
cerebellar nuclei (Hongo, Jankowska, & Lumberg, 1969; Lundberg,1970).
One could then postulate that this inhibition: 1) is normally suppressed
during the isometric contraction which precedes the onset of the movement;
and 2) is released after the onset of the movement by a central action
which is triggered by an appropriate input signal. While this problem
will be considered when we will deal with the logic of the control system
which comprises the cerebellum, it is pertinent to note here that input
data from the tendon organs are obviously available during the silent period of the agonist since the muscle tension in the biceps decays slowly at
the end of the EMG activity, the duration of the twitch of individual
muscle fibers (Buchtal & Schmalbruch, 1970) lasting more than 200 msec.
It shall be emphasized, however, that the duration of the silent periods of
the biceps appear to be independent of the value of the resistive force to
be overcome to initiate the movement, and therefore of the initial muscle
tension. Moreover, the activity of the biceps is completely suppressed in
man even when the resistive force is extremely small (a few hundred grams).
Therefore, no quantitative relation can be demonstrated between muscle
tension and silent period. This difficulty, however, could be overcome if
one were to postulate a facilitation of the inhibitory action of tendon af-
ferences upon the alpha motoneurons by the intervention of the central
control system which is disrupted by cerebellar hemispheric lesions. A
demonstrable relationship between the tendon organs' input and the parameters of the silence period would no longer be required in this case, because not only the magnitude but also the duration of the silent periods
could be determined centrally. The subject will be further considered
when the data obtained in trained monkeys will be presented.

Moving now to complete the discussion of sensory inputs which may
be involved in the shaping of the motor pattern we are considering, we
shall mention only briefly the activity of the biceps which was termed
"first burst of the agonist". The possible origins of this activity were

extensively discussed by Alston et al. (Alston, Angel, Fink, & Hoffman, 1967), and linked by these authors to a resumption in the activity of the primary ending via the gamma loop. Other possibilities, however, exist although its reflex nature cannot be doubted. In fact, this activity can occur within 20 msec after an ongoing and ballistically initiated movement is mechanically arrested shortly after its onset. This time is close to that of the transport delays for the human stretch reflex of the arm (Llinas, 1969).

Only the bursts of activity of the triceps remain to be considered. The presence and magnitude of the first burst of this muscle is dependent on the peak value of the acceleration and it occurs near to or at the peak of this parameter. Owing to the dynamic characteristics of the primary endings we mentioned above, this first burst of the triceps could be supported by input data generated by its stretch. However, the absence of such burst in cerebellar patients strongly suggest that a supraspinal control, by means of biasing actions upon the pertinent motoneurons' populations, is normally required for its presence (see below). Note that this burst can only provide to decelerate the movement but is inadequate to bring the motion to a halt. The triceps activity which is responsible for this behavior occurs, instead, at the peak of the velocity of the motion. The conditions under which this activity is injected into the antagonist, in normal subjects, are revealed, we believe, by comparing data from trials such as those which were presented in Figs. 3 and 6. It will be noted that when the velocity of the movement is zero at the time at which the second burst of the biceps causes the value of the inertial torque to return positive (as in trials B and C), then no activity is injected into the antagonist. Indeed, the value of the second peak of the acceleration is quite modest. Instead, activity is constantly injected into the triceps, even by modest accelerations causing a stretch of this muscle, when these accelerations occur while the velocity at which the triceps is stretched is still high (2nd burst of trial B; 2nd and 3rd bursts of trial A) or is increasing starting from a negative value (as for the 4th burst of trial A).

The prolonged bursting activity of the antagonist when the motion is not temporarily arrested is suggestive of a sampling process initiated centrally by the control system which comprises the cerebellum and could represent preferential times at which intentional actions may eventually intervene to modify the ongoing movement.

Can We Begin to Specify Some of the Functions of the
Control System Which Comprises the Cerebellum?

From the data presented under results it can be argued that whatever
sensory inputs are reaching those structures of the brain responsible for intentional motor outputs, these inputs are largely ineffective to control fast
movements after cerebellar lesions. We are referring here not only to the
segmental reflex activities but also to the known afferents to the sensory-
motor cortex and in particular to the data of the literature which indicate
the possibility of influencing unit activity within the motor area by changing limb position (Albe-Fessard & Liebeskind, 1966) and, more generally,
to the organization of activities of the motor cortex on the basis of sensory
information (cf. Brooks & Stoney, 1971, for a review).

Although the paucity of cerebellar patients we examined and the
impossibility of knowing exactly the extent of the lesions (including secondary degenerations) prevent us from defining specific sites (we believe,
however, that the cerebellar hemisphere and its nuclei are essentially involved) it is possible, on the basis of the data presented above, to suggest that the cerebellum contributes to the control of forearm movements
in man by:

1) suppressing the intentional motor commands to the agonist muscle
at the onset of a ballistically initiated movement, even when the resistive
force to be overcome to initiate this movement is modest;

2) determining the presence, timing and amount of the activity injected into the antagonist which is responsible for the unintentional deceleration, and eventually, the temporary arrest of the ballistically initiated
movement;

3) programming the time at which intentional actions can intervene
to modify an ongoing fast movement, whether these actions are directed
to accelerate or to arrest this movement;

4) focusing the intentional motor commands on the agonist muscle
when the initiation of the flexion movement requires near the maximal
force that the subject is capable of and during alternating movements of
flexion and extension;

5) bringing about the reciprocal behavior of agonist and antagonist
during: a) the automatic control of fast movement; b) the intentional and
sudden arrest of a fast movement.

A discussion of the ways and mechanisms by which each of the above actions may be accomplished would bring us to consider the logic of the control system which comprises the cerebellum and the operations which may be used in implementing this logic. It is not our aim to pursue here this subject for each of the points stated above. Indeed, only for some of these points pertinent data are available in the literature to permit the formulation of specific hypothesis, which can eventually be tested experimentally. Instead we would like to conclude this paper with a general consideration about the role of the system which comprises the cerebellum in regulating fast movements by utilizing sensory input data. The experimental findings pertinent to this point are: i) The effective unintentional arrest of the ballistically initiated movement is accomplished whenever the activity of the triceps approximately overlaps in time the velocity curve; ii) when an ongoing movement is intentionally arrested, a reciprocally organized motor output to the antagonist and the agonist is instated, which is dependent upon the automatic control system. These motor outputs are essentially in phase with the velocity of the movement, as shown quantitatively elsewhere (Viviani & Terzuolo, 1973); iii) during fast but not ballistically initiated movements the antagonist is automatically activated in phase with the velocity, the activity of the agonist being simultaneously diminished or suppressed (Terzuolo, Soechting, & Viviani, 1973); iv) in normal human subjects (and monkeys) the motor output is causally related and dependent upon sensory input data generated by the motion (Soechting, 1973); v) any such dependence was found to be absent in the three cerebellar patients we examined (Soechting, 1973); vi) the input-output analysis used to establish points iv) and v) above also demonstrates that changes in the inertial load do not affect such relationship.

It can therefore be concluded that the time relation between input data and motor output described above is dependent on cerebellar activities and the hypothesis can be put forward that cerebellar activities contribute to control the ongoing movement in the following way. The timing of the biasing actions imposed by the control system upon segmental mechanisms (by acting directly upon the alpha motoneurons and/or via the gamma loop) is such that information on the rate of the displacement are essentially utilized in controlling automatically fast movements, except that at the onset of a ballistic movement where higher derivatives are also contributing. Since the motion is dependent upon variables which are extrinsic to the nervous system – in particular the inertial load – the automatic control system has also the task of maintaining constant the relation between motor output and the parameters of the motion by utilizing sensory input data.

ACKNOWLEDGMENTS

This work was supported by Public Health Service Grant NS-2567. Computer facilities were made available by the Air Force Office of Scientific Research, AFSC (Grant AFOSR-1221).

The authors are deeply grateful to the subjects who participated in the experiments and to Dr. Shelley Chou, Department of Neurosurgery of the University of Minnesota, for the help and collaboration given in connection with the 3 cerebellar patients. Thanks are also due to Mr. J. Kerkes for the design of equipment and for the computer programming pertinent to the logging routine. To Mrs. Mary Robinson, for her unfailing assistance during many years, one of the authors (C.T.) likes to express his deep and sincere gratitude.

REFERENCES

ALBE-FESSARD, D. & LIEBESKIND, J. Origine des messages somato-sensitifs activant les cellules du cortex moteur chez le singe. Exp. Brain Res. 1:127-146, 1966.

ALSTON, W., ANGEL, R.W., FINK, F.S., & HOFFMAN, W.W. Motor activity following the silent period in human muscle. J. Physiol. London, 190:189-202, 1967.

ALTENBURGER, H. Untersuchungen zur Physiologie und Physiopathologie der Koordination die Willkürlichen. Einzelbewegungen bei Kleinhirn läsionen. Zeitschd. ges. neur. und Phych. 124:678-713, 1930.

ANGEL, R.W., EPPLER, W., & IANNONE, A. Silent period produced by unloading of muscle during voluntary contraction. J. Physiol. London, 180:864-870, 1965.

ARRIGO, A. Valore semeiologico del tempo silente. Sist. Nerv. 15: 280-292, 1963.

BERTHOZ, A., ROBERTS, W.J., & ROSENTHAL, N.P. Dynamic characteristics of stretch reflex using force input. J. Neurophysiol. 34: 612-619, 1971.

BROOKS, V.B. & STONEY, S.D. Motor mechanisms; The role of the pyramidal system in motor control. Ann. Rev. Physiol. 33:337-392, 1971.

BUCHTAL, F. & SCHMALBRUCH, H. Contraction times and fiber types in intact human muscle. Acta Physiol. Scand. 79:435-452, 1970.

CHAION, F., CHERMITTE, F., & SCHERRER, J. Exploration de l'activite motorice chez l'homme normal. Rev. Neurol. 105:330-343, 1961.

CHEN, W.J. & POPPELE, R.E. Static fusimotor effect on the sensitivity of mammalian muscle spindles. Brain Research, 54:244-247, 1973.

ECCLES, J.C., ITO, M., & SZENTAGOTHAI, J. "The Cerrebellum as a Neuronal Machine". Berlin: Springer-Verlag, 1964.

GRANIT, R. "The Basis of Motor Control". London: Academic Press, 1970.

HANSEN, K. & HOFFMANN, P. Weitere Untersuchungen uber die Bedentung der Eigenreflexe fur unsere Bewegungen. I. Anspannungs und Entspannungsreflexe. Z. Biol. 75:293-304, 1922.

HANSEN, K. & RECH, W. Beziehungen des Kleinhirns zu den Eigenreflexen. Dt. Z. Nervheilk. 87:207-222, 1925.

HENATSCH, H.D. Structural and functional aspects of fusimotor mechanisms in mammalian muscle spindles. In Drischel, H. & Dettmar, P. (Eds.) "Biocybernetics" Vol. IV. Berlin: G.F. Verlag Jen, 1972, pp. 170-180.

HIGGINS, D.C. & LIEBERMAN, J.S. The muscle silent period: variability in normal man. Electroenceph. Clin. Neurophysiol. 24:176-182, 1968.

HOFFMAN, P. Die physiologischen Eigenschaften der Eigenreflexe. Ergebn. Physiol. 36:15-108, 1934.

HOLMES, G. The cerebellum of man. Brain, 62:1-30, 1932.

HONGO, T., JANKOWSKA, E., & LUMBERG, A. The rubrospinal tract: II. Facilitation of interneuronal transmission in reflex paths to motoneurons. Brain Res. 7:365-391, 1969.

JANSEN, J.K.S. & RUDJORD, T. The silent period during twitch contraction of the soleus of the decerebrate cat. Acta Physiol. Scand. Suppl. 213, 59:69-70, 1963.

KENNEDY, W.R. & POPPELE, R.E. Sensory activity of human muscle spindles. (Submitted for publication).

LENNERSTRAND, G. & THODEN, U. Muscle spindle responses to concomitant variations in length and in fusimotor activation. Acta Physiol. Scand. 74:153-165, 1968.

LIEBERMAN, J.S. & HIGGINS, D.C. Delayed termination of the muscle silent period in cerebellar disorders. Electroenceph. Clin. Neurophysiol. 25:53-57, 1968.

LIPPOLD, O.C.J., REDFEARN, J.W.T., & VUCO, J. The rhythmical activity of groups of motor units in the voluntary contraction of muscle. J. Physiol. London, 137:473-487, 1957.

LLINAS, R. (Ed.). "Neurobiology of Cerebellar Evolution and Development". Chicago: Am. Med. Assn. Educ. and Res. Fdn., 1969.

LLOYD, D.L. On reflex action of muscular origin. Ann. Rev. Nerv. Ment. Dis. 30:48–67, 1952.

LUNDBERG, A. The supraspinal control of transmission in spinal reflex pathways. In Widen, L. (Ed.) "Recent Advances in Clinical Neurophysiology". Electroenceph. Clin. Neurophysiol. Suppl. 25, pp. 35–46.

MARSHALL, J. & WALSH, E. Physiological tremor. J. Neurol. Neurosurg. Psychiat. 19:260–267, 1956.

MATTHEWS, P.B.C. & STEIN, R.B. The sensitivity of muscle spindle afferents to small sinusoidal changes. J. Physiol. London, 200: 723–743, 1969.

McCALL, W.D. & WILLIAMS, W.J. Dynamic analysis of cat knee joint receptors. Fed. Proc. 30:709, 1971.

MERTON, P.A. The silent period in a muscle of the human hand. J. Physiol. London, 114:183–198, 1951.

POPPELE, R. & BOWMAN, R. Quantitative description of the linear behavior of mammalian muscle spindles. J. Neurophysiol. 33:59–72, 1970.

POPPELE, R.E. & TERZUOLO, C. Myotatic reflex: Its input–output relation. Science, 159:743–745, 1968.

ROBERTS, W.J., ROSENTHAL, N.P., & TERZUOLO, C. A control model of the stretch reflex. J. Neurophysiol. 34:620–634, 1971.

ROSENTHAL, N.P., McKEAN, T.A., ROBERTS, W.J., & TERZUOLO, C.A. Frequency analysis of stretch reflex and its main subsystems in the triceps surae muscles of the cat. J. Neurophysiol. 33:713–749, 1970.

SCHWERIN, O. Untersuchungen uber den Entlastungsreflex des menschen. Dt. Z. Nervheilk. 140:240–244, 1936.

SOECHTING, J.F. Modeling of a simple motor task in man: motor output dependence on sensory inputs. (Submitted)

SOECHTING, J.F. & ROBERTS, W.J. Transfer characteristics between EMG activity and muscle tension under isometric conditions. (submitted).

SOECHTING, J.F., STUART, P.A., HAWLEY, R.H., PASLAY, P.R., & DUFFY, J. Evaluation of neuromuscular parameters describing human reflex motion. J. Dynamic Systems, Measurements and Control, 93:221, 1971.

SOMMER, J. Der Entlastungsreflex des menschlichen muskels. Dt. Z. Nervheilk. 150:83–92, 1939.

STRUPPLER, A. & SCHNECK, E. Der sogennante Entlastungsreflex bei zerebellaren und anderen Ataxien. Fortschr. Neurol. Psychiat. 26:421–429, 1958.

STRUPPLER, A., LANDAU, W.M., & MEHLS, H. Analyse des Entlas-
tungsreflexes (ER) am Menschen. Pflugers Arch. ges. Physiol.
279:18-19, 1964.

TERZUOLO, C., SOECHTING, J.F., & VIVIANI, P. Studies on the
motor control of some simple motor task. I. Relations between
the parameters of the movement and EMG activities. Brain Res.
(in press).

TERZUOLO, C., SOECHTING, J.F., & VIVIANI, P. Studies on the
control of some simple motor tasks. II. On the cerebellar control
of movements in relation to the formulation of intentional commands. Brain. Res. (in press).

TERZUOLO, C., SOECHTING, J.F., & PALMINTERI, R. Studies on
the control of some simple motor tasks. III. Comparison of the
EMG pattern during ballistically initiated movements in man and
squirrel monkey. (Submitted).

VALLBO, A.B. Muscle spindle response at the onset of isometric voluntary contractions in man. Time difference between fusimotor and
skeletomotor effects. J. Physiol. London, 218:405-431, 1971.

VIVIANI, P., SOECHTING, J.F., & TERZUOLO, C. Influence of
mechanical properties on the relationship between EMG activity
and torque. (Submitted).

VIVIANI, P. & TERZUOLO, C. Modeling of a simple motor task in
man: Intentional arrest of an ongoing movement. (Submitted).

MODULATION OF SPONTANEOUS AND EVOKED CHLORALOSE MYOCLONUS BY CEREBELLAR STIMULATION IN THE CAT (RELATION TO RAMSEY HUNT SYNDROME)

Robert R. Myers and Reginald G. Bickford
Department of Neurosciences
University of California, San Diego

La Jolla, California

There exists both experimental and clinical evidence that the cerebellum has significant inhibitory influence at a variety of neuronal levels ranging from the cortex to the brain stem. The former is attested by much evidence in the literature demonstrating suppression of seizures and seizure discharges by electrical stimulation of the cerebellum (Snider & Cooke, 1953; Dow & Moruzzi, 1958; Dow, Fernández-Guardiola, & Manni, 1962). Clinical evidence of cerebellar involvement in seizure mechanisms is implied by the existence of the Ramsey Hunt Syndrome (Hunt, 1922), a severe form of myoclonic epilepsy associated with degenerative changes in the cerebellum. This syndrome can be interpreted on the basis of animal work as resulting from a removal of the usual inhibitory influence of the cerebellum on seizure areas.

The recent observations of Cooper (Cooper, 1973; Gilman & Cooper, 1973) that the frequency of seizures in selected patients can be greatly reduced or eliminated by electrical stimulation of the cerebellar hemisphere, is very important in demonstrating that the cerebellar inhibitory drive can be harnessed for therapeutic purposes. This discovery opens up a significant new approach to treatment in patients who are uncontrolled by medication. In spite of previous work, the mechanism of the therapeutic effect is poorly understood.

In reviewing Dr. Cooper's patients, we were particularly impressed by the case of severe action myoclonus, a sequel of cerebral anoxia, whose myoclonic symptoms have virtually disappeared with long continued cerebellar stimulation. Further research on the mechanism of this

217

suppressive effect demands an animal model showing long continued myoclonus with properties that resemble the clinical condition. We have used
the chloralose myoclonus model for this purpose both because of the great
deal of work that has already been done to investigate its mechanism
(Adrian & Moruzzi, 1939; Moruzzi, 1941a, b. c; Terzuolo, 1954; Stenhouse, 1970) and because some of its properties of stimulus and startle
sensitivity match those frequently encountered in post-anoxic encephalo-
pathy, in the Ramsey Hunt Syndrome, and in other myoclonic syndromes
such as diffuse neuronal degeneration, Jakob-Creutzfeldt Disease, etc.
This report describes our preliminary observations on suppression and augmentation of this type of myoclonus by cerebellar stimulation in a cat
with a discussion of the relevance of this model to the myoclonic phenomenon observed in a patient with Ramsey Hunt Syndrome.

ANIMAL EXPERIMENTS

Method

Six adult cats have been prepared following intraperitoneal injection
of 50 mg/kilogram of alpha chloralose. When unconscious, a venous catheter was inserted, the animal was curarized and placed in a stereotaxic
instrument under artificial ventilation. The skull was exposed and small
stainless steel screws were inserted in the frontal and occipital regions
bilaterally for EEG recording. A reference electrode was placed in the
midline frontal region over the frontal sinus.

The cerebellum was then exposed using sub-occipital craniotomy and
flat 2 mm. mobile metal discs with epoxy covering on one side were slid
onto the surface of the cerebellum for stimulation. We have used placements that simulate as far as possible those employed by Cooper in his
patients as follows:

1. Paleo Cerebellar stimulation of Cooper. The electrodes were
placed on the superior surface of the anterior lobe bilaterally.

2. Neo Cerebellar stimulation of Cooper. Same electrodes were
placed bilaterally and symmetrically on the lateral extremities of the
cerebellum. To obtain optimal placement, these electrodes were shifted
in the course of stimulation to maximize the suppressive effects on myoclonus. When maximal effect was obtained in the "paleo" or "neo" positions, subsequent observations were usually made from this position. A
few stimulation observations were made with a multi-contact depth electrode in which an attempt was made to arrest the myoclonus by probing

at various steps and directions during stimulation. In general, these experiments were unsuccessful in suppressing myoclonus are not further reported.

After the surgery had been completed, curare administration was stopped and myoclonus was allowed to manifest itself again.

EEG. The EEG was recorded on a Beckman-type CE 8 channel with a 0.3 second time constant and a high frequency filter cutoff at 70 Hz. EMG electrodes were placed in the limb muscles to record the activity on an EEG channel with time constant of 0.03 seconds.

Electrical stimulation of the cerebellum was carried out using a constant current stimulator (Shipton-Iowa design) which produces square wave pulses (1 millisecond duration) of frequencies ranging from 1 to 500 Hz. A stimulus isolation unit was employed to minimize artifact and the current and voltage of the stimulus were measured oscillographically across a small resistor in series with the stimulating electrodes.

Sensory Stimulation. Initial experiments used the click of a metal strip monitored by microphone pickup. Later experiments used a tone pip of 1000 Hz, 10 milliseconds duration, applied through a microphone close to the animal's ear. The sound level was approximately 70 db. Photic stimulation was applied with a Grass PS2 stimulator (I=8) placed eight inches in front of the animal's eyes. Since EMG recordings alone were found to give an inadequate picture of the character and distribution of the myoclonus, visual data were recorded by means of a videotape and camera. These recordings were made in control periods and during and after cerebellar stimulation.

RESULTS

General Observations - Chloralose Myoclonus

Following an intraperitoneal injection, the animal usually shows signs of trembling and incoordination in about 10 minutes. The cat rapidly becomes unconscious, lies on its side with continuous myoclonic jerks and some slight degree of extensor tonus. Myoclonic jerks were widespread and synchronous and have a slightly predominent flexor direction. These animals were often exquisitely sensitive to low intensity sounds in the environment which produce a generalized jerk. Touching the animal, stroking or moving limbs will likewise result in violent jerking as does photic stimulation as indicated in Figure 1. The spontaneous myoclonus

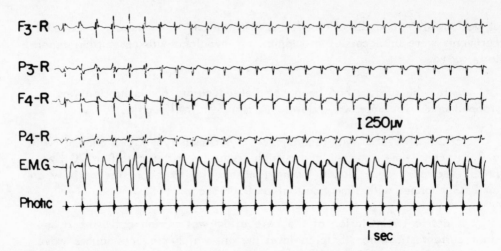

Fig. 1. Entrained myoclonic response of the chloralose cat to photic stimulation. Note the regularity of the EMG response and the evoked responses appearing in the cortex. The amplitude and at times the waveform of the cortical response does, however, undergo some systematic changes.

has a repetition frequency ranging from 0.5 to 2 per second and the myoclonus can be driven accurately by a repetitive stimulus, such as sound, touch, movement or light. No evidence of habituation to this stimulation has been noted though there is some apparently random variation in the amplitude of the muscle response during a stimulus train.

EEG. The EEG is dominated by almost continuous and widely synchronized discharges which consist of mono, di, or multiphasic transients-- the predominant component of which is usually negative. The complexes have an amplitude ranging from 100–500 microvolts and a duration of 100–300 milliseconds. Several different types of discharges can be distinguished while the largest and highest amplitude are usually associated with the myoclonic jerk. With photic stimulation, the cortical response can be entrained and this results in a considerable change in its waveform (Fig. 1). At slow rates (below 3 per second) a jerk is associated with each flash and the cortical response, though stereotyped when compared with a no stimulus situation (Figure 2), shows considerable modulation in amplitude and as can be seen in F3-R recording in Figure 1.

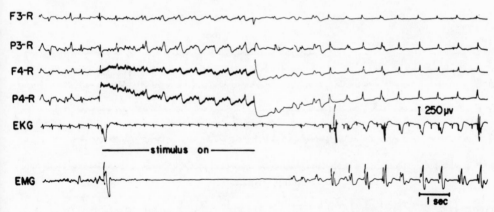

Fig. 2. Changes in EEG and myoclonus with stimulation of the anterior lobe of the cerebellum. Frequency 200, 2.0 milliamps. During stimulation the EEG becomes more regular, the random pattern present in the unstimulated cat tending to disappear. Myoclonus also disappears during stimulation and for one to two seconds following, during which there is some randomization of the EEG followed by a period of markedly increased regularity of EEG discharge associated with spontaneous myoclonus (rebound effect).

Cerebellar Stimulation. Anterior lobe (paleo cerebellar stimulation of Cooper). In the first two cats, there was clear suppression of spontaneous myoclonus during the stimulation period at frequencies of 100-200 per second. These effects were not seen at low rates of stimulation from 1-10 per second. During stimulation, there is suppression of myoclonus with a remarkable increase in the myoclonus at the end of the stimulation period (rebound effect). When stimulation was continued longer than 20 seconds, there was usually evidence of an escape phenomenon in which the myoclonus began to reappear. In these instances, the usual facilitation followed cessation of the stimulus. As can be seen from Figure 3, the stimulus (sound) induced myoclonus is likewise suppressed by cerebellar stimulation.

Suppression of myoclonus was also produced when the electrodes were shifted to the neocerebellar position in the lateral surface but these effects were usually less marked than those obtained from the anterior position.

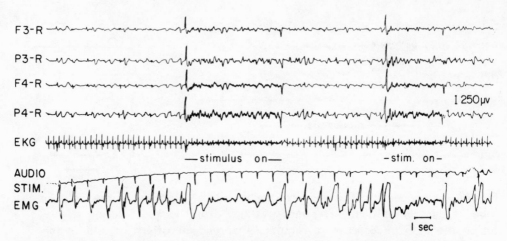

Fig. 3. Effect of neocerebellar stimulation on sound-induced myoclonic response. Sound stimulus (metallic click) produces an entrained mylconic response during control periods. Cerebellar stimulation (stim on); frequency 200; pulse duration, 1 millisecond; current, 2.0 milliamps; suppresses myoclonic response which is reestablished for five seconds following cessation of stimulation and the response is again suppressed on reapplication of cerebellar stimulation.

In the last two cats investigated, there has been difficulty in reproducing the suppressive effects of cerebellar stimulation seen in the earlier preparations. Instead, in both instances, facilitation of myoclonus both spontaneous and evoked by sensory stimulation has been encountered. An example of this is shown in Figure 4. At the present time, we are uncertain as to the origin of these differences since stimulus waveform, wave shape, chloralose level and general preparation seem to have been similar in all preparations.

Patient Data. The patient with Ramsey Hunt Syndrome, whose EEG is illustrated in Figure 5, is presented for comparison with the chloralose myoclonus model just described. The patient syndrome is most comparable to an animal under relatively light levels of chloralose anesthesia. In both conditions, there is spontaneous myoclonus though in the patient this was not usually a marked feature since the jerks that occurred could usually be related to environmental circumstance. In their sensitivity to

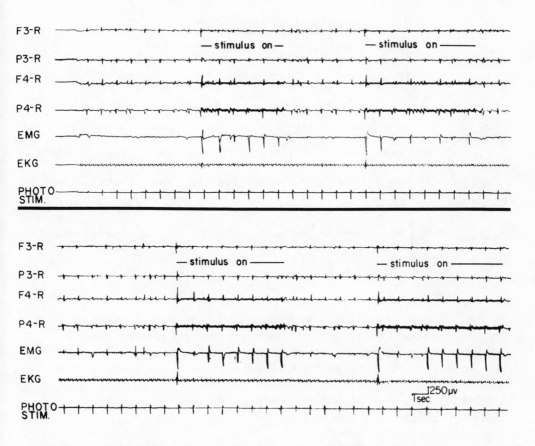

Fig. 4. Facilitatory effects of anterior lobe cerebellar stimulation on myoclonus during photic stimulation--Cat 9. During cerebellar stimulations, stimulus on; frequency, 200; pulse duration, 1 millisecond; current, 2.0 milliamps; there is marked facilitation of the myoclonic response and a disappearance during the interval between periods of cerebellar stimulation with reappearance of a myoclonic response on the second stimulation period. In the lower part of the illustration, some myoclonic response was present in the control period but this was always markedly increased during cerebellar stimulation.

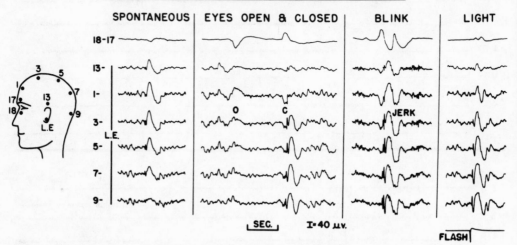

COMPARISON OF SPONTANEOUS, BLINK, AND LIGHT INDUCED DISCHARGES

Fig. 5. Patient, aged 30, with Ramsey Hunt Syndrome (dyssynergia cerebellaris myoclonica). Patient has had frequently severe myoclonic jerking with progressive cerebellar involvement for 10 years. No intellectual impairment. Marked light, sound and startle sensitivity causing generalized myoclonus. Limb movement also causes myoclonus as does elucidation of tendon reflexes. Patient was incapacitated by jerks caused by blinking and eye closing.

Jerks are associated with a single spike-wave or multiple spike wave complex occurring bilaterally and synchronously throughout all head regions. The occurrence of a spontaneous complex associated with a jerk is shown on the left. The occurrence of myoclonus on eye closing but not on eye opening is shown in next section. The blink induced myoclonus and cerebral response which was the patient's major disability is illustrated in the third column while the last column shows the response to a single flash of light.

afferent stimuli, there is a close resemblance and both patient and animal
can be driven regularly by a variety of afferent stimuli--sound, light,
etc.--producing entrained myoclonus so long as the repetition rate remains
relatively low (approximately 1-2 stimuli per second). Note that in the
patient, eye closing was always more effective than eye opening and only
the latter was normally associated with a jerk. Blinking was more effective than eye closing. The effect of eye opening and closing cannot be
modeled in the cat because of the effect of anesthesia. There is also a
rather close resemblance in the EEG insofar as widespread synchronized
discharges present in both patient and animal and was produced both spontaneously and with an afferent stimulus. In the human, however, the response is a more stereotyped single spike-wave than in the animal where
the slow component is not very evident. A similar finding of light sensitivity in a patient with this syndrome has also been reported by Christophe
and Remond (1951).

DISCUSSION

The animal experiments reported are preliminary and indicate that
surface cerebellar stimulation of both anterior cerebellar hemispheres and
laterally placed electrodes may produce suppression of spontaneous and
evoked myoclonus when relatively high stimulus rates are used. Little
effect was noted at the lower stimulus rates which Cooper has used for
suppression of other types of seizures. While stimulus currents were kept
as low as possible, spread of the stimulus to structures beyond the cerebellum cannot be altogether excluded either in these experiments or, in
fact, in the implanted stimulator observations of Cooper. It has already
been noted that our experiments have revealed both suppressive and facilitatory effects of cerebellar stimulation and that the precise difference
in animal or stimulus conditions producing these two opposing effects are
not yet evident. However, the findings are significant in indicating that
both facilitatory and inhibitory components exist in the cerebellar mechanism. This observation, if it can be applied to the human, would indicate
the need for continuing caution in applying the technique in case facilitatory effects are inadvertantly encountered.

While our initial goal was to investigate a model which reproduced
the suppressive effects of cerebellar stimulation on myoclonus, it is evident that this goal has not yet been reached. In Cooper's procedure, the
stimulation is longterm and requires chronic implantation of the stimulation
electrodes. Insofar as longterm stimulation in the present experiments
commonly resulted in escape and remanifestation of the myoclonus, this

finding would suggest that longterm suppression of chloralose myoclonus may not be attainable. To test the longterm hypothesis, however, we are implanting chronic stimulation electrodes in these animals which we hope will provide a more accurate simulation of Cooper's conditions. On the other hand, it is also possible that the chloralose model is not optimal and that an animal rendered myoclonic from anoxic damage and which manifests continuous myoclonus may be more appropriate. However, up to the present, we have not found it very easy to produce such a model in the cat.

SUMMARY

In a series of six cases with an acutely implanted cortical and depth cerebellar electrodes, it has been demonstrated that the cerebellar stimulation at a frequency of 200 per second can suppress spontaneous and stimulus induced myoclonus. These effects may well be produced at a brain stem level since there is relatively little change in the cortical EEG. The occurrence of facilitatory effects and the increase of myoclonus from cerebellar stimulation indicates that there are possible hazards insofar as cerebellar stimulation is used in the treatment of epilepsy.

A comparison is made with a case of Ramsey Hunt Syndrome and there are resemblances to the model in the widespread EEG, the widespread myoclonus and the sensitivity to afferent stimulation. On this limited evidence, it is reasonable to regard the patient syndrome as an example of cerebellar dysinhibition through destruction of cerebellar inhibitory systems.

ACKNOWLEDGMENTS

This work was supported by USPHS Grant number NS 08962 and the Epilepsy Foundation of America.

REFERENCES

ADRIAN, E.D. & MORUZZI, G. Impulses in the pyramidal tract. J. Physiol. 67:119-151, 1939.
CHRISTOPHE, M.J. & REMOND, A. Dyssynergia cerebellaris myoclonica de Ramsay Hunt. Etude clinique et electroencephalographique. Rev. Neurol. 84:256-262, 1951.

COOPER, I.S.   Effect of chronic stimulation of anterior cerebellum on neurological disease. Lancet, 1:206, January 1973.

DOW, R.S. & MORUZZI, G.   "The Physiology and Pathology of the Cerebellum".   Minneapolis: The University of Minnesota Press, 1958.

DOW, R.S., FERNANDEZ-GUARDIOLA, A., & MANNI, E.   The influence of the cerebellum on experimental epilepsy. Electroenceph. Clin. Neurophysiol. 14:383-398, 1962.

GILMAN, S. & COOPER, I.S.   The effect of chronic cerebellar stimulation upon epilepsy in man.   Program of the American Neurological Association 98th Annual Meeting, June 11-13, 1973, Montreal, Canada.

HUNT, J.R.   Dyssynergia cerebellaris myoclonica--primary atrophy of the dentate system: A contribution to the pathology and symptomatology of the cerebellum.   Brain, 44:490-538, 1922.

MORUZZI, G.   Sui rapporti fra cervelletto e corteccia cerebrale. I. Azione d'impulsi cerebellari sulle attivita corticali motrici dell'animale in narcosi cloralosica.   Arch. Fisiol. 41:87-139, 1941a.

MORUZZI, G.   Sui rapporti fra cervelletto e corteccia cerebrale. II. Azione d'impulsi cerebellari sulle attivita motrici provocate dalla stimolazione fradica o chimica del giro sigmoideo nel gatto. Arch. Fisiol. 41:157-182, 1941b.

MORUZZI, G.   Sui rapporti fra cervelletto e corteccia cerebrale. III. Meccanismi e localizzazione delle azioni inibitrici e dinamogene del cervelletto.   Arch. Fisiol. 41:183-206, 1941c.

SNIDER, R.S. & COOKE, P.M.   Cerebellar activity in relation to the electrocorticogram before, during and after seizure states.   Electroenceph. Clin. Neurophysiol. 5, suppl. 3:78, 1953.

STENHOUSE, D.   Suppression of chloralose jerk responses by stimulation of the anterior lobe of the cerebellum.   Brain Research, 17: 148-152, 1970.

TERZUOLO, C.   Influences supraspinales sur le tetanos strychnique de la moelle epiniere.   Arch. Internat. de Physiol. 62:179-196, 1954.

CEREBELLAR CORTICAL STIMULATION EFFECTS ON EEG ACTIVITY AND SEIZURE AFTER-DISCHARGE IN ANESTHETIZED CATS

George Dauth, Daniel Carr, and Sid Gilman

Department of Neurology, Columbia University College of
Physicians and Surgeons
New York, New York

INTRODUCTION

It has been known since the turn of the last century that stimulation of the cerebellar cortex can suppress tonic motor activity. Loewenthal and Horsely (1897) and Sherrington (1898) found that high-frequency stimulation of the cerebellar cortex alleviated the limb rigidity of decerebrate animals. Subsequently, Moruzzi (1941a, b) found that cerebellar stimulation depressed the movements resulting from direct cerebral cortical stimulation and reduced the myoclonic twitches of the limbs resulting from application of strychnine to the cerebral cortex. Moruzzi later suggested that seizure discharges originating in the cerebral cortex may trigger suppressor mechanisms of the cerebellum which, in turn, may be a factor in the termination of a seizure (Moruzzi, 1950). In testing directly the influence of cerebellar cortex upon the cerebral cortex, Cooke and Snider (1953) found that stimulation of various parts of the cerebellum resulted in an alteration of the pattern of electroencephalographic (EEG) activity. Thereafter, Cooke and Snider (1955) and Iwata and Snider (1959) demonstrated that electrical stimulation of various portions of the cerebellum can modify seizure discharges evoked by electrical stimulation of the cerebral cortex or hippocampus. In most of these observations, cerebellar stimulation shortened the duration of seizure discharge, but occasionally the discharge was prolonged.

Cerebellar stimulation has also been shown to modify seizure discharges resulting from application of various chemical agents to the cerebral cortex. Dow, Fernández-Guardiola, and Manni (1962) found that

229

cerebellar stimulation suppressed the seizures resulting from application of cobalt to the cerebral cortex of the rat. Steriade (1960) and Hutton, Frost, and Foster (1972) found that cerebellar stimulation suppressed the seizure activity resulting from the recent application of penicillin to the cerebral cortex in the cat. The foregoing observations provided the rationale for attempting to control seizure activity by chronic cerebellar stimulation in humans with intractable epilepsy (Cooper, 1973; Cooper & Gilman, 1973; Cooper, Amin, & Gilman, 1973). The favorable results obtained in these patients provide a basis for further use of cerebellar stimulation in other patients with uncontrolled seizures. However, this new therapeutic approach raises a multitude of problems which require solution. Among the most immediate problems are to determine for human subjects 1) the most appropriate sites for cerebellar electrode implantation in the various types of epilepsy; 2) the optimal type of electrode to deliver current efficiently while producing minimal tissue damage; and 3) the most effective, least noxious stimulus characteristics. Experiments in animals provide a convenient and rapid means of resolving some of these problems, particularly those related to stimulus characteristics and tissue damage with protracted stimulation.

Further animal experiments are also indicated to resolve certain dilemmas which have been found in experimental studies of the effects of cerebellar stimulation. Although high-frequency stimulation diminishes muscle rigidity in decerebrate animals, low-frequency stimulation accentuates it (Sherrington, 1898; Moruzzi, 1950). This finding is congruous with the current concept that the output of the cerebellar cortex, mediated by the Purkinje cells, is purely inhibitory (Eccles, Ito, & Szentágothai, 1967). It is also in keeping with the demonstration that low-frequency stimulation of cerebellum results in total inhibition of Purkinje cell action potentials (Andersen, Eccles, & Voorhoeve, 1964), which would depress tonic cerebellar inhibition. However, the finding is incongruous with the finding that low frequency stimulation is as effective as high frequency stimulation in attenuating seizures evoked by cerebral cortical stimulation (Cooke & Snider, 1955) or with the finding in human subjects that stimulation at low frequency is more effective than that at high frequency in reducing the incidence of epileptic attacks. Further experimentation is also needed to understand the interspecies differences in the effects of cerebellar stimulation upon experimental epilepsy. For example, Dow, Fernández-Guardiola, and Manni (1962) found cerebellar stimulation effective in attenuating cobalt-induced epilepsy in the rat, but Reimer, Grimm and Dow (1967) found it ineffective in the cat. In addition, Steriade (1960) found that cerebellar stimulation depressed the spike discharge resulting from the recent application of penicillin to the cerebral cortex, but enhanced the discharge emanating from older, well-established penicillin foci.

The present report represents a preliminary statement of our studies using animal models to resolve some of the problems. The results presented will be restricted to our observations of the optimal parameters of cerebellar stimulation required to alter EEG activity and cortically-evoked seizure after-discharge in anesthetized cats.

METHODS

Thirty-six adult cats were used in these experiments. Twenty-four were anesthetized by intraperitoneal injection of sodium pentobarbital 30 mg/kg, the remainder with intravenously injected alpha-chloralose, 40 mg/kg. The chloralose was prepared by heating to 70-80°C a mixture of 500 mg alpha-chloralose (Fisher Scientific) in 50 cc of 0.9% saline. After the drug dissolved the solution was cooled to 55°C, filtered, and then injected after cooling to body temperature.

After induction, a catheter was introduced into the femoral vein, a tracheotomy was performed, and the ear canals were filled with 2% viscous lidocaine. The animal was then placed in a stereotaxic device. The left post-cruciate and supra-sylvian cortices and the right paramedian lobule of the cerebellum were exposed. The dura was removed and a constant drip of mineral oil warmed to body temperature was directed over the exposed brain tissue. The body temperature was maintained at 38°C throughout the experiment. Prior to recording, most cats were paralyzed with gallamine triethiodide (Flaxedil) and artificially ventilated. In some of the earlier experiments, paralysis was not induced so that we could observe limb movements resulting from cerebral or cerebellar stimulation.

Recordings were made on a standard ink-writing electroencephalograph 5 to 6 hours after administration of anesthesia. The recording electrode consisted of a fixed montage of stainless steel screws embedded in the calvarium. Four pairs of screws were placed bilaterally 3 mm lateral to the midline. The first pair was placed on the coronal suture with each succeeding pair located 5 mm more caudally. Stimulation was provided by a two-channel square-wave stimulator through stimulus isolation and constant current units. The stimuli were capacity-coupled via 0.22 μF capacitors. The bipolar electrode consisted of 0.02-inch diameter platinum wire shaped to form a smooth curved tip. The electrode area in contact with the cortex was approximately one square mm. The tip separation for post-cruciate and supra-sylvian sites was 3 mm. For the paramedian lobule the separation varied from 3-5 mm depending upon the number of folia spanned.

Several precautions were taken to avoid spreading depression (Leão, 1972): 1) Cerebral sites were stimulated no more frequently than every 15 min; 2) exposed cortex was constantly protected by warm mineral oil; and 3) care was taken to avoid excessive pressure or damage to the cortex from the electrodes.

In determining the parameters of cerebellar stimulation most effective in altering spontaneous EEG activity, we first obtained a preliminary set of stimulus parameter values that appeared effective, and then varied separately the current frequency, pulse duration, and train duration. As each parameter was varied, the others were kept constant at optimal values. In the cats anesthetized with chloralose, only the latter two parameters were varied, and these in a systematic fashion from low to high values. In the cats anesthetized with pentobarbital, one parameter was varied in a random fashion during each series of observations, so that high and low values of that variable were tested in a non-sequential fashion. The major effect on the EEG in all preparations was a change from high-voltage slow wave activity to low-voltage fast activity, as described by Cooke and Snider (1953). We will refer to this change as "suppression". The duration of EEG activity suppression was scored according to arbitrary guidelines. In the chloralose-anesthetized cats, it was gauged as the time between the cessation of cerebellar stimulation and the reappearance of EEG activity with a consistent average amplitude in excess of 120 μV. In pentobarbital-anesthetized cats, suppression was scored as the length of time for the peak amplitude envelope of the EEG activity to return to one-half of the value observed during the 5 sec preceeding cerebellar stimulation.

In examining the effect of cerebellar stimulation on electrically-induced after-discharge in the cerebral cortex, we employed stimulus parameter values to cerebral cortex derived from Ajmone-Marsan's recent review (1972). Current intensity was then adjusted to attain the lowest value consistent with a stable, reproducible after-discharge. Each time the cerebral cortical stimulating electrodes were moved to a new site, the intensity of stimulation was adjusted as described. The key observation was whether the duration of after-discharge induced by cerebral cortical stimulation was reduced when the cerebellum was stimulated. It soon became clear that the duration of the "control" after-discharge (i.e., without cerebellar stimulation) varied to some degree between successive trials, so that a stimulation protocol of control-experimental-control was adopted to be certain that a valid effect had been obtained from the cerebellum. Finally, various time relations between cerebral and cerebellar stimuli were explored, ranging from cerebellar stimulation halting before the onset of cerebral stimulation, to the opposite situation, with varying gradations in between.

RESULTS

Effect of Cerebellar Stimulation on Background EEG Activity

In animals anesthetized with chloralose, the EEG pattern consisted of high-amplitude slow waves with superimposed low-amplitude fast activity, as well as frequent "chloralose spikes" (Fig. 1). As shown in Fig.

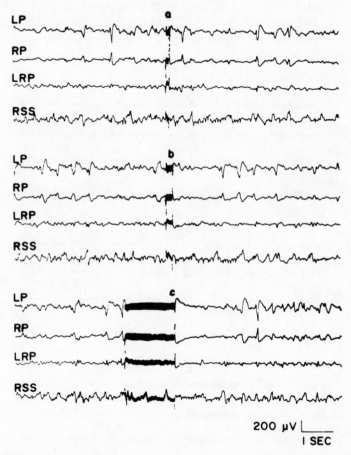

200 μV

I SEC

Fig. 1. Effects of stimulating at various train durations the right paramedian lobule of cerebellum on EEG activity in a cat anesthetized with chloralose. Cerebellar stimulation applied with pulse duration of 1.0 msec, frequency of 200 Hz, current of 5 mA, train durations of (a) 0.1 sec; (b) 0.2 sec; (c) 1.6 sec. Note suppression of slow wave and spike activity in b and c. EEG montage: LP=left posterior (i.e., 10 and 15 mm caudal to coronal suture); RP=right posterior; LRP=left-right posterior; RSS=right supra-sylvian.

1a, cerebellar stimulation with a train duration of 0.1 sec (using 5 mA, 200 Hz, 1 msec pulse width applied to the paramedian lobule) had no effect on the EEG activity. However, increasing the train duration to 0.2 sec while maintaining the other parameters fixed resulted in the brief loss of both the spikes and the high amplitude slow wave activity, with persistence of low voltage fast activity (Fig. 1b). Further increase of the train duration to 1.6 sec lengthened the duration of the EEG suppression (Fig. 1c). To some extent, it was possible to compensate for one ineffective parameter value by increasing the value of another. An example of this finding appears in Fig. 2, which contains records taken from the same experiment as those shown in Fig. 1. In Fig. 2a, a train

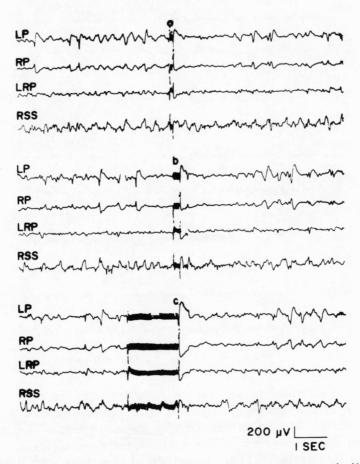

200 µV

I SEC

Fig. 2. Same preparation as in Fig. 1 except for use of cerebellar stimulation with pulse duration of 2.0 msec. Note suppression of slow wave and spike activity even with train duration of 0.1 sec (a).

duration of 0.1 sec results in a clear suppression of EEG activity when applied with a pulse width of 2 msec (rather than 1 msec as in Fig. 1a), the other parameters remaining the same as in Fig. 1. Similarly, the durations of suppression in Figures 2b and c are slightly longer than those in Figures 1b and c.

In animals anesthetized with pentobarbital, the background EEG pattern consisted of large amplitude slow waves with some low-voltage fast activity. Cerebellar stimulation converted this pattern into one of low-voltage fast activity exclusively (Fig. 3). The most remarkable effect appeared in the anterior cerebral leads contralateral to the side of cerebellar stimulation. Thus, stimulation of the right paramedian lobule influenced maximally the EEG activity recorded from the left frontal cerebral cortex. Similar focal effects were observed in the animals anesthetized with chloralose, but these effects were not as clear as in those anesthetized with pentobarbital. The effects of cerebellar stimulation upon EEG activity were completely abolished by undercutting the paramedian lobule to ascertain that the effects were mediated by the cerebellum and did not result from current spread into the brainstem.

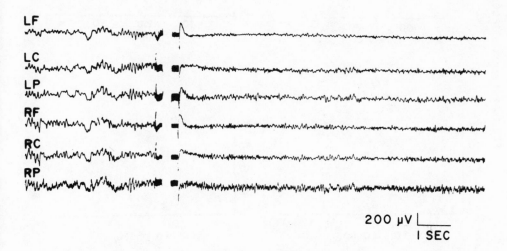

LF

LC

LP

RF

RC

RP

200 µV |____

I SEC

Fig. 3. Effects of stimulating the right paramedian lobule of cerebellum on EEG activity in a cat anesthetized lightly with pentobarbital. Stimulation parameters: pulse duration 2.0 msec; frequency 200 Hz; current 3 mA; train duration 10 sec. EEG montage: F = frontal; C = central; P = posterior; L = left; R = right. Note the suppression of the slow wave activity.

There was a clearcut relationship between the parameters of cerebellar stimulation and the duration of EEG suppression in animals anesthetized with pentobarbital (Fig. 4). Sigmoid curves were obtained for stimulus frequency, train duration, and probably also pulse duration. The inflection points were around 90 Hz for frequency, 2.5 sec for train duration, and 1 msec for pulse duration. However, it should be emphasized that 1) smaller values also resulted in some suppression; and 2) increasing these parameters above the optimal values did not prolong suppression appreciably. However, increasing the stimulation current appeared to increase the duration of EEG suppression in a roughly linear fashion (Fig. 4).

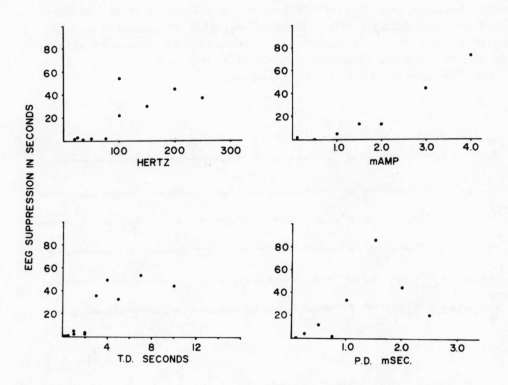

Fig. 4. Effects of varying cerebellar stimulation parameters on duration of EEG suppression in the cat under light pentobarbital anesthesia. Standard parameters are: pulse duration = 2.0 msec; frequency = 200 Hz; current = 3.0 mA; train duration = 10 sec. As one parameter was varied at random, the others were kept constant at the standard values.

Effect of Cerebellar Stimulation on Seizure After-Discharge Evoked by Cerebral Cortical Stimulation

As mentioned in the Methods section, variations in the duration of after-discharge evoked by cerebral cortical stimulation were sufficient to require a protocol of control (i.e., cerebral cortical stimulation alone)-- experimental (i.e., cerebral cortical plus cerebellar cortical stimulation)-- control. It proved possible to shorten appreciably the duration of after-

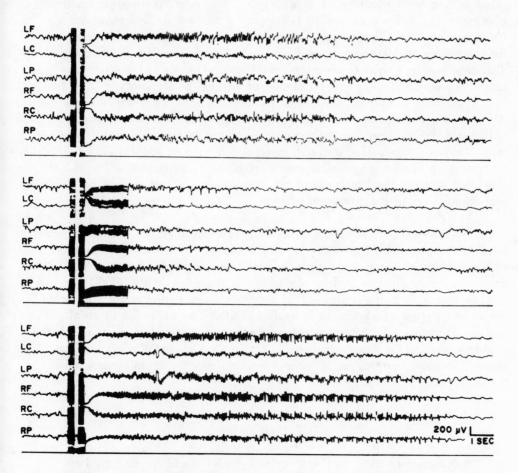

Fig. 5. Shortening of after-discharge by cerebellar stimulation in a cat under light nembutal anesthesia. Upward deflection of stimulus marker indicates left supra-sylvian cortex stimulation; downward deflection indic- ates stimulation of the right paramedian lobule. Stimulation parameter values for supra-sylvian cortex: 2.0 msec pulse duration, 50 Hz, 4 sec train duration, 2 mA current; cerebellum: 1 msec pulse duration, 100 Hz, 4 sec train duration, 2 mA stimulus current. Abbreviations same as Fig.3.

discharge in animals anesthetized lightly with pentobarbital but not in animals anesthetized with chloralose. An example of one experiment showing marked shortening of after-discharge by cerebellar stimulation appears in Figure 5. In these experiments, it was possible to apply the stimulus to cerebellum prior to the onset of cerebral cortical stimulation, during the application of cerebral stimulation, or after the offset of cerebral stimulation, and to shorten the after-discharge to essentially the same degree. In most of the experiments, cerebellar stimulation was applied with a train duration of 4 to 6 sec. The other parameters usually consisted of a pulse duration of 1-2 msec, a current of 2-5 mA, and a frequency of 100-200 Hz. We were unable to study optimal parameters for shortening of after-discharge because of the variability of the after-discharge within single experiments, a tendency for the after-discharge to shorten progressively in the absence of cerebellar stimulation, and the highly variable effects of cerebellar stimulation upon after-discharge. Although we never observed a prolongation of after-discharge from cerebellar stimulation, the shortening effect was highly variable and inconsistent. Indeed, cerebellar stimulation produced marked suppression of EEG activity in a number of animals anesthetized with pentobarbital or chloralose, but had no consistent effect on the after-discharge evoked by cerebral stimulation in the same experiments.

An incidental finding observed in 3 cats anesthetized with pentobarbital is illustrated in Figure 6. In the upper set of records, stimulation of the post-cruciate cortex results in prolonged cortical after-discharge and, simultaneously, an arrhythmia which is recorded in the EKG lead (bottom trace). In the lower set of records, the arrhythmia fails to occur during the period of cerebellar stimulation after the offset of cerebral cortical stimulation. After cessation of cerebellar stimulation, the arrhythmia appears, but is shorter in total duration than during the control run. There is a good correlation between the duration of after-discharge and the duration of the arrhythmia.

DISCUSSION

It is apparent that no single animal model could be expected to simulate the wide variety of naturally-occurring seizures in humans. Nevertheless, animal experimentation is vitally important in a continuing effort to improve the therapy of epileptic attacks in humans. The recent finding that chronic stimulation of cerebellum in humans with epilepsy may provide a new therapeutic tool makes further animal experimentation essential. Although it may prove necessary to determine the proper parameters of stimulation in each patient individually, experiments in animals may provide guidelines as to the most suitable ranges for the various parameters. Chronic experiments in animals are therefore vitally needed to determine the long-term effects of electrode contact and stimulation upon the

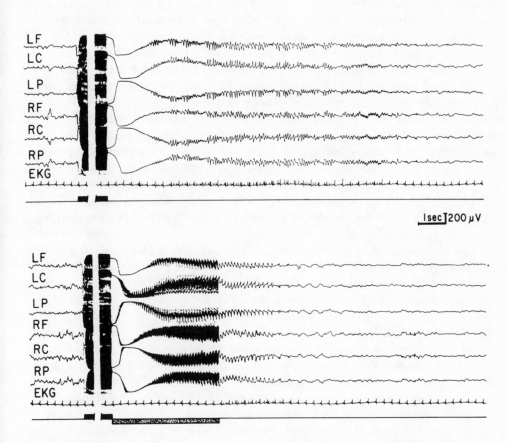

Fig. 6. Shortening of after-discharge and alteration of EKG abnormalities by cerebellar stimulation in a cat under light nembutal anesthesia. Up-ward deflection of the stimulus marker indicates stimulation of the left post-cruciate cortex; downward deflection indicates stimulation of the right paramedian lobule. Stimulation parameter values for post-cruciate cortex: 2.0 msec pulse duration, 50 Hz, 4 sec train duration, 5.0 mA current; cerebellum: 2.0 msec pulse duration, 50 Hz, 4 sec train dura-tion, 5.0 mA current. The abbreviations are the same as those in Fig.3.

morphology of the cerebellum.   In addition, it is necessary to explore
the chronic effects of cerebellar stimulation upon the biochemical and
physiological properties of the cerebellum as well as the psychological
functions of the organism as a whole.

The present study represents a pilot attempt to verify, and to place
on a firmer quantitative basis, two previously reported consequences of
cerebellar stimulation and their interrelation: first, the effect on background EEG activity, and second, the effect on electrically-evoked after-
discharges.   These experiments were designed in preparation for chronic
stimulation studies using primates, a study that is now underway.   The
most clearcut and reproducible findings in the present pilot study were
the effects of cerebellar stimulation upon EEG activity.   The findings confirmed the previous observations of Cooke and Snider (1953) that cerebellar
stimulation results in a characteristic EEG pattern of low-voltage fast
activity, here termed "suppression", and that the effect is most marked
over portions of the cerebral cortex known to have connections with the
site of cerebellum stimulated.   We found this effect in animals anesthetized with either pentobarbital or chloralose; previous investigators (Cooke
& Snider, 1953; Iwata & Snider, 1959) found essentially the same EEG
effect in unanesthetized paralyzed animals.   Our experiments demonstrated
that these EEG effects do not result from spread of the stimulating current
into the brainstem, as the effects were abolished by undercutting the region
of cerebellum stimulated.   The EEG changes were sufficiently clearcut and
reproducible to make it possible to study quantitatively the parameters of
stimulation most effective in altering the EEG pattern.   The findings of
sigmoid curves for stimulation frequency, train duration, and probably
pulse duration, indicate that there exist optimal values for each of these
parameters.   Increase above a certain value in any of these parameters
produces no greater benefit with the exception of the finding that an increase in one parameter pulse duration (cf. Figs. 1 and 2), may 'compensate' for a deficiency in another parameter (train duration).   Although we
have no evidence that the EEG suppression observed in these experiments
provides a valid working model for the human with a seizure disorder, the
findings do suggest that there may exist optimal parameters of stimulation
in humans also, and that exceeding particular values may provide no greater benefit to the patient.   Thus, it may be possible to minimize the stimulation parameters to the patients and thereby keep to a minimum any
adverse side effects as well as the power demands of the stimulation unit.

The data concerning the relationship of stimulating current to the
duration of EEG suppression were remarkably different from those obtained
from studying the other stimulation parameters.   There was an essentially

linear relationship between current and duration, suggesting that progressively larger currents recruit progressively larger populations of neurons. The present data do not permit us to comment on the site of the effect, but presumably the effects are mediated, at least in part, by Purkinje cells in cerebellar cortex. Thus, the implication of the present finding is that greater stimulus currents recruit greater numbers of Purkinje cells. However, the currents doubtless engage other elements within the cerebellar cortex, so that further experiments will be required to determine the cellular basis of this finding. The clinical implication of this finding is that stimulation current, unlike the other parameters, may provide progressively greater effects as the value is progressively increased. Thus, stimulating current may be the most important variable to regulate when attempting to determine optimal stimulation parameters in individual patients. Stimulation current is also a crucial parameter in that excessive current application has the capacity to destroy neuronal tissue. Future experiments will be required to study tissue tolerance of various current values, particularly in the chronic animal using the same electrodes as have been employed in humans.

The present experiments were successful in corroborating the finding of Cooke and Snider (1955) that cerebellar stimulation is capable of shortening the duration of after-discharge resulting from cerebral cortical stimulation. However, we found the effect to be so variable that it was not possible to study parameters properly. Our difficulties may have been due to the use of anesthetic agents in conducting these experiments. Consequently, it will be necessary to pursue these investigations further using an awake preparation, preferably a primate restrained in a chair with chronically implanted electrodes. It is worth calling attention to one finding of interest in the present studies, which was the development of a cardiac arrhythmia from cerebral cortical stimulation and its interruption by cerebellar stimulation. We found it difficult to reproduce the arrhythmia consistently, so that we were unable to study it fully. However, from the present observations it seems apparent that the cerebellar effect on the arrhythmia was due to an action at the level of the brainstem. Further experiments to pursue this finding will require production of cardiac disorders from hypothalamic stimulation, which is known to provide a reliable, reproducible model (Ban, 1966). Frequently in the present experiments we found that cerebellar stimulation altered background EEG patterns but failed to shorten after-discharge. This finding was particularly evident in chloralose-anesthetized animals, in which EEG patterns were consistently altered but after-discharge was never shortened. Thus, there is probably a good correlation between the parameters required to alter EEG activity and those to shorten seizure after-discharge, but the present experiments were not designed to answer this question.

SUMMARY

In cats anesthetized lightly with pentobarbital or alpha-chloralose, electrical stimulation of the paramedian lobule of cerebellum resulted in a change of EEG pattern. Prior to stimulation the pattern consisted of high-amplitude slow waves with superimposed low-amplitude fast activity. In addition, the EEGs of animals anesthetized with chloralose showed "chloralose spikes". Immediately following brief cerebellar stimulation the slow wave activity and spikes disappeared, leaving only low-voltage fast activity. The effect was most pronounced in the contralateral leads from the rostral portions of the cerebrum. Study of the parameters most effective in evoking this effect revealed that stimulation frequency, train duration, and probably pulse duration affected the duration of suppression in a sigmoid fashion, with inflection points at approximately 90 Hz, 2.5 sec, and 1 msec, respectively. Above threshold values, stimulation current showed an approximately linear relationship to duration of EEG suppression.

The after-discharge resulting from focal electrical stimulation of the cerebral cortex could be shortened by electrical stimulation of the paramedian lobule. The effect was essentially the same when cerebellar stimulation preceded, occurred during, or followed the cerebral cortical stimulation. The great variability of the after-discharge resulting from cerebral cortical stimulation as well as the variability of the effects of cerebellar stimulation made it impractical to study systematically the parameters optimal for shortening after-discharge. Such a study will require use of an awake, preferably partially restrained animal with electrodes chronically implanted.

ACKNOWLEDGMENTS

Supported, in part by USPHS grant NS 05184 from the National Institute of Neurological Diseases and Stroke and by grants from the Parkinson's Disease Foundation Sandoz Pharmaceuticals and the Office of the Dean, College of Physicians and Surgeons.

REFERENCES

AJMONE-MARSAN, C. Focal electrical stimulation. In Purpura, D., Penry, J., Tower, D., Woodbury, D., & Walter, R. (Eds.) "Experimental Models of Epilepsy". New York: Raven Press, 1972, pp. 147-172.

ANDERSEN, P., ECCLES, J.C., & VOORHOEVE, P.E. Postsynaptic inhibition of cerebellar Purkinje cells. J. Neurophysiol. 27:1138-1153, 1964.

BAN, T. The septo-preoptico-hypothalamic system and its automatic function. In Tokizane, T. & Schade, J.P. (Eds.) "Progress in Brain Research: Correlative Neurosciences, Part A. Fundamental Mechanisms". Amsterdam: Elsevier, 1966, pp. 1-43.

COOKE, P.M. & SNIDER, R.S. Some cerebellar effects on the electrocorticogram. Electroenceph. Clin. Neurophysiol. 5:563-569, 1953.

COOKE, P.M. & SNIDER, R.S. Some cerebellar influences on electrically-induced cerebral seizures. Epilepsia, Series III, 4:19-28,1955.

COOPER, I.S. Effect of chronic stimulation of anterior cerebellum on neurological disease. Lancet, 1:206, 1973.

COOPER, IS., AMIN, I., & GILMAN, S. The effect of chronic cerebellar stimulation upon epilepsy in man. Trans. Amer. Neurol. Assn. 98: (in press), 1973.

COOPER, I.S. & GILMAN, S. Chronic stimulation of the cerebellar cortex in the therapy of epilepsy in the human. In Fields, W.S. (Ed.) "Neural Organization and its Relevance to the Prosthetics". (In Press), 1973.

DOW, R.S., FERNÁNDEZ-GUARDIOLA, A., & MANNI, E. The influence of the cerebellum on experimental epilepsy. Electroenceph. Clin. Neurophysiol. 14:383-398, 1962.

ECCLES, J.C., ITO, M., & SZENTÁGOTHAI, J. "The Cerebellum as a Neuronal Machine". New York: Springer-Verlag, Inc., 1967.

HUTTON, J.T., FROST, J.D., & FOSTER, J. The influence of the cerebellum in cat penicillin epilepsy. Epilepsia, 13:401-408, 1972.

IWATA, M. & SNIDER, R.S. Cerebello-hippocampal influences on the electroencephalogram. Electroenceph. Clin. Neurophysiol. 11: 439-446, 1959.

LEÃO, A.A.P. Spreading Depression. In Purpura, D., Penry, J., Tower, D., Woodbury, G., & Walter, R. (Eds.) "Experimental Models of Epilepsy". New York: Raven Press, 1972, pp. 173-196.

LOEWENTHAL, M. & HORSELY, V. On the relation between the cerebellar and other centres (namely cerebral and spinal) with special reference to the action of antagonistic muscles. Proc. Roy. Soc. Med. 61:20-25, 1897.

MORUZZI, G. Sui rapporti fra cervelletto e corteccia cerebrale.
II. Azione d'impulsi cerebellari sulle attivita motrici provocate
dalla stimolazione faradica o chimica del giro sigmoideo nel gatto.
Arch. fisiol. 41:157-182, 1941a.

MORUZZI, G. Sui rapporti fra cervelletto e corteccia cerebrale.
III. Meccanismi e localizzazione delle azioni inibitrici e dinamogene del cervelletto. Arch. fisiol. 41:183-206, 1941b.

MORUZZI, G. "Problems in Cerebellar Physiology". Springfield:
Charles C. Thomas, 1950.

REIMER, G.R., GRIMM, R.J., & DOW, R.S. Effects of cerebellar
stimulation on cobalt-induced epilepsy in the cat. Electroenceph.
Clin. Neurophysiol. 23:456-462, 1967.

SHERRINGTON, C.S. Decerebrate rigidity and reflex coordination of
movements. J. Physiol. 22:319-332, 1898.

STERIADE, M. Mechanisme de facilitare si inhibitie in epilepsia
penicillinica focale corticale. Stud. Cercet. Neurol. 5:463-471,
1960.

THE EFFECT OF VARYING THE FREQUENCY OF CEREBELLAR STIMULATION UPON EPILEPSY

I. S. Cooper and R. S. Snider

St. Barnabas Hospital, Bronx, New York and

Center for Brain Research, Rochester, New York

The pioneering studies of Moruzzi (1948, see 1950 review) established the concept that frequency of electrical stimulation of the cerebellum can control the threshold effect of responses. Inhibition of postural reflex activity resulted from fast frequency (50 to 300/sec) of stimulation to the anterior lobe of the cat while slow frequency (10/sec) stimulation induced facilitation of postural tone. Nulsen, Black and Drake (1948) studying cortical induced movements in the monkey found facilitation resulting from fast frequency stimulation and inhibition of movements with slow frequencies. Snider and Magoun (1949) tried unsuccessfully to resolve the controversy by pointing to a species difference in that inhibition was the dominant result in the monkey. There was also an additional difference. Moruzzi (1948) was primarily interested in postural reflex activity while Nulsen et al. (Nulsen, Black, & Drake, 1948) were studying cerebellar effects on cortical induced movements. Terzuolo (1954) also saw reversal of cerebellar inhibition by lowering the rate of stimulation. Moruzzi and Pompeiano (1957) reported that lesions of rostral nucleus fastigii reversed the frequency of stimulation reversal effect. Iwata and Snider (1959), studying hippocampal seizures, failed to find a difference between slow and fast frequencies of cerebellar stimulation. Dow, Fernandez-Guardiola and Manni (1962) preferred fast frequencies rather than slow for alteration of cobalt induced seizures. Manzoni, Sapienza and Urbano (1968) reported that low frequency fastigial stimulation (5-15/sec) can induce electrocortical synchronization, which is occasionally accompanied by drowsiness, whereas fast stimulation (200-300/sec) can either block this or induce arousal. In a preliminary report (1973) Cooper et al. reported that slow frequency stimulation (10/sec) was more effective than fast in controlling

245

seizures in the human. The present report is a collaborative study on monkey and man to determine the efficacy of stimulation frequency.

RESULTS IN MAN

The effect of varying the frequency of stimulation of cerebellar cortex in 2 patients with epilepsy was observed during our efforts to determine the therapeutic parameters of chronic cerebellar stimulation.

The first use of chronic cerebellar stimulation in humans was for treatment of intractable spasticity. Our clinical experience confirmed Moruzzi's laboratory experience. That is, high frequency stimulation, 200 Hz, was required to lessen muscular hypertonicity. However, no worsening of spasticity was observed when low frequency stimulation, 10 Hz, was employed.

On the basis of experience with spastic patients we employed high frequency stimulation in our first patient with epilepsy. This patient, W.A., is reported in detail elsewhere in this monograph. Consequently, we will cite only the experience germane to this report.

W.A. suffered auras of epigastric sensation which he described variously as anxiety, tenseness, nausea, heat, or uneasiness. Stimulation of right anterior cerebellum at 200 cps and 10 volts repeatedly reproduced such subjective epigastric sensation which subsided promptly when stimulation ceased. On one occasion stimulation produced an epigastric aura which did not cease when the stimulation was terminated. Rather, the aura continued and within a minute was followed by a psychomotor seizure characterized by absence, eye blinking and mastication. Immediate stimulation at 10 cps and 10 volts arrested the seizure.

W.B., who suffered left sided focal seizures reported tingling in the left hand, developed staring and lip-smacking, followed by extension of the thumb, typifying his usual seizure pattern onset, when right anterior cerebellum was stimulated at 200 cps and 10 volts. These signs disappeared when the frequency of stimulation was changed to 10 cps.

Electroencephalographic evidence of seizure arrest employing low frequency stimulation in this patient (W.B.) is presented elsewhere (Cooper, Amin, Gilman, & Waltz) in this volume.

In order to determine whether a difference between slow and fast frequencies of cerebellar cortical stimulation might have different effects on experimental seizure discharge, the following series of experiments was carried out in monkey.

METHODS

Six Macaca mulatta monkeys were used in these experiments, four of which form the basis of this report. The cerebrum and cerebellum were quickly exposed under ether anesthesia. The animal was placed in a stereotaxic instrument, a tracheal cannula inserted, and the animal was given I.P. Flaxedil (10-20 mg/Kg). 1% Novocaine was carefully injected adjacent to incised areas and the animal was attached to a positive and negative pressure respirator. Four bipolar concentric recording stainless steel electrodes were placed in the ventral thalamus and surface recording electrodes were placed on cerebellar vermis and cerebral hemisphere. A bipolar side-by-side stimulating electrode was placed in nucleus fastigii and bipolar silver-silver chloride stimulating electrodes were placed on pial surface of cerebral hemisphere and cerebral vermis. Supplemental I.P. injections of Flaxedil were given when muscular twitchings appeared. Subcutaneous injections of normal saline and 5% glucose were usually given at hourly intervals. Care was taken to maintain good aeration of the animal, and to keep the body temperature between 35° and 38°C.

Seizure induction was accomplished via biphasic pial surface 40 to 60/second biphasic electrical pulses ranging between 60 and 90 volts applied to various cerebral sensory and motor areas (see legends of figures for additional details). In all cases, we attempted to limit stimulation to 5 seconds in order to obtain seizures which consistently endured for an average of 30 seconds.

Four groups of cerebellar stimulations were used: a) 8-12 per second and b) 150-300 per second biphasic pulses applied to cerebellar cortex, c) 8-12 per second, and d) 150-300 per second biphasic pulses applied to a cerebellar nucleus, usually nucleus fastigii. From 0.5 to 3.0 milliampere applied for 5 seconds were used. The usual value was 2.0 ($\pm$ 0.5) milliamperes. Higher values were commonly employed on cortical as compared with nuclear areas. Care was taken by means of control stimulations applied to nearby structures as a means to monitor for unwanted spread of current.

In all cases of depth recordings, for example, in diencephalic structures and depth stimulations in cerebellar nuclei, histological verification of electrode sites were made via Nissl stained sections.

RESULTS

A. Studies on Monkeys

In each of the EEG records shown below, the prestimulatory tracings are shown on the left. Then 5 seconds of electrical stimulation (60 to 90 volts) is applied to the pial surface in order to induce seizure activity that is consistent in wave form and duration before stopping spontaneously (CBR). A five second sample of the seizure is included and then the cerebellar cortex or nucleus (CBL or NI-NF) is stimulated for 5 seconds and the post stimulatory activity monitored in order to determine the effects of the cerebellar stimulation on the abnormal discharges. A companion series of tracings are included in order to allow comparison with EEGs which are not altered by electrical stimulation of the cerebellum. They are labeled (NO) or (O).

Figure 1 shows representative tracings taken from pial surface of temporal lobe (Temp-m) and ventral thalamic nuclei (VA, VL, VP) before, during and after seizure activity induced in cerebral hemisphere by electroshock. Series A records show electrical excitation of lobulus (LS-TV) simplex - tuber vermis with 10 pulses per second (2.0 milliamperes) stops the seizure activity within the 5 second interval. On the other hand, if the cerebellum is not stimulated (NO) the seizure continues for 29 seconds. However, if the frequency of LS-TV stimulation is increased to 200/second (2.0 milliamperes) seizure activity continues for 50 seconds.

Figure 2 records are similar to those shown in Figure 1 except the electroshock was applied to postcentral gyrus (CBR) instead of temporal gyrus and a different cerebellar area (crus II-paramedian) was stimulated. As shown in the series A control record there was 9 seconds of seizure activity which continued longer in cerebral areas than in the thalamus. However, when crus II-PM was stimulated with 200 pulses/second (2.0 milliamperes) the duration of the seizure was almost doubled (series B) whereas by using 10/second (2.0 milliamperes) stimuli and applying them as above the seizure activity was terminated within the 5 second stimulatory period (series C). From this we have concluded that slow frequency of cerebellar cortical stimulation is more effective than fast frequency in stopping seizure activity that starts in a cerebral sensory area. Furthermore, the records show that fast frequency of cerebellar stimulation can prolong the duration of the discharges.

Figure 3 EEG tracings are similar to those shown in Figure 1 and 2

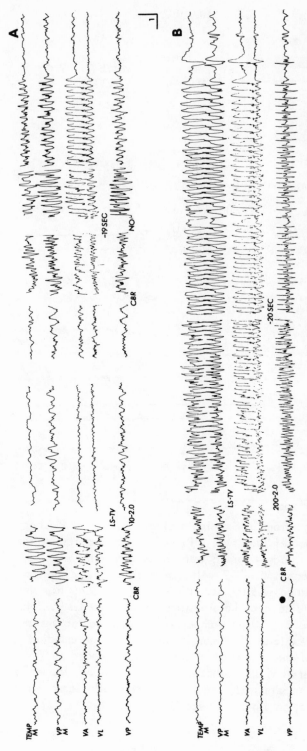

Fig. 1. EEG tracings taken from left cerebrum and ventral thalamic nucleus. Monopolar and bipolar recordings were used. The left temporal lobe was stimulated with 65 volts for 5 seconds at 60 pulses per second to induce seizure activity (CBR). Cerebellar stimulation of lobulus simplex–tuber vermis (LS–TV) with 2.0 milliamperes, 10 pulses per second for 5 seconds stopped the seizure as shown in series A. However, if cerebellum stimulation is not used the seizure activity continues for 29 seconds. Note that 19 seconds of the record has been removed. Records shown in series A should be compared with those shown in series B which were obtained after induction of seizure discharges (see above) but LS–TV stimulation was changed to 200/second (2.0 milliamperes). Other stimulation and recording conditions remain unchanged. Note that the seizure activity continued for 50 seconds. (20 seconds of the record has been removed).

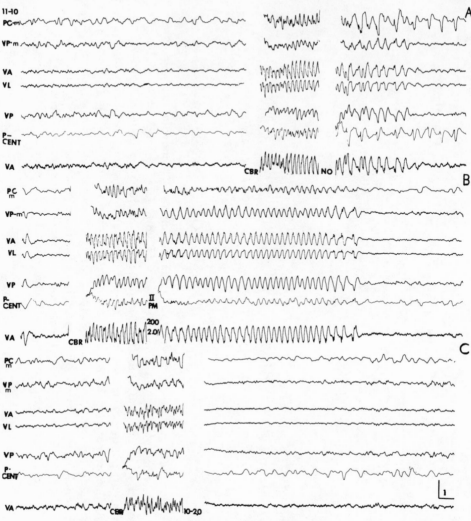

Fig. 2. EEG tracings taken from left postcentral gyrus (PC and P–Cent) and left ventral thalamic nuclei (VA, VI, VP) before, during, and after seizure stoppage. The left areas 4 and 6 were surgically removed five months previous. For 5 seconds (CBR) 7 volts (50/second) were applied to left temporal lobe to induce seizure activity which as shown in series A then continued for 9 more seconds before stopping spontaneously. However, if 200 pulses per second (2.0 milliamperes) are applied for 5 seconds to left cerebellar cortex (crus II – margin adjacent to paramedian lobule) then the duration of the abnormal discharges is extended to 7 seconds. The records in series C show that the seizure can be stopped by 10/second pulses (2.0 milliamperes) applied to same cerebellar area for 5 seconds. Horizontal calibration line = 1 second; vertical line = 0.1 millivolt.

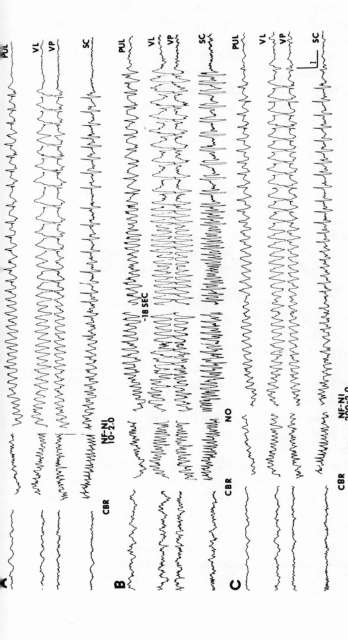

Fig. 3. EEG tracings taken from left thalamus and superior colliculus of monkey under Flaxedil medication. Bipolar recording seizure activity was induced by stimulating left temporal lobe at 50 pulses per second (70 volts) for 5 seconds (CBR). 10/second pulses at 2.0 milliamperes were applied at margin between left nucleus fastigii (NF) and (NI) nucleus interpositus. A seizure activity stopped after 20 seconds whereas in the control tracings B in which there was no cerebellar stimulation the seizure activity continued for 40 seconds. The tracings in series C show that NF-NI stimulation with 200/second pulses at 2.0 milliamperes can induce seizure stoppage within 20 seconds. In each series the preseizure, seizure and post seizure records can be compared. Note that 18 seconds of record have been removed from series B. Horizontal calibration line is one second and vertical one is 0.1 millivolt.

except the cerebellar nuclei and not the cerebellar cortex was stimulated. As shown in the control tracings in series B the seizure activity continued for 40 seconds whereas it only continues about half that interval when there is unilateral nucleus interpositus-nucleus fastigii stimulation at a frequency of 10/second for 5 seconds (2.0 milliamperes). However, as shown in series C increasing the stimulation frequency to 200/second does not increase the duration beyond that induced by the 10/second stimulation as long as the current remains the same. When the data shown in Figures 2 and 3 are compared it can be concluded that fast cortical stimulation can prolong seizure activity but this has not been found during studies with nuclear stimulation. However, it has been possible to shorten the duration of seizure discharges by electrical activation of nuclei fastigii and interpositus.

DISCUSSION

The data on the human and monkey which have been collected in this preliminary study strongly suggest that slow frequency electrical stimulation (8 to 12/second) is effective in suppressing seizure discharges whether they arise from natural causes or, in the case of the monkey, by electroshock. Furthermore, within the confines of the present study fast frequency stimulation (100-300/second) can prolong and/or worsen the abnormal discharges. Nulsen, Black and Drake (1948) in preliminary studies reported that slow frequency stimulation of the monkey anterior lobe inhibited cerebral motor activity while fast frequencies facilitated it. Manzoni, Sapienza, and Urbano (1968) observed that low frequency fastigial stimulation (5-15/sec) induced electrocortical synchronization whereas fast (200-300/sec) stimulation blocked this and often induced arousal. Snider and Mitra (1970) reported that slow frequency (10/sec) stimulation of nucleus fastigii induced long after discharges of slow frequency corresponding to the stimulation frequency, whereas 100/second stimulation induced long runs of abnormal fast discharges lasting for several seconds. Recently, Cooper et al (Cooper, Amin, Gilman, & Waltz, 1973) have reported that slow frequency stimulation of anterior cerebellar structures is more effective than fast (100-200/sec) in suppressing the clinical signs of epilepsy. On the other hand, Moruzzi (1948) and Terzuolo (1954) observed that slow stimulation frequencies facilitated reflex motor responses and Dow et al (Dow, Fernandez-Guardiola, & Manni, 1962) reported that fast rather than slow frequencies were more effective in stopping cobalt powder induced discharges in the rat. At this time it is not possible to explain these discrepancies.

Speculation may be warranted on the cerebellar mechanisms which are involved when slow stimulations are used to alter and/or stop seizures in higher centers. Eccles and associates (Eccles, Ito, & Szentagothai, 1967) have convincing evidence that cerebellar Purkinje cells exert inhibitory influences on areas of termination of the axons. Anderson, Eccles, and Voorhoeve (1964) were the first to describe a well delimited inhibition of P cells by basket (B) cells which endured approximately 100 msec. As indicated by repetitive stimuli ranging from 0.5 to 10/second P cells can recover from B cell inhibition before the next pulse but there is continued silence when faster stimuli are used. Therefore, the possibility exists that a similar mechanism is being activated during slow stimulations in the present experiments whereas fast stimulations by imposing continuous inhibition on P cells prevent the powerful inhibition of these cells from reaching extrinsic centers. However, the effect of fast stimulation of cerebellar cortex upon spasticity would seem to be contrary to this hypothesis. Although additional inhibitory roles of stellate and Golgi II cells exist which are especially prominent on the afferent volley to the P cell, the mechanisms which are involved are more obscure than is the case for the B cell. Nevertheless, the present report argues strongly for the existence of frequency modulation in the cerebellar cortex although an explanation of how this is accomplished must remain speculative.

Questions arise as to how the cerebellum becomes involved with seizures which are clearly initiated in the cerebrum. The most obvious answer is by way of the cortico-ponto-cerebellar system since this has long been accepted as a major afferent cerebellar system in all higher animals and is especially large in primates including man. Mitra and Snider (1973) have shown that it is prominently involved in cortical penicillin foci induced seizures spreading to the cerebellum. These workers by means of single unit studies have confirmed the work of Julien and Halpern (1972) which shows that the two types of paroxysmal discharges arising from the cortex produce enduring changes in rate of P cell firing which may be projected forward to higher centers.

A possible interpretation of cerebellar control of cerebral seizures arises from these observations on frequency of stimulation. For example, the 10/second stimuli applied to cerebellar cortex is sufficiently slow to allow P cells to escape from inhibition by B or S cells and G II cells and thus exercise a 10 ($\pm$2) per second burst of inhibition into the cerebellar nuclei which in turn is projected forward to diencephalic centers. This burst activity may be adequate to desynchronize the abnormal seizure frequencies. For example, Fernandez-Guardiola at this conference has shown there is burst activity in the dentate and red nucleus during seizure arrest. This would be the expected result if there was periodic escape of P cell inhibition from the influences of B and G II cells. The observations of Julien and Halpern (1972) may be relevant to the above discussion since they saw a heavy increase of P cell activity during initial stages of generalized seizure activity resulting from penicillin applied to cerebral cortex. We have observed that 10/second stimulations applied to cerebellar cortex can arrest cerebral discharges but it has not been possible to stop the seizure discharges when they have endured and become generalized. This state may be comparable to the later so called silent period of P cells which Julien and Halpern (1972) have seen.

This period has also been seen by Mitra and Snider (1973). The silence of P cells would allow the nuclear cells to continue activity and the cerebral seizure would endure. A fundamental question arises: What causes the continued P cell silence? Since it occurs after many minutes if vigorous synchronized seizure activity impinging on the cerebellum from higher centers and since there is a prominent increase of P cell activity during this period (see Julien and Halpern, 1972, and Mitra and Snider, 1973), then it might be argued that a fatigue like syndrome would result and the cerebro-cerebello-cerebral loop would continue without the inhibitory control of the P cells. Under such circumstances the seizure would continue until other mechanisms, perhaps neuronal fatigue in some yet to be designated higher center, interrupted it. Microelectrode studies on the cerebellar cortex are in progress to determine whether or not B, S and G II cells inhibition play an active or passive role in this P cell silent period. Such data are crucial if one is to answer the question: Is it pooling of inhibitory transmitter and/or fatigue which prolongs the reduced P cell firing rate?

No matter which mechanism prolongs the period of reduced P cell firing during a seizure, the prosthetic mobilization of potential P cell inhibition by chronic stimulation appears to be a rational approach to seizure arrest or prevention.

CONCLUSIONS

1. Chronic electrical stimuli applied to human cerebellum can arrest epileptiform seizures.

2. Slow frequency (10/sec) stimulations are more effective than fast (100-200/sec) in suppressing these abnormalities. Preliminary data indicate that fast frequency stimulation may be contraindicated in epilepsy,

although it has proved effective in alleviating generalized myoclonus and spasticity.

3. Experimental data from the monkey indicate that slow frequency (10/sec) stimulation to cerebellar cortex can arrest neocortical and/or hippocampal electroshock induced seizures while fast frequencies may prolong them.

4. A possible cerebellar mechanism to explain this phenomenon is presented along with data on the action of the cerebellar cortex during seizure discharges.

REFERENCES

ANDERSON, P., ECCLES, J.C., & VOORHOEVE, P.E. Postsynaptic inhibition of cerebellar Purkinje cells. J. Neurophysiol. 27:1138-1153, 1964.

COOPER, I.S., CRIGHEL, E., & AMIN, I. Clinical and physiological effects of stimulation of the paleocerebellum in humans. J. Amer. Geriatr. Soc. 21:40-43, 1973.

DOW, R.S., FERNÁNDEZ-GUARDIOLA, A., & MANNI, E. The influence of the cerebellum on experimental epilepsy. Electroenceph. Clin. Neurophysiol. 14:383-398, 1962.

ECCLES, J.C., ITO, M., & SZENTÁGOTHAI, J. "The Cerebellum as a Neuronal Machine". New York: Springer-Verlag, 1967.

IWATA, K. & SNIDER, R.S. Cerebello hippocampal influences on the electroencephalogram. Electroenceph. Clin. Neurophysiol. 11: 439-446, 1959.

JULIEN, R.M. & HALPERN, L. Effects of dipheylhydantoin and other antileptic drugs on epileptiform activity and Purkinje cell discharge rates. Epilepsia, 13:387-400, 1972.

MANZONI, T., SAPIENZA,S., & URBANO, A. EEG and behavioral sleep like effects induced by the fastigial nucleus in unrestrained, unanesthetized cats. Arch. Ital. de Biol. 106:61-73, 1968.

MITRA, J. & SNIDER, R.S. Effects of cerebral seizure activity on single unit activity in cerebellum. Fed. Proc. 32:420, 1973.

MORUZZI, G. Nuove ricerche singli effetti paleocerebellari aumentatori del tono. Ball Soc. Ital. bio. Spec. 24:753-755, 1948.

MORUZZI, G. "Problems in Cerebellar Physiology". Springfield: Charles C. Thomas, 1950.

MORUZZI, G. & POMERIANO, O. Effects of vermal stimulation after fastigial lesions. Arch. ital de biol. 95:31-55, 1957.

NULSEN, F., BLACK, S., & DRAKE, C. Inhibition and facilitation of
    motor activity by the anterior cerebellum. Fed. Proc. 7:86-87,
    1948.
SNIDER, R.S. & MAGOUN, H. Facilitation produced by cerebellar
    stimulation. J. Neurophy. 12:335-345, 1949.
SNIDER, R.S. & MITRA, J. Cerebellar influences on units in sensory
    areas of cerebral cortex. In Fields, W.S. & Willis, Jr. W.D.
    (Eds) "The Cerebellum in Health and Disease". St. Louis:
    W. H. Green, 1970, pp. 319-331.
TERZUOLO, G. Influences supraspinales sur le tetanos struchnique de la
    moelle espiniene. Arch. int. Physiol. 62:179-196, 1954.

THE EFFECTS OF CEREBELLAR STIMULATION ON THE

AVERAGED SENSORY EVOKED RESPONSES IN THE CAT

Stephen C. Boone, Blaine S. Nashold, Jr., and
William P. Wilson
Department of Surgery, Division of Neurosurgery and the
Department of Psychiatry, Duke University Medical Center,
and Department of Psychiatry, Durham Veterans Administration
Hospital, Durham, N.C.

INTRODUCTION

Although photic, auditory and somatosensory evoked responses can be recorded on the cerebellum (Snider & Stowell, 1944), and stimulations of the cerebellum can produce evoked responses in the sensory areas of the cerebral cortex (Henneman, Cooke, & Snider, 1950), it is not clearly understood what effect, if any, the cerebellum might have on the perception of sensory information at the cerebral cortical levels. Vague sensations have, however, been produced by stimulating with chronic depth electrodes in the cerebellum of awake humans (Nashold & Slaughter, 1969).

In studying the mechanisms of auditory and photic activation in epileptic rats, Dow, Fernández-Guardiola, and Manni (1962) observed that cerebellar stimulations could inhibit the cerebral photic and auditory evoked responses. Snider and Sato (1958), Snider, Sato, and Mizuno (1964), and Steriade and Stoupel (1960) have also shown that cerebellar stimulation in the cat alters the auditory evoked responses in the auditory cortex. Comparisons were made between single evoked responses to cerebellar stimulations carried out prior to, during, and after the sensory stimulus.

The use of the averaging computer in present experiments has allowed a sampling of groups of cells in the sensory cerebral cortex. The computer has provided a means of studying the effect of simultaneous

257

cerebellar stimulations on a series of repetitive sensory evoked responses
in the cerebral cortex, the mesencephalic reticular formation, and the
lateral geniculate body.

Cerebellar stimulations in the cat have been observed to inhibit
the photic and somatosensory averaged evoked responses. This inhibition
can be obtained if the voltages of cerebellar stimulation are raised. Indirect evidence suggests that these inhibitory impulses arise in the fastigial
nucleus and exit from the cerebellum either via the direct fastigiobulbar
pathway or the uncinate fascicle. The photic evoked response in the
lateral geniculate body was inhibited by ipsilateral cerebellar stimulation,
thus suggesting that sensory inhibitory impulses from the cerebellum produce
their effect at a thalamic level.

MATERIALS AND METHODS

Seventeen adult female cats weighing from 2.0 to 3.5 Kg were
used in these acute experiments. The cats were anesthetized with ether,
a tracheotomy was performed and the cat was placed on constant ventilation with a Harvard Apparatus animal respirator. An intravenous catheter
was inserted and Flaxedil at 6.0 to 10.0 mg/kg was given in interval
doses to provide neuromuscular blockade. The cat was then placed in an
animal stereotactic frame after all pressure points were anesthetized with
1% xylocaine. A heating pad was placed beneath the cat to provide a
constant temperature. The scalp was anesthetized with 1% xylocaine and
then both cerebral hemispheres were exposed. Following this, the right
cerebellar hemisphere was exposed through a suboccipital craniectomy with
removal of the bony tentorium cerebelli.

Silver ball electrodes, 2 mm in diameter, were used for the cortical
recording. Stainless steel epoxylite coated electrodes with a 0.4 mm diameter were used for both stimulating and recording within the cerebellum
and the brain stem. Both monopolar and bipolar recording and stimulation
were carried out. Stimulating and recording sites in the cerebellum and
brain stem were determined using the atlas of Snider and Niemer (1961).

Photic evoked responses were produced with a photic stimulator at
an intensity setting of 8 at one flash/second, the duration of each flash
being 10 microseconds. The cat's pupils were dilated with 0.5% Mydria-
cyl and the eyelids were held open, and the cornea moistened to prevent
drying. The visually evoked responses were recorded over the visual cortex with ball electrodes (Fig. 1). The exact location of the cortical
electrodes was adjusted until evoked responses with the highest voltage

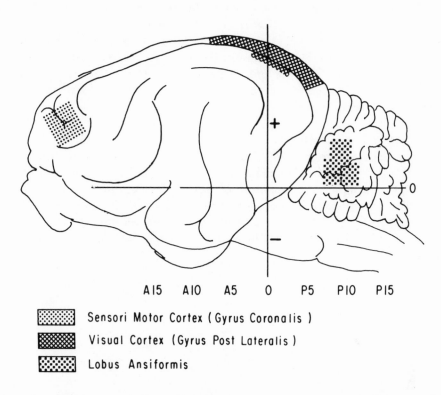

A15   A10   A5   0   P5   P10   P15

▓▓▓▓ Sensori Motor Cortex (Gyrus Coronalis)

▓▓▓▓ Visual Cortex (Gyrus Post Lateralis)

▓▓▓▓ Lobus Ansiformis

Fig. 1. Locations of Sensory Evoked Responses and Cerebellar Stimulation: The somatosensory evoked responses produced by shocks to the
sciatic nerve were recorded in the gyrus cornoalis.   The photic evoked
responses were recorded in the gyrus posterior lateralis.   Cerebellar
stimulation, both cortical and dentate nucleus, was carried out at 8.5
mm behind the stereotaxic zero point (Snider & Niemer, 1961) in the
region of the lobus ansiformis.

were obtained.   Responses evoked by photic stimulation were also recorded
with the stainless steel electrodes in the mesencephalic reticular formation
and the lateral geniculate body.

Cortical somatosensory responses (Fig. 2) were evoked by bipolar
stimulation of the exposed intact sciatic nerve.   The responses evoked
in this manner were also recorded from the mesencephalic reticular
formation.

We used the following coordinates in our experiments. In Fig. 1 the perpendicular lines cross at the stereotaxic zero point as used in the stereotaxic atlas of Snider and Niemer (1961). Coordinates for the cerebellar dentate nucleus were posterior 8.5 mm, lateral 6.0 mm and depth of -1.0 mm. Coordinates for the mesencephalic reticular nucleus were: anterior 4.0 mm, lateral 2.5 mm and depth of -1.0 mm. Coordinates of the lateral genicular nucleus were: anterior 6.5 mm, lateral 11.0 mm and depth of +5.0 mm.

All electrical stimulations were made by a Grass S8 stimulator. The evoked responses were amplified using Grass P5 preamplifiers, recorded on a FR1300 Ampex tape recorder and averaged on a Nuclear Chicago 7100 averaging computer. An average of 50 to 100 evoked responses were displayed on a storage oscilloscope (Tektronic RM564). The average of the evoked responses was then printed out on an X-Y plotter (Nuclear Chicago 7590ARS). A schematic illustration of the recording arrangements is shown in Figure 2.

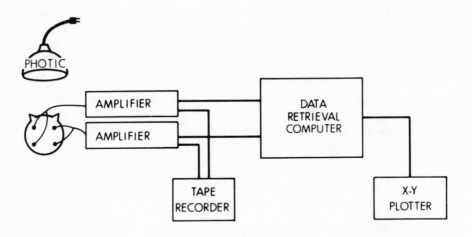

Fig. 2.   Schematic Representation of the Averaged Evoked Response Recording Design: Amplifiers (Grass Instrument Company, P511 preamplifiers), FM tape recorder (Ampex FR1300), Data retrieval computer (Nuclear Chicago 7100), and X-Y plotter (Nuclear Chicago 7590ARS).

The location of stimulating and recording sites were confirmed histologically by producing a small (0.5 mm. to 1.5 mm.) coagulative lesion. The brains were fixed in 10% formaldehyde and serial sections through the areas in question were made with a freezing microtome.

RESULTS

In the majority of the experiments, the right dentate nucleus was arbitratily used as a site of cerebellar stimulation. As experimentation progressed it became obvious that photic evoked responses in the visual cerebral cortex were inhibited by simultaneous cerebellar stimulation. In Figure 3, it is seen that an increase in the voltage caused progressively greater inhibition of the cortical evoked responses. At 2.0 volts complete ipsilateral inhibition was obtained while only partial contralateral inhibition of the photic response was seen. At 4.0 volts complete bilateral inhibition was observed.

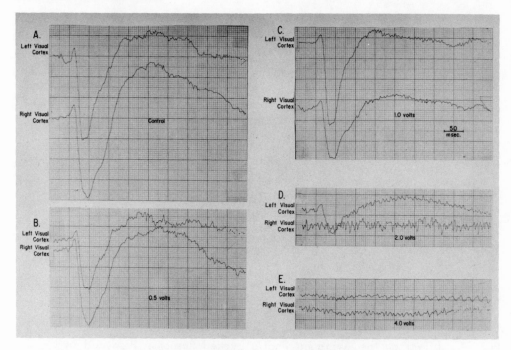

Fig. 3. Effect on the Averaged Photic Evoked Response Produced by Simultaneous Stimulation of the Cerebellum with Increasing Voltages: With the stimulus held constant at 0.5 milliseconds duration and 300 Hz, the voltage was increased from zero (control) to 1.0, 2.0, and 4.0 volts. The right dentate nucleus was the site of cerebellar stimulation.

Varying frequencies of right dentate nucleus stimulation were then tested with a constant setting of 0.5 msec duration and 2.0 volts. As the frequency of cerebellar stimulation increased, the amount of inhibition of the cortical photic evoked responses increased. Partial inhibition was seen at 60 Hz while at 300 Hz complete inhibition of the photic evoked response was noted in the ipsilateral visual cortex and partial inhibition was seen in the contralateral visual cortex.

With the voltage at a constant 2.0 volts and the frequency constant at 300 Hz, varying durations of cerebellar stimulation were then tested (Fig. 4). Again it is seen that complete inhibition of the photic evoked response is achieved at a smaller stimulus duration on the ipsilateral side than on the contralateral side. These voltage, frequency and duration curves all suggest that ipsilateral inhibition of the cerebral photic evoked response by cerebellar stimulation is more specific than the contralateral inhibition since higher values are always needed for contralateral inhibition.

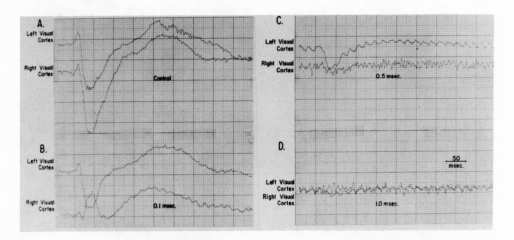

Fig. 4. Effect on the Averaged Photic Evoked Response Produced by Simultaneous Stimulation of the Cerebellum with Increasing Stimulus Duration: With the stimulus held constant at 2.0 volts and 300 Hz the stimulus duration was increased from zero (control) to 0.1, 0.5 and 1.0 millisecond duration. The right dentate nucleus was the site of cerebellar stimulation.

The above voltage, frequency and duration experiments were all performed using monopolar stimulation with the indifferent electrode in the
nasion. The same results were obtained with bipolar stimulation except
that the voltage required for complete ipsilateral inhibition varied from
6.0 to 10.0 volts. It was noted that at low frequency cerebellar stimulation, no facial or lingual movements occurred during times when it was
obvious that the Flaxedil was wearing off, suggesting that there was no
significant spread of nonspecific electrical stimulation to the brain stem.

Evoked responses in the sensorimotor cortex were obtained by contralateral sciatic nerve stimulation. In Figure 5 it is demonstrated that
the evoked response in the left sensorimotor cortex produced by right
sciatic nerve stimulation is easily inhibited by ipsilateral (left) cerebellar
stimulation.

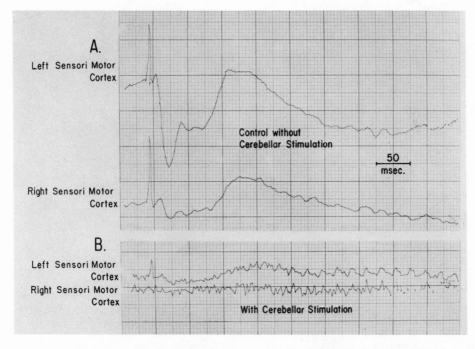

Fig. 5. Effect on the Averaged Somatosensory Evoked Response Produced
by Simultaneous Cerebellar Stimulation: The evoked responses were produced by right sciatic nerve stimulation 7.5 volts, 1 Hz., 1.0 msec
duration. A. The control evoked responses were recorded from the sensorimotor cortex bilaterally. B. The evoked response seen in the left
sensorimotor cortex was completely inhibited by simultaneous monopolar
left dentate stimulation at 2.0 volts, 300 Hz., 0.5 msec duration.

Although cerebellar stimulation inhibits both photic and somatosensory evoked cortical responses, the photic and somatosensory evoked responses in the medial mesencephalic reticular formation are not affected by dentate nucleus stimulation (Figs. 6 & 7). It would appear from these observations that cerebellar stimulation does not affect the mesencephalic reticular formation. It is also shown in Figures 6 and 7 that the sensory evoked response is recorded from the cortex approximately 10 msec prior to that recorded from the mesencephalic reticular formation.

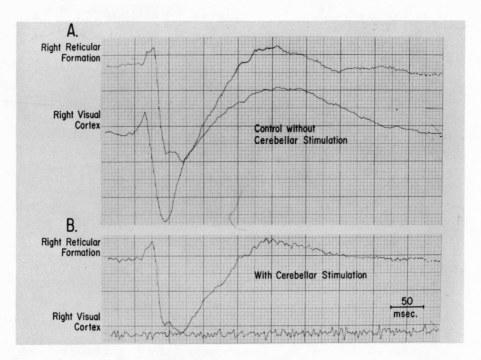

Fig. 6. Effect of Simultaneous Cerebellar Stimulation on the Averaged Photic Evoked Response in the Right Visual Cortex and Right Mesencephalic Reticular Formation: A. Control. B. With monopolar right dentate nucleus stimulation 4.0 volts, 300 Hz., and 1.0 msec duration.

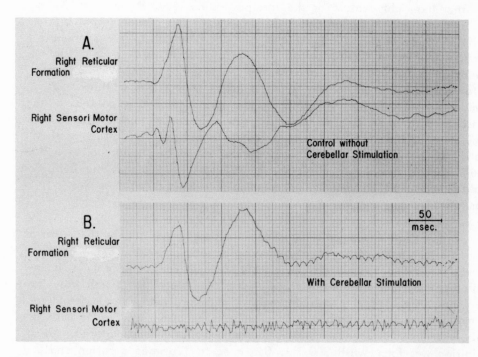

Fig. 7. Effect of Simultaneous Cerebellar Stimulation on the Averaged Somatosensory Evoked Response in the Right Sensorimotor Cortex and the Right Mesencephalic Reticular Formation. A. The control was produced by left sciatic nerve stimulation at 7.5 volts, 1.0 msec duration. B. Simultaneously with left sciatic nerve stimulation the right dentate nucleus was stimulated with a monopolar electrode at 4.0 volts, 300 Hz., and 1.0 msec duration.

In an attempt to localize the source of inhibition within the cerebellum, all deep nuclei and the cerebellar cortex overlying the dentate nucleus were stimulated and their effects on the photic evoked responses measured. The photic evoked responses in the visual cortex were inhibited by simultaneous stimulation of each of the three cerebellar nuclei. Stimulating with a monopolar electrode at 300 Hz, 0.5 msec and 3 volts in either the right dentate or the interpositus nucleus, it was possible to inhibit completely the photic evoked response in the visual cortex bilaterally. When the right fastigial nucleus was stimulated, it was possible to achieve bilateral inhibition of the photic evoked response at a slightly lower voltage of 2.5 volts, at 300 Hz, 0.5 msec duration. When the cortex of the lobus ansiformis, 7.0 mm laterally from the midline, was stimulated only a partial inhibition of the photic evoked response was obtained at 300 Hz, 0.5 msec and 3.0 volts. Thus, it appears that the stimulation of the deep nuclei produced more complete inhibition of the photic evoked response than did stimulation of the cerebellar cortex. Although the difference was minimal, it was also observed that the inhibition could be produced at lower voltages when the fastigial nucleus was stimulated.

Stimulation and ablation studies were done to determine the route of the inhibitory pathway to the mesencephalic reticular formation. Stimulation of the mesencephalic reticular formation was less consistent in its inhibitory effect than cerebellar stimulation. Ipsilateral inhibition was, however, predominent. The same frequency, duration, and voltage found to be most inhibitory in cerebellar stimulation were also found to be most inhibitory when the mesencephalic reticular formation was stimulated. Peak inhibition was found with 300 Hz, 0.5 msec to 1.0 msec duration and 5 to 8 volts of bipolar stimulation. These results suggest that an inhibitory pathway passes from the cerebellum near the mesencephalic reticular formation. Unilateral mesencephalic reticular ablation did not prevent the cerebellar stimulation from inhibiting the photic evoked responses but bilateral reticular lesions did prevent the cerebellar inhibitory effect.

The effects of pentobarbital on the inhibitory mechanism was also studied since barbiturates inhibit multisynaptic pathways and in particular the ascending reticular formation (King, Naquet, & Magoun, 1957). Intravenous sodium pentobarbital (30 mg/kg) completely prevented cerebellar inhibition of the photic evoked response both in the visual cortex and in the lateral geniculate body.

In an effort to determine where in the optic pathways cerebellar stimulation exerted its inhibitory effect, the photic evoked response in the lateral geniculate body to cerebellar stimulation was studied. Right dentate nucleus stimulation inhibited the photic response in the right lateral geniculate body but not in the left lateral geniculate body.   Figure 8 illustrates the photic evoked responses in the right lateral geniculate body and right visual cortex.   Stimulation of the right dentate nucleus

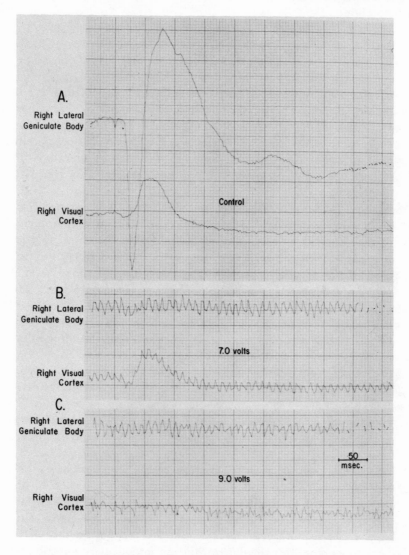

Fig. 8.   Effect of Simultaneous Cerebellar Stimulation on the Averaged Photic Evoked Response in the Right Lateral Geniculate Body and the Right visual Cortex.   A. Control without cerebellar stimulation.   B. Simultaneous bipolar right dentate nucleus stimulation at 7.0 volts, 300 Hz, and 1.0 msec duration.   C. Simultaneous bipolar right dentate stimulation at 9.0 volts, 300 Hz, 1.0 msec duration.

at 7 volts produced complete inhibition of the photic evoked response in the right lateral geniculate body but only partial inhibition was seen in the right visual cortex. Stimulation using 9 volts totally inhibited the photic evoked response in both the right lateral geniculate body and the right visual cortex.

DISCUSSION

Moruzzi (1950) has shown that the rigidity in precollicular cats can be inhibited by paleocerebellar stimulation. This inhibition is primarily ipsilateral and the optimum frequency of cerebellar stimulation is 300 Hz. Similar results were also noted in this study in that inhibition of either the photic or somatosensory evoked responses was always greater with ipsilateral cerebellar stimulation and occurred maximally at 300 Hz.

Cooke and Snider (1955) stimulated the cerebellar cortex at 40 volts, 300 Hz for 5 seconds and inhibited electrically induced cerebral cortical seizures. Snider and Sato (1958) were able to inhibit 20-60 db auditory evoked responses in the cerebral cortex with a 2-15 volt stimulus to the auditory area of the cerebellar cortex. In cats, Snider, Sato, and Mizuno (1964) and Steriade and Stoupel (1960) were also able to inhibit auditory evoked responses with cerebellar stimulation at 4-15 volts using bipolar electrodes. In rats, Dow, Fernández-Guardiola, and Manni (1962) were able to inhibit cerebral cortical photic and auditory evoked responses with cerebellar stimulations of 1 to 5 volts at 200 to 400 Hz. These voltages and frequencies necessary for inhibition of seizures and photic and auditory evoked responses are very similar to results seen in the present experiments. When monopolar stimulations were used, 2 to 4 volts caused bilateral suppression of the photic evoked response while 5 to 10 volts were necessary if bipolar stimulation was used.

It has been suggested that stimulation of the cerebellum at 10 volts or more may cause a nonspecific current spread to the brain stem, thus making it impossible to determine the specificity of the cerebellar stimulation (Dow, Fernández-Guardiola, & Manni, 1962; Dow & Moruzzi, 1958). Mutani, Bergamini, and Doriguzzi (1969) suggested that if the voltages used in cerebellar stimulation did not produce movement of the muscles innervated by the brain stem nuclei, then no current spread from the cerebellum to the brain stem has occurred. During the present experiments when it was obvious that the Flaxedil was wearing off and the animal was beginning to move, cerebellar stimulation, both at high frequencies and at 1 Hz, never produced facial or lingual movements. The observation in our experiments that cerebellar stimulation does not inhibit the averaged photic response in the mesencephalic reticular formation suggests that the inhibitory effects seen at the level of the lateral geniculate body and the cerebral cortex were not the result of a nonspecific spread of current through the cerebellum into the brain stem.

The site of exit of the sensory inhibitory impulses from the cerebellum remains unknown but our experimental results suggest they may exit by fastigial pathways. The dentate and interpositus nuclei are not thought to be the origin of the inhibitory effects because their projections are predominantly contralateral instead of ipsilateral. The direct fastigiobulbar fibers, however, pass via the ipsilateral juxtarestiform body to the ipsilateral vestibulbar nuclei and bulbar reticular formation. If the fastigial nucleus was the origin of the sensory inhibitory impulses then perhaps a nucleus was the origin of the sensory inhibitory impulses then perhaps a more specific response would be expected when different areas of the cerebellum were stimulated. However, as observed sensory inhibition occurred with stimulation of all the cerebellar nuclei although the fastigial nucleus did seem slightly more sensitive.

The uncinate fascicle, after its decussation in the cerebellum, crosses the contralateral fastigial and interpositus nucleus and prior to its two pronged exit from the cerebellum lies adjacent to the dentate nucleus (Cohen, Chambers, & Sprague, 1958; Thomas, Kaufman, Sprague, & Chambers, 1956; Voogd, 1964). The efferent output from the fastigial nucleus is illustrated in Figure 9. It is possible that the uncinate fascicle was stimulated with the macroelectrodes placed in the fastigial, interpositus or dentate nucleus. The brain section in Figure 10 illustrates that the electrode in each of the cerebellar nuclei was near the dorsal surface and could have also stimulated the uncinate fascicle. Ito, Udo, and Mano (1967) have shown that the uncinate fascicle is frequently unavoidably stimulated when stimulations of the interpositus nucleus are attempted. This idea would explain the seemingly nonspecificity produced by cerebellar stimulations at different locations. Although the uncinate fascicle is a crossed tract. It is possible that it was stimulated beyond the decussation in the cerebellum. The ascending limb of the uncinate fascicle passes dorsally to the brachium conjunctivum but enters the mesencephalon adjacent to it (Voogd, 1964) and does not cross at the decussation of the brachium conjunctivum. These uncinate fibers continue ipsilaterally through mesencephalic reticular formation and terminate on a multitude of thalamic nuclei (Cohen, Chambers, & Sprague, 1958; Thomas, Kaufman, Sprague, & Chambers, 1956; Voogd, 1964). Termination of the uncinate fascicle on the lateral geniculate body has not been described in the literature. As the uncinate fascicle ascends in the midbrain approximately 25% of

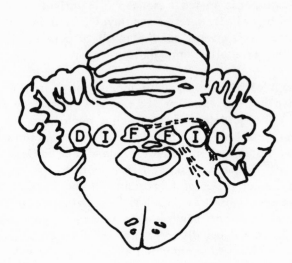

Fig. 9. Efferent Projections from the Fastigial Nucleus: The ipsilateral projection is the direct fastigiobulbar tract. The uncinate fascicle decussates within the cerebellum. Dentate (D), Interpositus (I), Fastigial (F) nuclei.

the fibers have been observed to cross to the opposite side via the peri-aqueductal gray and the posterior commisure (Cohen, Chambers, & Sprague 1958; Voogd, 1964). This could explain why certain cerebellar stimulations cause a partial contralateral inhibition of sensory evoked responses.

At what level in the CNS do cerebellar impulses inhibit the photic and somatosensory impulses? Our results suggest that the inhibition occurs at a thalamic level and it would appear that none occurs at the level of the reticular formation since results in Figures 6 and 7 show that while the photic and somatosensory averaged responses are completely inhibited at the cortical level, they are not affected at the mesencephalic reticular formation level. The cerebellar inhibitory effect is also noted at the level of the lateral geniculate body. Snider, Sato, and Mizuno (1964) have observed that cerebellar stimulation inhibits the auditory evoked responses in the medial geniculate body. Snider, Sato, & Mizuno (1964) have observed that cerebellar stimulation inhibits the auditory evoked response in the medial geniculate body.

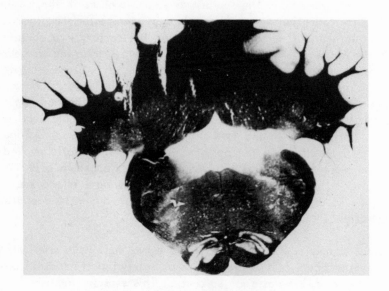

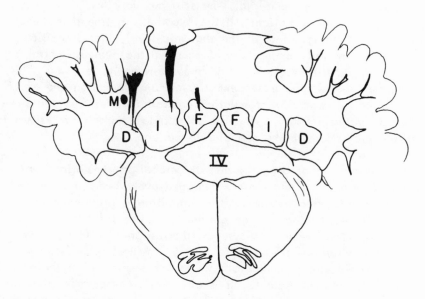

Fig. 10. Location of the Cerebellar Nuclear Electrodes: A. Myelin stained section showing the electrode tracts to each cerebellar nucleus. B. Tracing of the section in A further illustrating the electrode tracts into each nuclear area. Dentate (D), Interpositus (I), and Fastigial (F) nuclei, and Right Marker (M).

As previously observed, the sensory evoked responses in the mesencephalic reticular formation were not blocked by cerebellar stimulation. In control studies without cerebellar stimulation the sensory evoked response in the mesencephalic reticular formation always followed the evoked response at the cortical level by at least 10 msec. It is proposed that the sensory evoked response recorded at the mesencephalic reticular formation and the cerebral cortex arrive there by completely different pathways. The photic evoked response recorded on the visual cortex is believed to travel via the optic tracts to the lateral geniculate body, synapse, and then project to the cortex via the optic radiations. The photic evoked response in the mesencephalic reticular formation is thought to exit the optic tracts rostral to the lateral geniculate body, synapse in the pretectal area, the superior colliculus and eventually in the mesencephalic reticular formation.

Electrical shocks applied to the sciatic nerve must have stimulated all of the afferent fibers. It is proposed that cerebellar stimulation blocks the sensory input from the posterior columns. This sensory pathway passes through the brain stem as the medial lemniscus has very few, if any, synapses with the reticular formation. If the hypothesis is true that the cerebellum has its inhibitory effect at the thalamic level, then inhibition of the somatosensory evoked response should occur in the nucleus ventral posterior lateralis. Experiments to test this hypothesis are under way. The evoked responses seen in the mesencephalic reticular formation and which are not inhibited by cerebellar stimulation are felt to arise from the slower conducting spinothalamic pathways. The spinothalamic tracts are known to have multiple projections to the reticular formation.

In conclusion, it has been shown that cerebellar stimulation can suppress both photic and somatosensory averaged evoked responses at their respective cerebral cortical regions. This inhibition is preferentially ipsilateral but by increasing the voltage of the cerebellar stimulation, bilateral inhibition occurs. Mainly because of the ipsilateral effects, it is thought that the inhibitory effects arise from the contralateral fastigial nucleus, but are stimulated ipsilaterally in the cerebellum after their decussation as the uncinate fascicle. It is also possible, however, that the fastigial nucleus itself is being stimulated ipsilaterally and the inhibitory impulses exit the cerebellum through the direct fastigiobulbar pathway in ipsilateral juxtarestiform body. After reaching the ipsilateral brain stem the sensory inhibitory impulses are felt to travel in a multisynaptic pathway near the reticular formation to the thalamus. The photic evoked responses can be inhibited at the lateral geniculate body. Voogd (1964) has observed that the ascending limb of the uncinate fascicle has many endings in the reticular and intralaminar nuclei of the thalamus. It is thus speculated that these thalamic intralaminar and reticular nuclei project to the lateral geniculate body, the medial geniculate body and the nucleus ventralis posterior lateralis to modulate the visual, auditory, and somatosensory perception respectively.

SUMMARY

Cerebellar stimulation has been observed to inhibit cortical responses to both photic and somatosensory stimuli. Peak inhibition is obtained when the cerebellum is stimulated at 300 Hz. The sensory evoked responses are inhibited bilaterally with unilateral cerebellar stimulation but ipsilateral inhibition is clearly predominant. It is suggested that the cerebellar inhibitory impulses arise in the contralateral fastigial nucleus and enter the brain stem via the uncinate fascicle which decussates within the cerebellum prior to its exit. Following its decussation the uncinate fascicle passes adjacent to the fastigial, interpositus and dentate nuclei before leaving the cerebellum adjacent to the brachium conjunctivum. Since sensory inhibitory impulses were obtained from all three cerebellar nuclei, it is proposed that the uncinate fascicle was unavoidably stimulated at each nuclear area. The inhibitory impulses seem to travel ipsilaterally adjacent to the mesencephalic reticular formation to the thalamus. Experimentally it was observed that the photic evoked responses in the lateral geniculate body were inhibited by ipsilateral cerebellar stimulation, thus suggesting that the inhibition of sensory evoked responses may occur at a thalamic level. The data from the present experiments suggest that the cerebellum may play a role in sensory perception. Thus, it would appear that the cerebellum may be a central coordinator of both motor and sensory functions.

ACKNOWLEDGMENTS

Cooperation and assistance from Talmade L. Peele, M.D., Mr. Victor Hope and Mrs. Carolyn Barbee is acknowledged.

REFERENCES

COHEN, D., CHAMBERS, W.D., & SPRAGUE, J.M. Experimental study of the efferent projections from the cerebellar nuclei to the brain stem of the cat. J. Comp. Neurol. 109:233-259, 1958.

COOKE, P.M. & SNIDER, R.S. Some cerebellar influences on elec-
    trically induced cerebral seizures. Epilepsia, 4:19–28, 1955,
DOW, R.S., FERNANDEZ-GUARDIOLA, A., & MANNI, E. The
    influence of the cerebellum on experimental epilepsy. Electro-
    enceph. Clin. Neurophysiol. 14:383–398, 1962.
DOW, R.S. & MORUZZI, G. "The Physiology and Pathology of the
    Cerebellum". Minneapolis: University of Minnesota Press, 1958.
HENNEMAN, E., COOKE, P.M., & SNIDER, R.S. Cerebellar pro-
    jections to the cerebral cortex. Res. Publ. Assoc. Nerv. Ment.
    Dis. 30:317–333, 1950.
ITO, M., UDO, M., & MANO, S. In Eccles, J.C., Ito, M., &
    Szentigothai, J. (Eds.) "The Cerebellum as a Neuronal Machine".
    New York: Springer-Verlag, 1967.
KING, E.E., NAQUET, R., & MAGOUN, H.W. Alterations in
    somatic afferent transmission through the thalamus by central mech-
    anisms and barbiturates. J. Pharm. Exp. Therap. 119:48–63, 1957.
McDONALD, J.V. & OKAWARA, S. The effect of frequency changes
    and responses to electrical stimulation of the cerebellum in the
    unanesthetized cat. J. Nerv. Ment. Dis. 147:65–69, 1968.
MORUZZI, G. "Problems in Cerebellar Physiology". Springfield:
    Charles C. Thomas, 1950.
MUTANI, R., BERGAMINI, L., & DORIGUZZI, T. Experimental
    evidence for the existence of an extrarhinencephalic control of
    the activity of the cobalt rhinencephalic epileptogenic focus.
    Epilepsia, 10:351–362, 1969.
NASHOLD, B.S. & SLAUGHTER, D.G. Effects of stimulating or de-
    stroying the deep cerebellar regions in man. J. Neurosurg: 31:
    172–186, 1969.
SNIDER, R.S. & STOWELL, A. Receiving areas of the tactile, audit-
    ory, and visual systems in the cerebellum. J. Neurophysiol. 7:
    331–357, 1944.
SNIDER, R.S. & SATO, K. Some cerebellar influences on evoked
    cerebral auditory response. Fed. Proc. 17:152, 1958. Abstract.
SNIDER, R.S. & NIEMER, W.T. "A Stereotactic Atlas of the Cat
    Brain". Chicago: The University of Chicago Press, 1961.
SNIDER, R.S., SATO, I., & MIZUNO, S. Cerebellar influences on
    evoked cerebral responses. J. Neurol. Scien. 1:325–339, 1964.
STERIADE, M. & STOUPEL, N. Contribution a l'etude des relations
    entire l'aire auditive du cervelet et l'ecarce cerebral chez le
    chat. Electroenceph. Clin. Neurophysiol. 12:119–136, 1960.

THOMAS, D.M., KAUFMAN, R.P., SPRAGUE, J.M., & CHAMBERS, W.W. Experimental studies of the vermal cerebellar projections in the brainstem of the cat (fastigiobulbar tract). J. Anat. 90: 371-385, 1956.

VOOGD, J. "The Cerebellum of the Cat". Philadelphia: F.A. Davis Co., 1964, pp. 130-201.

THE EFFECT OF CEREBELLAR LESIONS ON EMOTIONAL
BEHAVIOR IN THE RHESUS MONKEY

A. J. Berman, D. Berman, and J. W. Prescott
Neurosurgical Research Unit, Department of Surgery, Jewish
Hospital and Medical Center of Brooklyn, Brooklyn, New
York; Department of Neurosurgery, Mt. Sinai School of
Medicine, New York, New York; Department of Psychology,
Queens College of the City University of New York, Flushing,
New York; and National Institute of Child Health and Human
Development, National Institute of Health, Bethesda, Mary-
land, respectively

Although the relationship between limbic system structures and emotionality is well known, the role of the cerebellum in the control of affective behavior is not usually appreciated (Berman, 1970a, b; 1971).
Involvement of the limbic system in the elaboration of emotional behavior
has been demonstrated by studies such as those of Kluver and Bucy (1939),
Pribram and Bagshaw (1953) and Weiskrantz (1956), in which a taming
effect was reported following amygdaloidectomy in the monkey. Reduced
emotionality in the monkey has also been reported following cingulectomy
(Glees, Cole, Whitty, & Cairns, 1950) and postero-medial orbital frontal
cortex ablations (Butter, Snyder, & McDonald, 1970).

Cerebellar participation in affective behavior has been indicated
through the demonstration of functional connections between cerebellar
and limbic structures. Anand, Malhotra, Singh, and Dua (1959), working
with dogs, showed that stimulation of posterior paleocerebellar structures,
including the flocculonodular lobe, evoked potentials in all limbic regions
from which recordings were taken. Stimulation of anterior paleocerebellum
evoked potentials mainly in orbital cortex, hippocampus and posterior hypothalamus. Heath (1972a), using evoked potential and mirror focus techniques, demonstrated numerous interconnections between cerebellar nuclei
and limbic system structures, including direct back and forth connections
between the fastigial nuclei and the septal region and hippocampus.

Clark (1939) was the first to show that electrical stimulation of the cerebellum in the unanaesthetized cat produced a cringe-like response with a kneading of the claws in a pleasure-like reaction occurring on occasion as a rebound effect. In addition, he noted what appeared to be a hypersensitivity to touch. Chambers (1947) found that stimulation of the midline vermis and fastigial nuclei resulted in hypersensitivity to sound and touch and in attempted escape. Chambers and Sprague (1955) and Sprague and Chambers (1959) reported that cerebellar ablations resulted in persistent pleasure reactions, as demonstrated by constant purring and kneading of the claws, while lesions of the fastigial nucleus resulted in lethargy. Peters (1969) and Peters and Monjan (1971) not only confirmed this work but also reported that squirrel monkeys which showed aggressive cage behavior before surgery became tame and tractable following lesions of the vermis.

One of the best established etiologies of aggression in the monkey is a lack of social interaction during development (Harlow & Harlow, 1962). Monkeys that are raised in individual cages, with visual and auditory contact but no bodily contact with each other, develop a number of bizarre behaviors. They indulge in a great deal of head or body rocking, sucking of body parts, and self-clutching. They are timorous of human approaches and, when placed with their peers, do not indulge in the usual social interactions of young primates. If such infants are maintained in partial isolation, then as adults they manifest violent aggressive behaviors directed at themselves and others.

Mason (1968) demonstrated that much of the abnormal behavior of partially isolated infant monkeys could be prevented by providing them with mobile rather than stationary surrogate mothers. Based on this finding, Prescott (1971) suggested that somatosensory and vestibular stimulation provided by the moving surrogate prevented the development of the abnormal behavior patterns. This interpretation parallels that of many human studies in which it has been suggested that children with autistic behaviors have suffered a lack of proprioceptive, labyrinthine, kinesthetic and tactile stimulation (Fraiberg & Freedman, 1964; Freedman, 1968; Klein, 1962). It is supported by the finding of Heath (1972b) that isolation-reared adult monkeys show electroencephalographic abnormalities in cerebellar nuclei concerned with these sensory inputs, as well as limbic structures.

Given this evidence linking lack of proprioceptive, tactile and vestibular input to the occurrence of so-called isolation behaviors in infant monkeys, and considering the abnormal discharge of relevant cerebellar nuclei in adult isolation-reared animals, we undertook to investigate the effects, if any, of various cerebellar lesions on the emotional behavior of the monkey. Some attempt was made to evaluate the effects of cerebellar lesions on the social interactions of juvenile M. rhesus, but our major attention was focused on the effects of such ablations on indices of aggression in adult male rhesus monkeys.

We received from Hazeltine Laboratories six juvenile monkeys, approximately eight months of age, which had been raised in partial social isolation and demonstrated the emotional and behavioral disorders consequent to such rearing. These animals were placed in a large observation chamber for a one hour period each month in order to observe their social interaction. Three walls and the ceiling of this enclosure were composed of cyclone fencing, to facilitate climbing, while one wall was of clear plastic for ease of monitoring and photographing group behavior. On each occasion, the six animals arranged themselves within the chamber so that little or no body contact occurred. Any that did occur appeared to be accidental and was not followed by any further interchange. In the main, each huddled or sat or rocked as though alone in the cage.

The adult animals used in this study were six highly aggressive ferally-reared male rhesus (Bishop, Love, Shiff, Diddle, Throck, and Anesthesia) that had been in our laboratory for several years and had been dropped from other experiments because of their aggressiveness toward laboratory personnel, who were unable to handle them. In addition, two violent, isolation-reared adult male rhesus (Ding and Dong) were contributed by Dr. Gary Mitchell. In studying these mature animals, we used the method of direct confrontation. This entailed placing two monkeys at a time in the observation cage, while recording their encounter on film for subsequent analysis. This technique resulted in a social response obviously synonymous with the complex of behaviors known as aggression, although several drawbacks to its use were recognized. These included a lack of behavioral control, risk to the animals and the impossibility of replication. Despite these limitations the method proved most rewarding. In each case, when two of these adult animals were placed in the observation chamber, violent fighting ensued and there was great difficulty in separating the animals. This response occurred even after several pairings of the same animals.

After the initial observations had been made, surgery was performed under endotracheal anesthesia with subjects in the sitting position. A suboccipital approach was used and a dural flap turned, exposing the posterior fossa. At this time Mannitol (2 mg. per kg. of body weight) was administered intravenously, resulting in marked shrinking of the brain, which allowed visualization of the anterior lobe of the cerebellum. It

was possible, in fact, with slight gentle retraction on the superior surface
of the cerebellum, to visualize the pineal gland and the superior quadri-
geminal body. The superficial cerebellar surface was then coagulated,
after which approximately 2-3 mm. of cortex was removed by suction.
Care was taken to avoid direct damage to the deep cerebellar nuclei.
Surgery was performed under 6X and 10X magnification with constant monitoring of vital signs. Drawings of the lesions were made before closure.

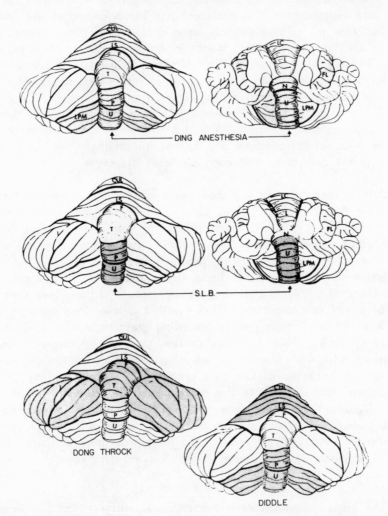

Fig. 1. Drawings of cerebellar lesions. Abbreviations: CUL=culmen;
F=folium vermis; FL=flocculus; L=lingula; LC=lobulus centralis; LPM=para-
median lobule; LS=lobulus simplex; N=nodulus; P=pyramis; T=tuber;
U=uvula.

Two of the juvenile animals (Wes and Betty) were operated at 11 months of age. In one (Wes), a lesion was made similar to that in Ding (see below) which included culmen, lobulus simplex, pyramis, paramedian lobule, uvula, and flocculonodular lobe. In the other (Betty), the lesion was similar to that in Dong (see below) and was confined to the neocerebellum. Two months after surgery, when placed in the observation chamber, these two animals began to interact. The initiation of each social contact was made by Wes, while Betty responded to his overtures. No such behavior was elicited from the remaining non-operated juveniles, who remained withdrawn and non-responsive.

A variety of lesions were made in the aggressive adult animals in an attempt to delineate cerebellar areas that might selectively alter emotional behaviors. In two cases (Ding, isolation-reared, and Anesthesia, ferally-reared), the superficial cortex of culmen, lobulus simplex, paramis, paramedian lobule, uvula and flocculonodular lobe, were removed. Two monkeys (Dong, isolation-reared, and Throck, ferrally-reared) received neocerebellar lesions and three ferally-reared animals (Bishop, Love and Shiff) had incomplete vermian lesions that included pyramis, uvula and part of nodulus. A final ferally-reared animal (Diddle) was subjected to resection of the cortex of culmen, lobulus simplex, pyramis, uvula and part of the nodulus.

Postoperatively, the two animals with the lesions which included culmen, lobulus simplex, pyramis, paramedian lobule, uvula and flocculonodular lobe demonstrated marked behavioral alteration. They became quite docile and showed no signs of aggression in the confrontation situation. They could be handled by the laboratory personnel with no difficulty. The three animals with incomplete vermian lesions continued to be as aggressive as before surgery. The animal in which the lesion was larger than in the previous three cases and included part of the anterior lobe of the cerebellum, however, became more tractable. All these animals showed a transient neurological deficit. The two monkeys with neocerebellar lesions remained as aggressive after surgery as they had been before, despite the fact that both were ataxic throughout the study period.

The difference in effect between a fairly complete midline lesion and one which was laterally placed was clearly seen in the two adult isolation-reared animals (Ding and Dong). Ding, whose lesions included culmen, lobulus simplex, pyramis, paramedian lobule, uvula and flocculonodular lobe was immediately tamed. He could be handled easily. When placed in the observation chamber with Dong (neocerebellar lesion) during the first postoperative month, little interaction between the two animals occurred. During this period, though, Dong was grossly incapacitated. His gait was extremely unsteady and there was marked ataxia, making it difficult for the animal to even feed itself. Three months after surgery, although still ataxic and unable to climb, Dong pursued Ding with fury. Ding would no longer remain on the ground once Dong entered the cage. Similarly, none of the laboratory personnel could be persuaded to enter the cage with him. Dong's neurological deficit gradually subsided, but his aggressiveness increased and has, in fact, persisted to the present time, three and one half years after surgery. Recently, another highly aggressive feral male, slightly larger and heavier than Dong, was placed in the encounter chamber with him. A violent fight ensued, from which it was difficult to extricate the animals. Although Dong emerged from this encounter a decided second best, two additional confrontations resulted in similar pugnacity.

The number of animals used in this study are too few to reach un-equivocal conclusions, but there does appear to be a differential effect on aggressive behavior between midline and neocerebellar lesions in the adult animal. The taming seen following midline cerebellar lesions was persistent and dramatic while no such effect resulted from neocerebellar lesions. The altered behavior of the two juvenile animals is difficult to interpret within the same framework, however, as a beneficial result seemed to occur in each, despite the fact that one had a vermian and the other a neocerebellar lesion. It should be noted, nevertheless, that the greater socializing effect was apparent in the animal with the midline vermian lesion.

Precise correlation of behavior with the lesions must of course await histological documentation. It is possible that the deep cerebellar nuclei might have been injured at the time of surgery, or subsequently as a re-sult of interference with blood supply. Notwithstanding these reservations, the present study suggests that vermian lesions of the cerebellum result in modification of aggressive behavior in adult rhesus monkeys and that this alteration in behavior is unrelated to any neurological deficit.

ACKNOWLEDGMENTS

Supported in part by National Science Foundation Grant GB30920.

REFERENCES

ANAND, B.K., MALHOTRA, C.L., SINGH, B., & DUA, S. Cerebellar projections to limbic system. Amer. J. Physiol. 188:451-457, 1959.

BERMAN, A.J. Somatosensory-cerebellar lesions and behavior. In (J.W. Prescott, Chairman) "Neural-behavioral ontogeny of violent-aggressive and autistic-depressive disorders". Symposium presented at Third Annual Winter Conference on Brain Research, Snowmass-at-Aspen, Colorado, January 1970.

BERMAN, A.J. Cerebellar decortication and the modification of aggressive behavior. In (A.H. Riesen, Chairman) "Maternal-social deprivation as functional somatosensory deafferentation in the abnormal development of the brain and behavior". Symposium presented at the 78th Annual Convention of the American Psychological Association, Miami, September 1970.

BERMAN, A.J. Cerebellar decortication and the modification of abnormal behavior in isolation-reared rhesus monkeys. In (J.W. Prescott, Chairman) "Neurobiological perspectives on parental, social and sensory deprivations". Harlow Memorial Symposium presented at the 79th Annual Convention of the American Psychological Association, Hawaii, September 1971.

BUTTER, C.M., SNYDER, D.R., & McDONALD, J.A. Effects of orbital frontal lesions on aversive and aggressive behaviors in rhesus monkeys. J. Comp. Physiol. Psychol. 72:132-144, 1970.

CHAMBERS, W.W. Electrical stimulation of the interior of the cerebellum in the cat. Amer. J. Anatomy, 80:55-94, 1947.

CHAMBERS, W.W. & SPRAGUE, J.M. Functional localization in the cerebellum. I. Organization in longitudinal cortico-nuclear zones and their contribution to the control of posture both extrapyramidal and pyramidal. J. Comp. Neurol. 103:105-129, 1955.

CLARK, S.L. Responses following electrical stimulation of the cerebellar cortex in the normal cat. J. Neurophysiol. 2:19-36, 1939.

FRAIBERG, S. & FREEDMAN, D. Studies in the ego development of the congenitally blind child. Psychoanalytic Study of a Child, 19:113-169, 1964.

FREEDMAN, D.A. The influence of congenital and perinatal sensory deprivations on later development. Psychonomics, 9:272-277, 1968.

GLEES, P., COLE, J., WHITTY, C.W.M., & CAIRNS, H. The effects of lesions in the cingular gyrus and adjacent areas in monkeys. J. Neurosurg. Psychiat. 13:178-190, 1950.

HARLOW, H.F. & HARLOW, M.K. The effect of rearing conditions on behavior. Bulletin of the Meninger Clinic, 26:213-224, 1962.

HEATH, R.G. Physiologic basis of emotional expression: Evoked potential and mirror focus studies in rhesus monkeys. Biol. Psychiat. 5:15-31, 1972a.

HEATH, R.G. Electroencephalographic studies in isolation-reared monkeys with behavioral impairment. Dis. Nerv. Syst. 33:157-163, 1972b.

KLEIN, G.W. Blindness and isolation. Psychoanalytic Study of the Child. 17:82-93, 1962.

KLÜVER, H. & BUCY, P.C. Preliminary analysis of functions of temporal lobes in monkeys. Arch. Neurol. Psychiat. 42:979-1000, 1939.

MASON, W.A. "Early Social Deprivation in the Non-Human Primate: Implications for Human Behavior in Environmental Influences". New York: The Rockefeller University Press and Russel Sage Foundation, 1968.

PETERS, M. A cerebellar role in behavior. Ph.D. thesis, University of Western Ontario, 1969.

PETERS, M. & MONJAN, A.A. Behavior after cerebellar lesions in cats and monkeys. Physiol. Behav. 6:205-206, 1971.

PRESCOTT, J.W. Early somatosensory deprevation as an ontogenetic process in the abnormal development of the brain and behavior. Medical Primatology, Basel: Karger, 1971.

PRIBRAM, K.H. & BAGSHAW, M. Further analysis of the temporal lobe syndrome utilizing fronto-temporal ablations. J. Comp. Neurol. 99:347-375, 1953.

SPRAGUE, J.M. & CHAMBERS, W.W. An analysis of cerebellar function in the cat as revealed by its partial and complete destruction and its interaction with cerebral cortex. Arch. Italiennes de Biologie, 97:68-88, 1959.

WARD, A.A. The cingular gyrus: Area 24. J. Neurophysiol. 11:12-23, 1948.

WEISKRANTZ, L. Behavioral changes associated with ablation of the amygdaloid complex in monkeys. J. Comp. Physiol. Psychol. 49: 381-391, 1956.

PSYCHOLOGICAL STUDIES OF CHRONIC CEREBELLAR

STIMULATION IN MAN

M. Riklan, K. Marisak and I. S. Cooper

Departments of Psychology and Neurologic Surgery
St. Barnabas Hospital
Bronx, New York

The structure, afferent and efferent pathways, and functions of the cerebellum have been the subject of numerous experimental studies in the past decades, and several reference sources, including recent textbooks, are readily available with respect to current data in this area (Dow & Moruzzi, 1958; Brookhart, 1960; Crosby, Humphrey, & Lauer, 1962; Eccles, Ito, & Szentagothai, 1967; Fox & Snider, 1967; Truex & Carpenter, 1969; Larsell & Jansen, 1972). Furthermore, other reports in the present symposium will consider such material in further detail (cf Snider, Dow, & Fernandez-Guardiola). Consequently, it is the purpose of this introduction to present only a brief summary of certain relevant factors with respect to cerebellar functions with particular implications for psychological studies.

The cerebellum is usually described as being concerned primarily with the coordination of somatic motor activity, equilibrium, and muscle tone. Afferent fibers projecting to the cerebellum originate from cell groups in the spinal cord and from specific brain stem nuclei which in turn relay impulses from the cerebral cortex, the reticular formation, and certain cranial nerves. The inputs, which eventually reach the cerebellar cortex, are supplied by tracts entering the cerebellum mainly via the inferior and middle cerebellar peduncles, and include specifically the spino-cerebellar, the cuneocerebellar, the reticulocerebellar, the olivo-cerebellar, the vestibulocerebellar, and the pontocerebellar tracts. The deep cerebellar nuclei, the dentate, emboliform, globose and fastigial, serve to integrate and convey afferent and efferent cerebellar impulses. In turn, the cerebellum is connected to the brain stem by the inferior, middle, and superior cerebellar peduncles. The afferent fibers which connect the cerebellum with the periphery convey primarily special proprioceptive impulses from the vestibular end organ and impulses from stretch receptors in muscles and tendons. In addition, exteroceptive impulses including tactile, auditory, and visual impulses also reach the cerebellum, although their tracts have not been fully delineated.

The principal efferent tracts of the cerebellum arise from the deep cerebellar nuclei. Fibers from the dentate, emboliform, and globose nuclei form the largest cerebellar efferent fiber system, the superior cerebellar peduncle. The majority of these fibers ascend to the contralateral red nucleus, the ventrolateral nucleus of the thalamus, and the cerebral cortex. In addition, some fibers of the superior cerebellar peduncle pass to the more rostral intralaminar thalamic nuclei. Other fibers descend and are distributed to parts of the vestibular nuclei and to portions of the reticular formation of the pons and medulla. Many of the structures receiving cerebellar impulses project fibers back to the cerebellum, to form a series of feedback systems. These systems include areas of the contralateral motor cortex, several thalamic nuclei, and portions of the lower brain stem reticular formation.

The variety of afferent, efferent, and feedback systems of the cerebellum, play a significant role in the coordination of somatic motor activity, the regulation of muscle tone, and mechanisms that influence and maintain equilibrium. In addition, afferent pathways convey impulses from a variety of receptors including the organs of special sense. The sensory impulses involving the cerebellum are concerned primarily with the conscious regulation of posture and equilibrium, and involve primarily the visual system and kinesthetic receptors. Investigations reviewed by Snider (1950), however, suggest that cerebellar influence is not related solely to the control of muscular coordination, but is exerted on practically all neural functions, both sensory and motor. For example, stimulation of the cerebellar "audiovisual" area (simple lobule and tuber) evokes responses in the cortical auditory area and in parts of the cortical visual area. This system of sensorimotor interactions led Snider (1950) to describe the cerebellum as the great modulator of neurologic function.

One of the most extensive recent reviews of the literature concerning a cerebellar role in sensation, and related areas, is that of Snider (1967) who assessed a series of anatomical, functional, ablation, and electrophysiological studies which demonstrate the wide influence of the cerebellum on sensory functions. He noted that Whiteside and Snider (1953) earlier had demonstrated extensive projections from the cerebellum not only to the thalamus and diencephalon, but also to a variety of thalamic nuclei. Moreover, cerebellar influences were found to be exerted on the midbrain and diencephalic reticular formation, both parts of the reticular activating system. These projections implied strongly that the cerebellum may influence sensory systems ascending to the cerebrum. Such findings substantiate the fact that the cerebellum sends sizable projections fo the ascending reticular formation and to some of the so-called sensory relay nuclei. Consequently, the cerebellum may be described as part of a generalized system going to the cerebrum to involve sensory as well as motor cortices. Furthermore, intrathalamic regulation of the cerebello-cerebral projection also exists.

Ablation studies undertaken by Chambers and Sprague (1955), who removed the tuber vermis and folium vermis, indicated that cats undergoing such surgery had difficulty in gauging distances properly and a diminution in "sensory attention". These authors also reported that responses to acoustic and visual stimuli were hypoactive following lesions of the tuber and folium while the same responses were hyperactive following lesions of the nucleus fastigii. Steriade and Stoupel (1960) proposed a dual cerebello-cerebral projection, one of which passes through the reticular formation and the other through the thalamus but not the medial geniculate nucleus. This study can also be interpreted to indicate that the cerebellum may function to help control "levels of excitability" in the ascending reticular formation.

In essence, the cerebellum has widespread ascending projections to the mesencephalic and diencephalic reticular formation, and when one considers both the ascending and descending connections of the cerebellum to the reticular formation then, with the exception of the major ascending systems it is difficult to find structures which have a more extensive input to the reticular formation (Snider, 1967). The implication is strong, according to Snider, that the cerebellum is one of the suprasegmental regulators of reticular activity. Furthermore, both a tonic and phasic influence could be exerted on the so-called "proprioceptive input" from the extremities. The tonic influence would be via the ascending reticular formation and the phasic influence via the so-called sensory relay nucleus of the thalamus. Snider concludes that it is not too early to ask about a cerebellar role in the mechanism of perception, and notes that speculations abound about a possible cerebellar role in the mechanisms of memory. With further respect to a possible role of the cerebellum in behavior, Marr (1969), in his theory of the cerebellar cortex, points out that it is possible that the cerebellum, in addition to somehow storing movements and gestures, may also provide visual cues and information about mood and related factors which in turn may provide a context to initiate an action.

While the output of the cerebellar cortex, conveyed solely by Purkinje cell axons, is inhibitory, this inhibition is exerted primarily upon
the deep cerebellar nuclei. In turn, their output tend to be excitatory,
suggesting that excitatory as well as inhibitory impulses reach them. Moreover, a series of studies indicate that both inhibition and facilitation can
be obtained by stimulation of the anterior lobe of the cerebellum (Dow &
Moruzzi, 1958). Low rates tend to increase muscle tone while higher
rates tend to produce relaxation of muscles. More specifically, according
to Deutch and Deutch (1966) stimulation of the anterior or posterior lobe
with high frequency (over 40 cps) impulses leads to a depression of muscular
tonus (hypotonus), while stimulation of the anterior lobe with lower frequency impulses leads to facilitation of muscular tonus or hypertonus. Consequently, frequency of cerebellar cortex stimulation plays an important
role in determining whether eventual physiological (and behavioral) inhibition or facilitation will occur. Through integration and organization of
information, both ascending and descending, the cerebellum appears to act
as a computer, according to Eccles, Ito and Szentagothai (1967) to modify
the control of movement and related functions.

It is of some interest to note that despite the vast amount of data
now available with respect to the anatomy, structure, and function of the
cerebellum, very little has been done directly with respect to the medical
or surgical therapy of this organ. In the laboratory, however, there has
been much recent interest with respect to the role of the cerebellum in
experimental epilepsy (Cooke & Snider, 1955; Dow, Fernández-Guardiola,
& Manni, 1962; Kreindler, 1962; Hutton, Frost, & Foster, 1972). In such
studies cerebellar stimulation was found generally to modify or inhibit experimentally induced cortical epileptic foci. In turn, Snider and his
associates (Snider, Sato, & Mizuno, 1967; Snider, Mitra, & Sudilovsky,
1970; Snider & Sinis, 1971) also have demonstrated influences on levels
of excitability in sensory areas of the cerebral cortex and on several thalamic nuclei, following cerebellar stimulation, with inhibition being predominant.

Some data are available with respect to the effects of ablation of
cerebellar nuclei or cerebellar cortex stimulation in man. Nashold and
Slaughter (1969) described five patients with involuntary movements in
whom cerebellar nuclei were stimulated or ablated. Stimulation (of several subcortical cerebellar regions) resulted in a variety of events, including ocular phenomenon, postural alterations, production of a variety of
sensations and changes in muscle tone. Sensations, mainly from brachium
conjunctivum stimulation, included dizziness, scared and unpleasant feelings. Lesions resulted primarily in reduction of tone and alterations of

abnormal posture, aside from transient effects. Such lesions have the ad-
vantage of "not altering memory or speech functions", according to
Nashold and Slaughter (1969, p. 184). Previously Snider and Wetzel
(1965), in perhaps the most extensive electrophysiological study in humans,
reviewed 26 cases in which EEG data were collected from the scalp following electrical stimulation of the cerebellum in patients undergoing
standardized procedures for pain alleviation, tumor removal and trauma.
In most instances changes were noted in frequency and amplitude of the
EEG, the usual alteration being from a normal or fast frequency to a
slower one, accompanied by an increase in voltage. The authors also
note that "disturbances of consciousness were not observed, nor were sensory alterations in the auditory and tactile spheres noted. Changes in
visual and proprioceptive sensations were not studied (p. 183)".

The experimental studies of Dow and Moruzzi and Snider and associates led Cooper (1973a, b, c) to implant electrodes in the paleo- and
neocerebellar cortex in individuals suffering from intractable epilepsy and
hypertonicity. Implantation was followed by chronic stimulation according
to pre-determined parameters of voltage, frequency, and time. These
studies, including details with respect to the surgical technique and results,
are being presented separately in this symposium (Cooper, Amin, Gilman,
and Waltz) and will not be considered here.

The purpose of the present study is to explore a variety of psychological and behavioral functions which may be altered as a result of chronic paleo- and neocerebellar cortical stimulation in man. A separate study
is now being undertaken with respect to acute stimulation, with an emphasis on visual sensation and perception. Since the preponderance of reports concerning the effects of such stimulation (and ablation) refer largely
to sensorimotor function, tone and coordination, very few data were
available to guide us in the selection of specific psychological and behavioral areas for assessment. However, as Snider (1967) noted "neurophysiological concepts of cerebellar function are broadening and behavioral studies are overdue (p. 331)". Consequently, primarily on an empirical basis,
a variety of integrative behavioral functions, in particular, perception,
perceptual-motor functions, cognition, memory, anxiety and emotion were
selected for initial assessment. It was hypothesized that the widespread
ascending and descending efferent cerebellar influences might result in one
or more aspects of such integrative functions being altered as a result of
chronic stimulation of either paleo- or neocerebellar cortex. Furthermore,
the earlier suggestions of Snider emphasizing sensory as well as motor functions for the cerebellum led us to expect that alterations in "higher" integrative functions may in turn result from changes in specific sensory-

motor factors. In turn, it was felt that an assessment of possible alterations in higher integrative functions might also provide clues to feedback
in developing further concepts concerning patterns of inhibition, facilitation, and integration ongoing in the cerebellum.

PROCEDURE

Subjects and Design of Study

The patient population consisted of 13 individuals either with seizure
disorders, or other neurologic abnormalities in which hypertonicity was
present (with one exception, case D.C.), who underwent a surgical procedure involving electrode placement, followed by chronic stimulation in
areas of the paleo- or neocerebellar cortex. Table 1 presents data on
sex, age, diagnosis, stimulation side and site(s) for this group.

TABLE 1

Sex, Age, Diagnosis, Stimulation Side and Site(s) for
Cerebellar Stimulation Group (N = 13)

Patient	Sex	Age	Diagnosis	Side	Site(s) Cerebellar Lobe
W.A.	M	24	Psychomotor Epilepsy	Right	Anterior
W.B.	M	23	Grand Mal Epilepsy	Right	Anterior
J.W.	F	29	Grand Mal Epilepsy	Right	Anterior
R.S.	M	24	Grand and Petit Mal Epilepsy	Right	Anterior
M.C.	M	16	Psychomotor Epilepsy	Right	Anterior & Posterior
M.B.	F	56	Grand and Petit Mal Epilepsy	Right	Anterior & Posterior
S.H.	M	18	Psychomotor Epilepsy	Right	Anterior & Posterior
J.G.	M	74	Left Cerebral Vascular Accident	Right	Posterior
B.M.	M	26	Basilar Artery Thrombosis	Left	Posterior
R.G.	F	58	Right Cerebral Vascular Accident	Left	Posterior
R.M.	M	12	Cerebral Palsy	Right	Posterior
D.C.	F	39	Intention Myoclonus	Right	Anterior
M.L.	M	21	Cerebral Palsy	Left	Posterior

As   noted in Table 1 seven patients were diagnosed as having epilepsy, either psychomotor, grand mal, or combined grand and petit mal.
This group consisted of 5 males and 2 females whose ages ranged from 16
to 56 years with a mean of 27 years.   For each of these patients electrodes were placed on the right cerebellar cortex and in all instances
involved the anterior lobe, with 3 patients having electrodes placed on
both the anterior and posterior lobes.   This group will subsequently be
referred to as the seizure group.   Six other patients represented a variety
of neurologic entities including cerebral vascular accident, basilar artery
thrombosis, cerebral palsy, and intention myoclonus.   This group consisted
of 4 males and 2 females whose ages ranged from 12 to 74 years with a
mean of 38 years.   For this group electrodes were placed on the left cerebellar cortex in 3 instances and on the right side for 3 others, with posterior lobe placement in all instances except for one patient with intention
myoclonus in which electrodes were placed on the anterior lobe.   For purposes of later data presentation and discussion this group will be referred
to as the hypertonic group, since in all instances (with the exception of
Mrs. D.C.) patients manifested spasticity among their presenting symptoms.
In addition, this group had posterior cerebellar cortex electrode placement
(again with the exception of Mrs. D.C.), and stimulation parameters involved similar frequencies.

Stimulation parameters, specifically voltage, frequency, and time on
and off, tended to vary slightly from patient to patient, and in some instances were altered somewhat during the course of stimulation.   However,
relatively stable norms were achieved for the patients described in Table 1,
particularly by the time of postoperative psychological testing and evaluation.   In all instances the stimulation voltage was in the range of 10 volts.
For the seizure disorder group the frequency was 10 cycles per second.
For the hypertonic group it was in the area of 200 cps.   With respect to
stimulation time on and off, for patients with single electrode sites the
pattern generally established was 10 minutes on and 10 minutes off, around
the clock, where feasible.   For patients with two stimulator sites (anterior
and posterior) the time parameters ordinarily involved   alternation of each
stimulator each 10 minutes (i.e., each stimulator on 10 minutes and off
10 minutes), around the clock where feasible.   Four patients had subsequent
additional electrodes placed, but psychological data to be presented were
collected prior to such placement and these latter electrodes will not be
taken into account, for the most part, in this report.

Two comparison groups were utilized.   The first consisted of 5 patients with seizure disorders who were tested on 2, and in several instances
on 3 occasions, with time between testing equivalent to that of the seizure

patient sample. A second group consisted of 8 individuals who had suffered strokes and concomitant spasticity, who were also tested on two occasions with time variables equivalent to the hypertonic stimulation group.
This latter comparison group was selected as representative of individuals
with neurologic disease, brain damage, and hypertonicity, and although
not fully matched with the hypertonic stimulation group, are considered
fairly equivalent.

The specific testing procedure involved administration of a battery
of psychological tests, as well as a clinical interview, to the stimulation
subjects immediately prior to surgery, after "short term" chronic stimulation. As previously noted, for the two comparison groups, either two or
three sets of psychological tests were administered with time sequences
equivalent to the shorter term and longer term cerebellar stimulation subjects. Table 2 summarizes the time sequences for the shorter and longer
range testing for the stimulation and comparison groups.

TABLE 2

Time Between Testing for Cerebellar Stimulation and
Comparison Groups

	Time Between 1st & 2nd Tests	Time Between 1st & 3rd Tests
Seizure Disorders – Stimulation (N = 7)	21.9 days	112.2 days
Seizure Disorders – Comparison (N = 5)	29.8 days	134.3 days
Hypertonic – Stimulation (N = 6)	32.8 days	129.3 days
Stroke – Comparison (N = 8)	19.2 days	_____

In all, 13 patients undergoing chronic cerebellar stimulation and 13 patients in the two comparison groups were tested. As indicated in Table 2, the time between first and second testing averaged 27.3 days for the combined stimulation groups and 24.5 days for the combined comparison groups. Time between first and third testing averaged 112.2 days for the seizure stimulation group, 129.3 days for the hypertonic stimulation group, and 134.3 days for the seizure comparison sample. No third set of data was available for the stroke comparison group.

For both the stimulation and comparison groups, patients were selected on the basis of testability and anticipated reliability of test scores. In general, both sets of subjects were individuals who were grossly alert and oriented, who could communicate adequately, and who manifested no significant cognitive deterioration, as based upon clinical interview. Wherever feasible, attempts were made to equate the stimulation and comparison groups on such variables as sex, age, general educational and social background, and type of disease and disability.

Time sequences for shorter term testing of the stimulation group were based upon reliability of testing. That is to say, sufficient time was allowed before such testing to permit for effects directly related to surgery such as stress and trauma of surgery, effects of anesthesia and edema, etc., to attenuate sufficiently. In addition, it was felt that at least several weeks of regular cerebellar stimulation should be permitted before testing, so that behavioral alterations, if any, would be based upon a sufficient duration of stimulation. Longer range testing was undertaken when patients appeared for follow-up neurological examination, with the comparison groups being called in for testing at essentially equivalent time intervals.

Tests Administered

As previously noted, the battery of psychological tests was selected partly on an empirical basis, in an effort to assess a variety of perceptual, perceptual-motor functions, cognition and memory. It was hypothesized, also, that if any specific sensory-motor functions were altered, such alterations might manifest themselves as well in changes in the "integrative" behavioral variables being assessed by the psychological test battery. The battery itself consisted of the following standardized psychological tests:

1. Wechsler Adult Intelligence Scale (WAIS - A standardized test of intellectual (cognitive and perceptual) functions, assessed through both

verbal and non-verbal means (Wechsler, 1958). The scale consists of 11 sub-scales and permits the derivation of a verbal, a performance, and a full-scale IQ. The following is a brief description of what the individual sub-tests measure:

Information (I) - Series of questions which tap store of general information, particularly everyday and educationally acquired information.

Comprehension (C) - Questions which tap ability to comprehend and evaluate situations and solve problems of a practical and social nature. Tests for a certain amount of practical information and a general ability to evaluate past experience, and to articulate responses.

Arithmetic (A) - Problems to be solved without written aid that test computational skills and general arithmetical reasoning. Memory, concentration, attention, and speed are also tapped.

Similarities (S) - List of paired words which test individual's ability to perceive the common elements of the terms he is asked to compare and, at higher levels, his ability to bring them under a single concept. Involves abstract reasoning, verbal comprehension, and expression.

Digit Span (DSp) - Task requiring the reciting of digits from memory, either forward (in order presented) or backwards (in reverse order). Taps concentration, short-term memory, new learning, and ability to change set.

Vocabulary (V) - List of words to define which tests general vocabulary, learning ability, fund of verbal information, general range of ideas, reasoning ability, and expressive abilities. Correlates highly with overall IQ.

Digit Symbol (DSy) - Task requiring the association of certain symbols with certain other symbols with speed and accuracy. Taps new learning ability and motor speed, while flexibility, visual acuity, and motor coordination are also involved.

Picture Completion (PC) - Series of incompletely drawn pictures for which the task is to discover and identify the missing part. Measures the perceptual and conceptual abilities involved in the visual recognition and identification of familiar objects, the ability to notice small details, and to differentiate essential from non-essential details.

Block Design (BD) - Series of cards with printed abstract designs that are to be reproduced with colored blocks. Tests non-verbal abstract reasoning, visual-motor coordination, the ability to perceive spatial patterns and to analyze the whole into parts.

Picture Arrangement (PA) - A series of pictures which, when placed in the right sequence, tell a story, are presented in a disarranged order to be properly arranged by the subject. Measures ability to comprehend and size up a total situation, to grasp the whole idea behind it and taps "social intelligence" and ability to comprehend human or practical situations.

Object Assembly (OA) - Form-board puzzle pieces to be assembled into familiar objects. Taps the ability to perceive and synthesize parts into wholes, integrative ability, and task persistence.

2. Wechsler Memory Scale - A standardized measure of orientation, current information, recent and remote memory, assessed through both verbal and perceptual means (Wechsler, 1945; Wechsler & Stone, 1959).

3. Bender-Visual-Motor Gestalt Test - A measure of visual-motor perception and integration, requiring the copying of a standardized series of designs while viewing the stimuli (Bender, 1938).

4. Critical Flicker Frequency Test (CFF) - A visual-perceptual test of cerebral function and efficiency. Accumulated data suggest that the CFF can be used as a useful behavioral correlate of what has been described, among other things, as "overall cerebral functioning" (Honigfeld, 1962; Misiak, 1967).

5. Tachistoscope - A test of visual perception in which stimuli can be presented at time intervals ranging from 1 millisecond to 900 milliseconds. Stimuli used were single words, single symbols, and combinations of words and symbols presented centrally, and in the left and right fields of vision. Figure 1 illustrates the words, symbols, and combinations of words and symbols used in the Tachistoscopic presentation. The same set of stimuli cards was used during the 1st, 2nd, and 3rd sets of testing, but were presented in random order in each instance.

In addition to the battery of standardized psychological tests, each stimulation patient was interviewed preoperatively, and on several occasions during chronic cerebellar stimulation, and behavioral observations

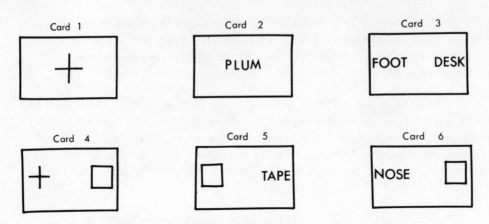

Fig. 1. Words and symbols used in Tachistoscope presentations.

were made. Furthermore, the patients' charts were reviewed, in particular daily nurses' notes and progress notes, and data were culled relevant to psychological or behavioral alterations which might be related to chronic cerebellar stimulation. Observations made by the staff as well as patient's subjective reactions and those of his family were noted.

RESULTS

The psychological findings will be presented under the following categories: psychological test results; shorter range findings; longer range findings; and individual case reports and observations.

A. Shorter Range Psychological Test Results

Initial data analysis will concern itself with the results of the standardized psychological tests previously described, and administered to stimulation patients and comparison subjects on two or three occasions. Before presenting such results certain delimitations and qualifications must be noted. In the first instance, there are relatively small numbers of patients in the stimulation and comparison groups, with numbers ranging from 5 to 8.

With such small groups, one must be cautious in interpreting any statistical findings. Moreover, each of the stimulation groups represents a
somewhat heterogeneous population itself. For example, those patients
described as "seizure" patients include epileptics with a variety of seizure
disorders including psychomotor, petit mal, and grand mal epilepsy, and
having different medical and neurological histories as well as different
social and educational backgrounds. In the case of the "hypertonic"
group, even more heterogeneity is present. As previously noted, 3 of
the group suffered strokes or thromboses, 2 were diagnosed as cerebral
palsy, and 1 as intention myoclonus. This group is held together primarily by the fact that 5 of the 6 manifested hypertonicity, although they
differ in age, educational and social background, as well as other medical and neurological variables. It must also be noted that although effort was made to select comparison patients as closely equivalent as possible to the stimulation group, definitive equivalency could not be achieved. For example, the "seizure" comparison group tended to have a
somewhat more limited educational background as well as lower intellectual functioning. In turn, the comparison group used for the hypertonic
stimulation group consisted of a fairly homogeneous sample of individuals
with cerebral vascular accidents. However, they cannot be considered
fully equivalent to the somewhat heterogeneous group included in the
hypertonic stimulation sample.

Because of the limitations just enumerated, it was felt that the
widest variety of intra and intergroup comparisons should be achieved.
From the 4 samples of stimulation and comparison groups the following
combinations were chosen for graphic presentation and statistical comparison:

1. Seizure stimulation vs seizure comparison group
2. Hypertonic stimulation vs stroke comparison group
3. Seizure stimulation vs hypertonic stimulation group
4. Both stimulation groups vs both comparison groups

The first involved the presentation of line graphs for each of the
comparisons noted above, particularly for the sub-tests of the Wechsler
Adult Intelligence Scale and the specific stimulus cards for the Tachistoscope. Secondly, the Mann-Whitney U Test was utilized as the primary
method of statistical comparison. This test was chosen as representative
of a relatively powerful, non-parametric test, useful for small numbers,
which requires ordinal measurement, and which can be used with independent samples (Seigel, 1956). Furthermore, since our primary interest

was in the possible test score changes which may occur following shorter or longer range chronic stimulation, an emphasis was placed upon "change" scores rather than upon the raw test data. The use of "change" scores also tends to reduce certain of the limitations noted above, particularly the lack of complete equivalency between the stimulation and comparison groups. By the combined methods of utilizing comparison groups, change scores and data presentation involving both graphic and statistical analysis, it was hoped that a sufficiently thorough presentation of the data could be achieved. Figure 2 shows WAIS change scores achieved by the seizure stimulation and seizure comparison groups.

As noted on Figure 2 both the seizure stimulation and comparison groups tend to increase in most sub-tests as well as in verbal, performance, and full-scale IQ, in the 2nd or shorter range postoperative testing, as compared with their baseline scores. However, with this general pattern, certain differences are apparent. First, it will be noted that the seizure

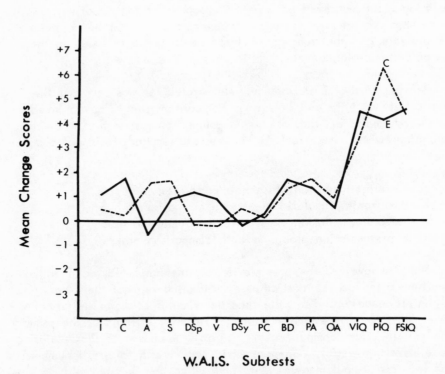

W.A.I.S. Subtests

Fig. 2. Wechsler Adult Intelligence Scale change scores - Scaled sub-test scores, Verbal IQ, Performance IQ, and Full-Scale IQ. Seizure stimulation group (E) vs seizure comparison group (C).

stimulation group tends to increase somewhat more in the information, comprehension, digit span, and vocabulary sub-tests than do the comparison subjects. Furthermore, the seizure stimulation group shows a somewhat greater increase in overall verbal IQ, whereas the comparison group demonstrates a greater increase in performance IQ sub-tests.

When a series of Mann-Whitney U tests were calculated, none of these differences quite achieved statistical significance at the p = .05 level, the commonly accepted criterion of statistical significance. However, several of the sub-test scores showed strong tendencies in the anticipated direction. In particular, comprehension (p = .12) and vocabulary (p = .15) come close to statistical significance, on the basis of a two-tailed test. One might thus infer that in these two tests involving comprehension, verbal facilitation and output, the seizure stimulation group showed a greater tendency to increase shorter range postoperatively than did the comparison group. This finding tends to be confirmed by the greater overall verbal IQ increase shown by the same group. In contrast, the seizure group, while improving in performance IQ, did so to a much lesser degree than the seizure comparison group. The overall suggestion here is that seizure stimulation tends to enhance some aspects of verbal outflow while perhaps depressing certain aspects of performance outflow or input, the latter of which involves a greater degree of perceptual and perceptual-motor functions. Figure 3 compares WAIS sub-test change scores between the hypertonic stimulation group and its stroke comparison group.

Observation of Figure 3 indicates that the hypertonic stimulation group tends to increase postoperatively in the comprehension sub-test to a higher degree than does the stroke comparison group, while the stroke comparison group improves during the second testing to a higher degree than does the hypertonic stimulation group in two performance sub-tests, picture arrangement and object assembly. The comprehension difference almost achieves statistical significance (p = .07), while the picture arrangement and object assembly sub-tests, although not reaching statistical significance, show definite trends in the direction expected from the figure. In addition, there is a slight trend for the stroke comparison group to improve moreso in the information sub-test than does the hypertonic stimulation group. As in the earlier comparison between the seizure stimulation group and its comparison group, the hypertonic stimulation group tended to increase somewhat moreso in verbal sub-tests while its comparison group tended to increase moreso in performance sub-tests. Neither of these changes, however, achieved statistical significance. Nevertheless, the pattern shown in Figures 2 and 3 are clearly suggestive of greater increases in some aspects of verbal facility for the stimulation group and greater

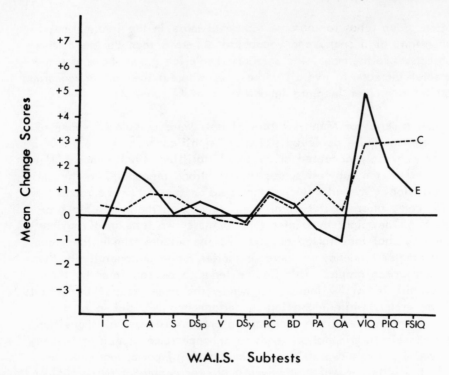

W.A.I.S. Subtests

Fig. 3. Wechsler Adult Intelligence Scale Change Scores - Scaled
sub-test scores, Verbal IQ, Performance IQ, and Full-Scale IQ.
Hypertonic stimulation (E) vs stroke comparison group (C).

increases in performance, or perceptual and perceptual-motor functions for
their comparison groups. One might also state the findings in a somewhat
different way, by noting that stimulation patients tend to increase in verbal sub-tests and not to increase in performance sub-tests. Their performance IQ increases seem due more to practice effects than to a "real"
change in the functions measured.

Figure 4 shows comparative short range change scores for the seizure
stimulation and hypertonic groups, on the WAIS sub-test.

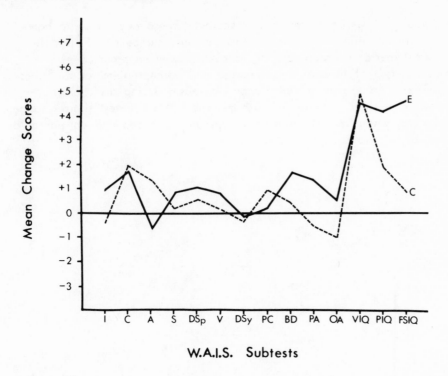

Fig. 4. Wechsler Adult Intelligence Scale Change Scores - Scaled sub-
test scores, Verbal IQ, Performance IQ, and Full-Scale IQ. Seizure
stimulation (E) vs hypertonic stimulation (C).

When the stimulation groups are compared one to another, several
observations of interest are to be noted. In the first instance, there appear to be no gross differences in overall functions with respect to change
scores. However, the information sub-test demonstrates a significant difference between the groups (p = .01), with the seizure stimulation patients
showing greater increases than the hypertonic group. With respect to performance scores the seizure group also tends to increase moreso in several
of the sub-tests, but in no instances achieving statistical significance or
near significance. However, overall performance IQ increases a full 2
points more for the seizure stimulation than the hypertonic group. Moreover, in three of the performance sub-tests the hypertonic stimulation

group actually shows decreases in test scores. These decreases, in combination with the relatively low increase in performance and full-scale
IQ for the hypertonic group suggest, particularly when practice effects
are considered, that in certain perceptual and perceptual-motor functions
the hypertonic group may actually show decreases during the shorter range
postoperative testing. Figure 5 illustrates the WAIS sub-test shorter range
change scores when both stimulation groups are combined and compared to
both comparison groups.

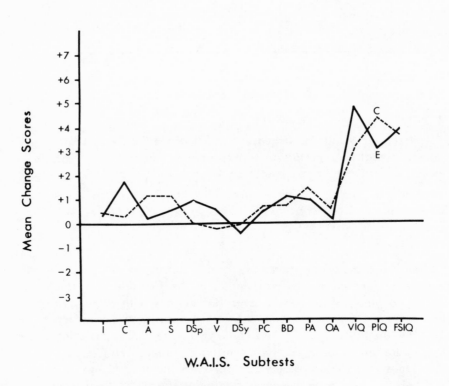

W.A.I.S. Subtests

Fig. 5. Wechsler Adult Intelligence Scale Change Scores - Scaled sub-
test scores, Verbal IQ, Performance IQ, and Full-Scale IQ. Both
stimulation groups (E) vs both comparison groups (C).

Statistical analysis of the data in Figure 5 showed that the stimulation groups in combination manifested statistically significant increases
in the comprehension sub-test (p = .02) as compared to the combined
control groups. This is the only sub-test manifesting a statistically significant difference, although vocabulary approaches statistical significance
(p = .10) in the same direction. Again, the trend is for the stimulation
groups to show greater increases in some tests of verbal function than do
their comparison non-stimulation groups. This is manifested by the greater
increase, although non-statistically significant, in the verbal IQ, for the
stimulation groups as compared to the comparison groups. Furthermore,
although again not statistically significant, there is a tendency for the
comparison groups to show greater increases in performance sub-tests than
do the stimulation groups.

Although but few of the differences in change scores between the
various combination of stimulation and comparison groups achieved statistical significance in shorter range testing, several patterns seem to emerge.
These may be summarized as follows:

1. Stimulation subjects appear to increase more in verbal sub-tests
than do their comparison counterparts, and comparison subjects seem to
increase more in performance tests than do the stimulation subjects. Indeed, when practice effects are taken into account, the stimulation groups
may actually show slight declines in performance scores.

2. Seizure stimulation patients tend to improve in overall verbal functions similarly to hypertonic stimulation patients, but tend to improve more
in performance sub-tests than do the hypertonic stimulation patients.
Moreover, the hypertonic stimulation group tends to decrease somewhat in
several performance sub-tests.

For the Tachistoscopic stimuli presentations a series of comparisons
were made between the stimulation and comparison groups and between
each of the stimulation groups, as was done for the WAIS sub-tests. These
findings were also graphically tabulated and a series of statistical tests were
undertaken to compare changes between the various comparison groups.
Figure 6 shows change scores achieved on the Tachistoscope test by the
seizure stimulation and seizure comparison groups. It is to be noted that
in this test plus scores indicate greater time taken to identify the stimuli,
and minus scores indicate less time taken.

Observation of Figure 6 indicates that the major differences between
the seizure stimulation and their comparison groups are in the combination

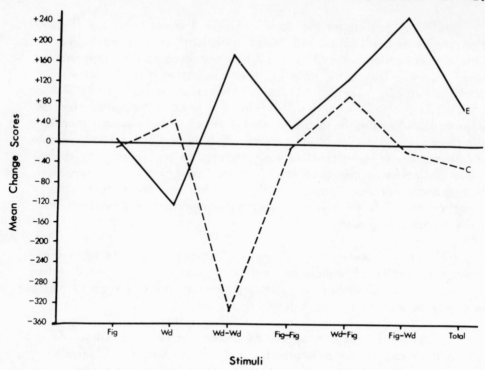

Fig. 6. Tachistoscope Change Scores (in seconds) for standard stimuli cards. Seizure stimulation group (E) vs seizure comparison group (C).

stimuli of word-word and figure-word. Statistical analysis indicates that each of these approach statistical significance (word-word, p = .13; figure-word, p = .08), with the seizure stimulation group tending to show increased time in identifying the stimulation cards in both instances, in contrast to a decreased time manifested by the comparison group. The pattern, consequently, is for the seizure stimulation group to take near significantly longer times to identify the combination stimuli, particularly in which a word is involved, during the shorter range period than does its comparison group. Figure 7 compares the hypertonic stimulation and and its stroke comparison groups on the shorter range Tachistoscopic changes.

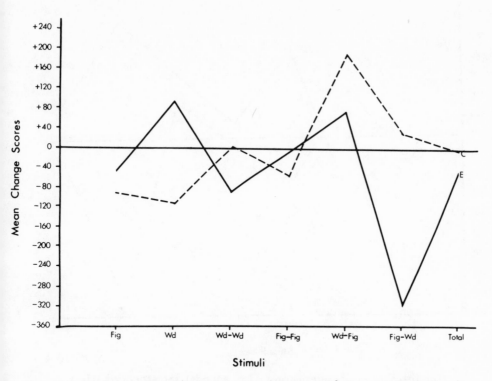

Fig. 7.   Tachistoscope Change Scores (in seconds) for standard stimuli cards.   Hypertonic stimulation (E) vs stroke comparison group (C).

Observation of Figure 7 indicates that the hypertonic group requires a longer time for correct identification of a single word than does the stroke comparison group, while in contrast it requires much less time for identification of the figure-word combination than does the comparison group.   The difference for the single word approaches statistical significance (p = .11) for a two-tailed test.   The pattern here is for the hypertonic stimulation group to worsen somewhat in the single word stimulus but to improve somewhat for the figure-word combination, in contrast to its comparison group.

Figure 8 shows Tachistoscope change scores for the seizure stimulation and hypertonic stimulation groups.

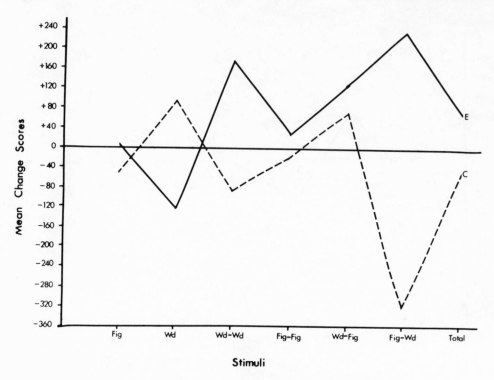

Fig. 8. Tachistoscope Change Scores (in seconds) for standard stimuli cards. Seizure stimulation (E) vs hypertonic stimulation (C).

Observation of Figure 8 indicates that the seizure stimulation group improves somewhat in identifying the single word stimulus, but regresses somewhat in identifying the word-word stimulus and moreso for the figure-word stimulus, with the hypertonic stimulation group showing essentially a reverse process. Only the single word difference achieves near statistical significance (p = .17). However, observation of the mean difference scores in Figure 8 clearly shows a trend for the seizure stimulation pat-ients to worsen in the shorter range testing, in particular when the word is on the right half of the visual field. This pattern was also seen to occur when the seizure group was contrasted to its comparison group, in which a similar pattern of findings was noted (cf Figure 6). Figure 9 shows the shorter range change scores when both stimulation groups are combined and compared.

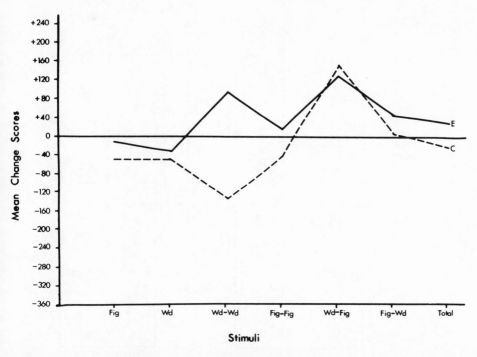

Fig. 9.   Tachistoscope Change Scores (in seconds) for standard stimuli cards.   Both stimulation groups (E) vs both comparison groups (C).

In comparing the stimulation patients with their comparison groups none of the stimulation card change response times achieved a statistical significance.   However, there is a tendency for the stimulation groups in combination to show a regression in the word–word identification whereas the control groups show some improvement.

With further respect to Tachistoscope findings, efforts were made to determine the side of the visual field in which performance might be most altered and whether the word or figure is most susceptible of such alteration.   Consequently, for the 6 seizure patients for whom data were available (all of these had electrodes placed on the right cerebellum, 3 anterior only and 3 anterior and posterior), and for the 2 hypertonic patients for whom data were available (both of whom had left posterior electrodes placed), comparisons were made as shown in Table 3.

TABLE 3

Pre and Shorter Range Postoperative Raw Score Response Times (in seconds) for Combined Word and Symbol Tachistoscope Cards for Seizure and Hypertonic Stimulation Groups

A. Seizure Group (N = 6) – All Right Anterior Electrodes

	Word	Word	Figure	Figure	Word	Figure	Figure	Word
Preoperative	67.5	57.2	4.0	3.8	60.8	25.8	35.7	44.3
Postoperative	184.8	253.0	38.0	1.0	193.3	2.8	277.0	228.0

B. Hypertonic Group (N = 2) – Both Left Posterior Electrodes

	Word	Word	Figure	Figure	Word	Figure	Figure	Word
Preoperative	77.5	50.0	13.0	15.0	17.5	7.5	110.0	92.5
Postoperative	102.5	87.5	37.5	15	140	12.5	15.5	20.0

For the seizure patients, observation of the Tachistoscope scores suggested that the group tended to worsen in performance during the shorter range postoperative testing on the word rather than the figure, and in particular when the word appeared on the right side of the visual field. This finding tends to confirm earlier impressions previously described. In essence, some form of visual-perception "inhibition" occurs for this group, primarily for word symbols presented on the right visual field.

For the 2 left posterior cerebellar cortex subjects (hypertonic group), the tendency was for an "inhibition" in response to occur primarily on the left field of vision, whether a word or figure appeared on that field. Although neither the seizure or hypertonic stimulation data were subjected to statistical analysis, primarily due to the small number in each group, a pattern emerges. In essence, patients whose stimulators are placed on the right cerebellar cortex tend to show a worsening in visual-perception for words in the right visual field whereas patients for whom stimulators are placed on the left cerebellar cortex tend to show a worsening in the left field of vision, for both words and figures. Considering the known decussation of cerebellar efferents in the ascending cerebellar tracts, this would seem to suggest a lateralized effect derived from cerebellar stimulation, not unlike the lateralization traditionally described for the cerebral cortex. This concept will be further considered later, in the discussion section.

A review of the shorter range changes in Tachistoscope identification when the stimulation groups and control groups are compared and contrasted shows the following pattern:

1. The seizure stimulation group tends to worsen, particularly in identifying the word-word and figure-word stimuli in contrast to its comparison group.

2. In general, the hypertonic group appears to improve equally or moreso than its stroke comparison group on all stimulus figures with the exception of the single word.

3. The seizure stimulation group tends to worsen in word-word and figure-word identification in comparison to improvements shown by the hypertonic stimulation group.

4. When both stimulation groups are compared to both control groups there is a slight tendency for the stimulation groups to worsen in the word-word stimulus when compared with the comparison groups.

5. A form of cerebellar lateralization seems to occur for verbal and spatial material analogous to concepts of cortical identification.

On the Critical Flicker Fusion test no statistically significant differences were found when the stimulation groups were compared with their controls individually or in combination, and when each stimulation group was compared with the other. There was a tendency, however, for the seizure stimulation group to improve somewhat in this function in contrast to its comparison group which remained essentially the same. With respect to the hypertonic stimulation group, no shorter range changes were noted, nor were shorter range changes in its stroke comparison group. Therefore, on the CFF test there is a slight tendency, not statistically significant, for the seizure stimulation group to improve in performance, in contrast to no alterations in the other three groups.

On the Wechsler Memory Scale the seizure stimulation group gained 6.3 points during shorter range testing as compared to a gain of 3.6 points for the seizure comparison group, indicating a tendency, not statistically significant, for memory scores to improve moreso for this group. No statistical comparisons were made between the hypertonic stimulation group and its comparison group on this test since too few patients were involved. However, practice effect may play a role in these changes. In addition, two specific sub-tests of the Wechsler Memory Scale, specifically Visual Reproduction and Associate Learning, were contrasted with respect to change scores for the various stimulation and control groups. Again, no significant differences were noted in any instance. However, when the hypertonic stimulation group was compared with its stroke comparison group a tendency was found for the hypertonic group to increase somewhat moreso than their comparison group in a test of verbal associate learning, although not statistically significant ($p = .13$) in a two-tailed test. Finally, no significant changes were noted between any shorter range change scores for the Bender-Gestalt test.

B. Longer Range Psychological Test Results

As previously noted, wherever feasible longer range psychological test data were collected both for the stimulation and comparison groups. However, only a portion of stimulation patients or comparison subjects were available for such testing. The largest portion of patients tested longer range were in the seizure stimulation group in which 7 individuals were tested preoperatively and in the short range assessment, and 5 of whom were seen for follow-up testing a mean of 3 months following chronic cerebellar stimulation. Consequently, some tabulated data are available for this group. Figure 10 shows the preoperative, shorter range, and longer range postoperative WAIS scaled sub-test scores for the seizure stimulation group.

Figure 10 shows that several of the sub-test scores showed progressive improvement from preoperative to shorter to longer range testing. These included information, comprehension, similarities, and vocabulary, and in turn the overall verbal IQ score increased from 93.3, to 97.9, to 101.4, for the pre, shorter and longer range subjects, respectively. With respect to overall performance IQ a similar increase was noted, although two of the performance tests failed to show such increases, picture completion and picture arrangement, both of which actually were lower in the longer range than in shorter range testing. It is likely that some of the improvement noted in these longer range test-retest measurements are due to practice effect, since they are based upon performance in the identical tests.

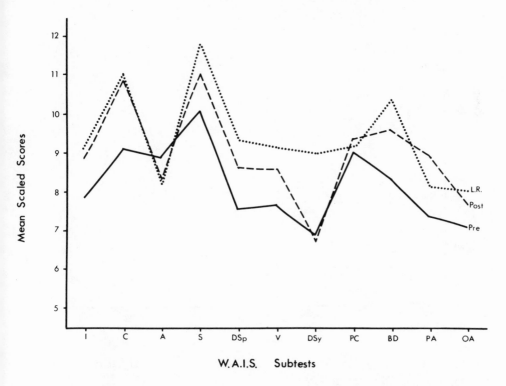

Fig. 10. Preoperative, shorter range and longer range scaled WAIS scores for seizure stimulation group.

Since very little in the way of comparison group scores is available for the longer range testing, one must be cautious in interpreting the findings. At best, one might conclude that little or no decrements occurred with the overall intellectual pattern showing improvements in large part related to practice effects, and that possibly progressive increments occurred in some tests of verbal output. Only the arithmetic sub-test showed a decrement in longer range as compared to preoperative score.

Figure 11 shows the preoperative, shorter, and longer range Tachistoscope time response scores for the seizure stimulation group.

Observation of Figure 11 indicates that preoperatively the seizure stimulation group (all right cerebellar placements) manifested longest time to identify the stimulus card for the word-word presentation. During the shorter range testing the time to identify the word-word stimulus card had increased somewhat, and the time to identify the figure-word stimulus card

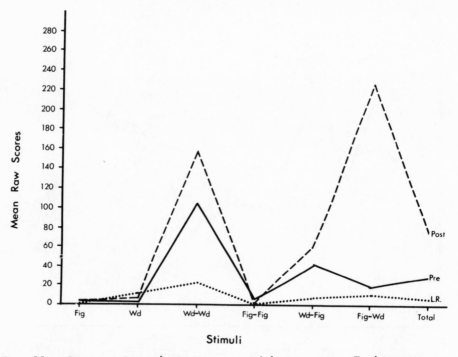

Fig. 11. Preoperative, shorter range and longer range Tachistoscope raw scores for seizure stimulation group.

had increased markedly. By longer range testing the group had returned at least to its preoperative level, or better, for all of the stimulus cards. The pattern here is a shorter range postoperative regression, particularly for stimulus cards in which a word is present, and more specifically where a word is present on the right side of the visual field, with an improvement in the longer range situation to a level at least equal to preoperatively. The role of practice effect, particularly, for the longer range testing cannot here be assessed due to the lack of adequate comparison-control data.

Table 4 shows the Critical Flicker Fusion test mean scores, pre, shorter range and longer range postoperatively, respectively, for the 3 groups for which such data are available.

TABLE 4

Pre and Postoperative Critical Flicker Fusion Mean Scores —
All Groups

	Seizure Stimulation	Seizure Comparison	Hypertonic Stimulation	Stroke Comparison
Preoperative (Baseline)	40.5 (N=6)	35.5 (N=5)	37.9 (N=5)	39.8 (N=8)
Shorter Range	43.2 (N=6)	33.9 (N=5)	38.3 (N=5)	39.5 (N=8)
Longer Range	48.1 (N=5)	37.5 (N=3)	42.9 (N=2)	——

Although these findings were not submitted to statistical analysis, because of the small number of subjects in each group, it is apparent from Table 4 that the seizure stimulation group improved in its performance in Critical Flicker Fusion from pre to shorter range to longer range postoperatively, to a degree apparently greater than that of the hypertonic stimulation group or the seizure comparison group. This test is minimally influenced by practice or learning effects. This suggests that overall "perceptual efficiency" may increase somewhat for the seizure stimulation group during the chronic cerebellar stimulation process. The small numbers involved and problems of adequate control, however, make this finding most tentative.

Table 5 presents preoperative, shorter range and longer range scores on the Wechsler Memory Quotient for the two groups for whom such data were available.

TABLE 5

Pre and Postoperative Memory Quotient Mean Scores –
Seizure Stimulation and Comparison Groups

	Seizure Stimulation	Seizure Comparison
Preoperative (Baseline)	89.6 (N = 7)	73.6 (N = 5)
Shorter Range	95.9 (N = 7)	77.2 (N = 5)
Longer Range	109.6 (N = 5)	90.0 (N = 3)

As noted in Table 5 memory quotients increase consecutively for the seizure stimulation group from pre to shorter to longer range postoperative testing with a total increase of 20.0 memory quotient points. This is in comparison to an increase of 16.4 memory quotient points for the seizure comparison group, and is not statistically significant. The trend is for both groups to increase equivalently in memory quotient, indicating no decrease for the seizure stimulation sample. Practice effect is probably most responsible for these changes.

The following statements summarize the situation of the seizure stimulation sample with respect to longer range psychological test findings:

1. Overall IQ scores tend to increase from pre to shorter to longer range testing, equivalently for the seizure stimulation patients and their seizure comparison group. The seizure stimulation group shows least gains in the arithmetic, picture completion and picture arrangement sub-tests and most gains in the verbal sub-tests of information, comprehension, similarities, and vocabulary.

2. Tachistoscopic scores worsen for word-word and figure-word during the shorter range postoperative period, with the right field of vision being primarily affected, but improve in the longer range status, to the degree where they are at least equivalent to preoperatively.

3. CFF and memory quotient scores tend to increase from pre to shorter range to longer range status for the seizure stimulation group, to a degree somewhat greater than the increases for the seizure comparison group, although the differences are not of a statistically significant degree.

C. Case Reports

As previously noted, in addition to administration of standard psychological tests preoperatively and during shorter and longer range cerebellar stimulation, efforts were made to secure other data not ordinarily sampled by such tests, which might provide cues to possible behavioral alterations. Consequently, daily nurses' notes and progress notes were reviewed. In addition, at stated times postoperatively patients were interviewed in depth in an effort to determine "subjective" impressions or feelings noted by patients at various times during cerebellar stimulation, and also to make relevant observations. The following case reports are presented to describe such data. Individual reports are presented for each seizure stimulation patient separately and are summarized for the hypertonic stimulation group.

Neurological, surgical, and seizure frequency data are kept to a minimum as they are documented elsewhere in this symposium (Cooper et al.):

W.A. - This 24-year old single male was initially admitted to St. Barnabas Hospital February 22 with a diagnosis of psychomotor epilepsy. According to the patient his seizures began approximately three and a half years previously, some months following being hit by a baseball. Over the years, and particularly in recent months, seizures had varied from one to five daily with brief intervals of time with no seizures. No therapy was recommended at that time but the patient was subsequently readmitted to the hospital October 30, 1972 at which time he reported that since his previous admission he had been totally incapacitated by his seizures which then involved from 2 to 20 auras a day, including a feeling of discomfort, anxiety, and nausea. At times these auras were followed by psychomotor seizures but not always. The longest recent period without seizures was three weeks. As a result the patient has been unable to work, drive a car, or engage in any social or extracurricular activities.

High school records indicated that the patient graduated high school in May of 1966, ranked 18th in a class of 31, and was essentially an average student, with most of his marks ranging in the 80's. The school reported that he was quite interested in art and sketching and was very active in extracurricular activities such as athletics and music.

On November 7 the patient underwent surgery at which time electrodes were placed on the anterior lobe of the right cerebellar cortex. During stimulation notable reduction in seizure activity was observed and during the first month following such stimulation medication was gradually reduced somewhat. He underwent psychological testing preoperatively, one month postoperatively, and again 4-1/2 months postoperatively. After one month of chronic cerebellar stimulation he had gained 8 points on an overall intelligence test, but at 4-1/2 months postoperatively he had returned essentially to his preoperative level, suggesting that the earlier gain was largely a practice effect. In contrast, the patient's Memory Quotient remained unchanged from pre to shorter range postoperatively, and then increased markedly, from 110 to 127 when tested 4-1/2 months after initial testing. At all times the patient's IQ and memory level remained in the bright normal or superior range.

Extensive psychological interviews were undertaken with this patient both during shorter and longer range stimulation times. The patient was articulate and was well able to verbalize his feelings, and to describe possible psychological changes which occurred during cerebellar stimulation.

During these interviews he reported that at all times postoperatively he felt well and energetic, particularly in contrast to his preoperative condition which he described as always involving feeling tired and inactive. He returned to his drawing which came easier and felt that his motivation had increased. He reported that he is "more confident" about himself and about his future. He believes his memory and thinking had improved. Before surgery he was "depressed" and this had become markedly reduced. He had become more outgoing as compared to having been "withdrawn" in the past several months. When last interviewed, 7 months following surgery, the patient's subjective condition remained essentially as just described.

W.B. – This 23-year old male suffered a right temporal lobe trauma at the age of 10 and since that time has had continuing and rather marked grand mal epileptic seizures, sometimes accompanied by aggressive behavior. In 1966 he underwent a right frontal lobectomy and in 1967 a right temporal lobectomy, neither of which provided significant improvement in seizures. In June of 1971 he underwent a right cryopulvinectomy at St. Barnabas which also failed to significantly reduce his seizures. Over the years the patient had been on a variety of anti-convulsive medications. He was readmitted to St. Barnabas on December 18, 1972 and the following day underwent electrode implantation on the right paleocerebellar cortex.

Reports from his high school indicated that because of his seizure disorder his program of studies was very light and it was also noted that his performance level was minimal. An IQ test administered in 1968 recorded an IQ score of 78.

The patient underwent psychological testing immediately prior to this operation and again some two weeks after continuing cerebellar stimulation. On preoperative psychological testing the patient scored a full-scale IQ of 88, and two weeks postoperatively scored 87, suggesting no gross changes in his performance. Indeed, a decline might be assumed inasmuch as practice effects would ordinarily be expected to raise such a score by several points. This decline was particularly notable in spatial-perception tasks. Moreover, the patient's Memory Quotient reduced from 87 preoperatively to 72 postoperatively due largely to his poor scores in performing spatial tasks from memory. It is also to be noted that during the first two weeks of cerebellar stimulation, although seizure frequency was reduced, the patient continued to manifest a pattern of grand mal seizures on an intermittent basis, but with no evidence of aggression during the ictal stage.

The patient was interviewed psychologically approximately one month following surgery. By that time his anti-convulsive medication had been reduced by approximately 50%. The patient reported that he felt a lot better and not as drugged as previously. He felt also more alert and "more chipper". Previously he tended constantly to lose his temper and disagree with people but did this much less following surgery. His spirits generally have been good although he has fluctuated in his mood, depending upon seizure frequency and other environmental factors such as being given "orders" by the nurses. The patient believed that his intelligence and thinking were quicker postoperatively and that he was able to respond more quickly to questions.

J.W. - This 29-year old female developed her first epileptic seizure at the age of 22. In the subsequent years the length and frequency of her seizures had increased and appeared to be intractable to such medication as dilantin, mysoline, and phenobarbital. The attacks generally start without an aura except for some changes in mood, and are composed of tonic-clonic movements which last from two to five minutes. On January 4, 1973 the patient had an electrode placed over the right paleocerebellar cortex. Stimulation at the rate of 10 volts and 10 cycles per second was undertaken for 10 minutes each hour, and gradually mysoline was discontinued. During her postoperative stay the patient was essentially free of seizures except for one incident during a week-end visit to relatives.

The patient underwent preoperative psychological evaluation and was retested two weeks after chronic cerebellar stimulation. On postoperative psychological testing the patient's IQ score had increased from 77 to 84 and her memory quotient had increased from 89 to 100. Both of these increases seem due at least in part to practice effect and possibly in part to the reduction in medication previously noted.

The patient was interviewed psychologically two weeks after chronic cerebellar stimulation and again five weeks later. During the initial postoperative interview she reported that she was able to think and talk better, although she complained of slight migraine headaches. She felt that her speech improvement was due in part to a decrease in medication. She also reported a decrease in depression and an improved "outlook". She felt less "shaky", less "tremulous", and very calm as compared to being "very anxious" for many months prior to surgery. When interviewed 5 weeks postoperatively she stated that she continued to feel better "like a better person". Depression and "despondency" continued to be diminished and an increase in energy was noted. She was more optimistic about the future as compared to a previous "pessimistic" outlook. In particular, the patient reported that she continued to feel much more relaxed and less tense than previously. She described herself as having always been so "uptight" over everything but now much less so, although she still continued to be a "sensitive" individual.

R.S. - This 24-year old male was admitted to St. Barnabas Hospital on January 4, 1973 with a diagnosis of grand and petit mal epilepsy dating from the time he was 7 years of age. The frequency of both the petit and grand mal seizures had increased over the years and were essentially intractable despite the fact that the patient had been on dilantin and phenobarbital for many years. According to the patient's history these seizures occurred most often when he was under stress, and averaged one grand mal seizure every 10 days, with intermittent petit mal seizures. School records indicated that the patient's IQ was essentially in the average range with scores ranging from 94 to 107 during the years 1957 to 1961.

On January 10, 1973 an electrode was placed on the right paleocerebellar cortex and on April 13, 1973 a second electrode was placed on the right neocerebellar cortex. Following initial (paleocerebellum) electrode placement the patient continued to manifest a pattern of seizures not dissimilar to his preoperative status. Following placement of the second stimulator with alternating stimulation between the paleo and neocerebellar cortex petit mal seizures decreased markedly and grand mal seizures decreased moderately. By the time of the hospital discharge on May 21 both grand mal and petit mal seizures had been markedly reduced, although occasional grand mal seizures continued to be present.

The patient underwent psychological testing several days before surgery, 12 days following chronic paleocerebellar stimulation, and again 4-1/2 months following this placement (i.e., 5 weeks following the additional placement of a neocerebellar stimulator). Preoperative psychological evaluation showed an IQ score of 104. Two weeks later it was 112, an increase probably largely due to practice effect. When tested 4-1/2 months after initial cerebellar electrode placement (i.e., 5 weeks after second electrode placement) his IQ score had reduced slightly to 108, a score which may be described as essentially equivalent to his presurgical level. In contrast, the patient showed a steady increase in Memory Quotient from 86 preoperatively to 112 twelve days after regular cerebellar stimulation, to 125 four and a half months after initial paleocerebellar stimulation (i.e., 5 weeks following placement of a second neocerebellar stimulator). This pattern of Memory Quotient increase is more than might be expected from practice alone.

The patient was interviewed psychologically on several occasions following initial placement of the paleocerebellar stimulator. A week following beginning of stimulation, the patient reported that his mental state was "excellent", which he felt might be due to a reduction in medication. However, he complained of occasional headaches, in addition to other somatic symptoms such as perspiration and chills. He stated also that he was optimistic about the future. Approximately one month after cerebellar stimulation the patient reported that his spirits remained "pretty good" and that he felt his thinking was better than before surgery, giving as an example the fact that he can play chess better and can think "in depth" better. He felt also that he is more relaxed and had increased "motivation". When interviewed some two months after chronic paleocerebellar stimulation the patient reported that he thought his "IQ" went up, inasmuch as he is still able to see problems better such as in playing chess as he previously noted. He felt also that he was more "forward" rather than shy as he was previously, and that his "anxieties and tensions" appeared to be less pronounced than preoperatively.

M.C. - This 16-year old male has a history of temporal lobe seizures dating from about the age of 8. Even prior to the development of seizures the patient was described as having had frequent episodes of violent behavior. Subsequently a pattern of seizures developed with episodes occurring once a week and lasting from 20 to 40 minutes. The frequency of these seizures had increased somewhat over the years despite the use of a wide variety of anti-convulsive medication. The patient's aura consists of blinking of the eyes. During the ictal stage a variety of peculiar movements of the limbs occurs, the patient wanders around meaninglessly, becomes violent, and makes frequent attempts to beat or attack others around him. The patient underwent implantation of right anterior and posterior cerebellar electrodes on January 16, 1973, followed by chronic stimulation which resulted in marked reduction of seizures during the following weeks.

The patient was administered standardized psychological tests several days before surgery, again two weeks postoperatively, and again three months postoperatively. On intelligence testing the patient's full-scale IQ scores for these three sets of tests were 70, 71, and 75, respectively, indicating no apparent change. Possibly a slight practice effect occurred resulting in an increase in longer range scores. However, the patient's Memory Quotient increased 5 points from 64 to 69 in pre to shorter range testing, and had increased 12 further points in longer range testing. This would appear to represent a significant increase in recent memory, with a particular gain in verbal memory (e.g., Associate Learning test).

The patient was interviewed 8 days following placement of cerebellar electrodes and again 3 weeks following surgery. In the initial interview the patient reported that he felt "good" because he knows he is going to get better. He felt that his thinking and mental functions were better and his spirits were "very good" as compared with before surgery. He noted also that he hasn't lost his temper once since surgery and didn't think he would lose his temper. It was observed that the patient had become more cooperative, more placid, and less aggressive than noted prior to surgery. In the latter interview the patient himself reported that he was "very mild" compared to preoperatively and that he continued to be in good spirits compared to "being down" prior to surgery.

M.B. - This 56-year old female has a history of grand and petit mal epilepsy with petit mal symptoms beginning at the age of 7, and grand mal seizures at the age of 13. These seizures had continued in the subsequent years despite medications which have included dilantin, phenobarbital, and valium. More recently seizures have occurred at least monthly with petit mal seizures ranging up to 6 to 12 per day and grand mal seizures occasionally reaching 4 per day. The patient was admitted to the hospital on February 22, 1973 and on February 26 electrodes were placed on the right neo- and paleocerebellar cortex. Following implantation and stimulation both petit mal and grand mal seizures were markedly reduced. At the time of her discharge late in May of 1973 she was essentially free of grand mal and showed marked reduction in petit mal attacks, although she manifested occasional myoclonic flexion movements of her arms.

School records indicated that the patient was an excellent student who maintained an A average in most of her subjects during her high school years. She was tested psychologically preoperatively, one month following chronic cerebellar stimulation, and again three months after surgery. In the shorter range testing no significant changes were noted in the patient's overall IQ score as compared to preoperatively, but her longer range IQ score of 105 was some 10 points higher than the initial score, which cannot necessarily be attributed to a practice effect due to the relatively long time between second and third testing. This increase, moreover, was probably not due to changes in medication, since the medication was essentially identical pre and postoperatively. The patient's Memory Quotient remained essentially the same from pre to shorter range testing, but increased 9 points from pre to three months postoperative testing.

In several interviews during the weeks of cerebellar stimulation the patient noted that she found no significant changes in herself, stating "I'm the same person". In contrast, progress and nurses' notes indicated that the patient appeared to be more calm and less anxious, and that her mood had improved.

S.H. - This 18-year old male has a history of psychomotor epilepsy dating from the age of 2 years and increasing during the subsequent years. His attacks were frequently associated with behavior disorders including violence and suicidal attempts. Prior to surgery the patient's seizures occurred from 15 to 30 times each month with time durations of 2 to 8 minutes. The aura consisted of feelings of lightness and weightlessness and a staring look. In the ictal stage the patient "looks ugly", grimaces, cries out, and makes noise. He loses consciousness. His parents described him as always having been aggressive, with poor self-control, frequently getting into fights. The patient had been on a variety of medication including dilantin, mysoline, phenobarbital, triaval, eskabarb, and philanton. Preoperatively he was on phenobarbital and dilantin. The patient underwent surgery on February 28, 1973, at which time right neo- and paleo-cerebellar electrodes were implanted. During the weeks following this implantation the patient was essentially free of seizures and auras. During this time progress notes described his behavior as "more docile, amiable, and sociable". He was discharged on April 12, 1973.

High school records indicate that the patient was a somewhat below average student in Junior High School, leaving in 1970 because of "lack of interest". An IQ test administered at about that time revealed an IQ score of 88. A note from the patient's 6th grade teacher described him as slightly below average in scholastic ability and noted that he experienced numerous seizures in the classroom and in the playground. She describes the patient as having an "inferiority complex" and one who needed much encouragement to achieve.

Psychological testing was administered to the patient preoperatively, 3 weeks postoperatively, and again 3 months postoperatively. From pre to shorter range postoperatively the patient's IQ score increased from 86 to 98, and was 94 in the longer range evaluation. The 86 IQ score is equivalent to that found in 1970 during school testing. The shorter range postoperative gain of 14 points may have been due in part to practice effect and in part to actual improvement in certain performances, but probably not related to medication, since no gross changes in medication were made during his postoperative course. Of further note, the patient's Memory Quotient increased from 86 to 105, a gain of 19 points, from preoperative testing to shorter range postoperatively, a change which cannot be fully attributed to a practice effect. In longer range testing his memory IQ score was 101, 15 points above his preoperative score.

The patient was interviewed psychologically 5 weeks following surgery. He noted then that he was not "as nasty" as he used to be, and
found that he could control his temper better. He has a different outlook,
is more optimistic, socializes more, and is less afraid to talk to others.
Emotionally he felt better with less depression, believed he spoke more
freely and no longer thought of suicide. He is more confident and has a
more positive image of himself. Soon after discharge the patient became
employed as a leather cutter, and according to the parents seems to have
"settled down". He was described by his parents as "considerate",
"shares things", and much more friendly than prior to surgery.

In addition to the 7 patients with seizure disorders whose histories
have been presented along with test results and their own responses during
chronic stimulation, comments made by several other patients undergoing
chronic stimulation with diagnoses other than seizure disorders appear
worthy of note. For example, Mrs. D.C. was interviewed three weeks
following right anterior cerebellar lobe implantation during which time
some improvement was noted in her intention myoclonus. She reported a
reduction in depression which she attributed directly to this symptom improvement. She was interviewed again some four months following surgery
during which time continuing symptomatic improvement occurred and reported at that time "I'm not as nervous as I was". She describes herself as
being less tense and having less fears and as being less depressed. She
noted also that prior to stimulation she frequently had "nightmarish dreams"
and has not experienced these in months.

B.M. – A 26-year old male with a diagnosis of basilar artery thrombosis with spasticity, was interviewed some three weeks following left posterior cerebellar cortex implantation and chronic stimulation. He noted
that he was less "emotional" and more outgoing. Clinical observations
indicated that prior to surgery he tended to be markedly labile with poor
emotional control, frequently breaking into uncontrollable and unprovoked
laughter. When seen three months following stimulation he laughed when
"appropriate" within more normal limits, and was better able to control
his emotions.

The mother of R.M., a 12-year old cerebral palsy patient, was
interviewed twice during the course of her son's right posterior chronic
cerebellar stimulation, the first time approximately one week after electrode placement and the second time approximately three weeks later.
In the first interview the mother reported that her son seems more happy,
but still in pain as a result of his cerebral palsy. No other changes in
the patient's overall behavior were then described .by the mother. In the

latter interview she reported improvement in her son's speech and breath-
ing.   He was described as less demanding and more self-reliant.   Much
of this may be as a result of improvement in spasticity and consequent
improvement in some functions.

It is of some interest also to note that several of the patients reported a variety of conscious sensations which they noted during cerebellar stimulation.   Such sensations were noted both by patients in the seizure group and some in the hypertonic group, while still other patients
reported no notice of any conscious sensation whatever.   For those who
noticed sensations they were described variously as involving a tingling,
itching, and sometimes a pain experience.   These sensations were noted
primarily during initiation of the stimulator, and lasted perhaps some moments, then became attenuated.   Several patients described a sensation
of a "tightness around the head" or a numbness.   Aside from this type of
sensation, no patients reported any unusual or any untoward responses in
any aspect of emotional, cognitive, perceptual, auditory, or visual function at any time during stimulation periods, when questioned in this respect.

The vast majority of behavioral changes noted by the stimulation
patients, both the seizure and hypertonic groups were of a positive nature.
Although individual differences were present, these reported changes may
be summarized as follows:

1. Reduction in anxiety, tension, and feelings of stress.
2. Improvement in thinking and fluency of speech; increased
   alertness.
3. Reduction in depression; increased feelings of optimism.
4. Reduced feelings of anger and reduction in outbursts of aggression associated with seizures and between seizures;
   improved emotional control.

DISCUSSION

Because of the varied and somewhat complex nature of the psychological findings, the discussion will be organized in the following manner:
1) Intellectual functions and memory, 2) Visual perception, 3) Emotional
functions (i.e., depression, anxiety, tension and arousal), and 4) Role of
side, site and frequency of stimulation.

1. Intellectual Functions and Memory

Psychological data with respect to intellectual functions and memory were derived primarily from standardized tests and to a lesser degree from subjective impressions of patients. Among the most salient findings, in this respect, is the fact that cerebellar stimulation, whether of seizure or hypertonic groups of patients, and whether of paleo- or neocerebellar cortex, does not eventuate in apparent decrements or deficits in any aspect of a variety of intellectual functions assessed, either during the shorter or longer range postoperative status. This particular finding stands in clear contrast to the reported effects of most surgical therapy, particularly in which brain lesion production is involved, in other neurological areas. For example, a series of studies by Riklan and his associates concerning the psychological effects of unilateral and bilateral ventrolateral thalamic surgery in parkinsonians, and using essentially the same techniques of assessment as described here, generally found significant declines in intellectual functions when patients were tested from 2 to 4 weeks postoperatively, although scores tended to return to their preoperative level when patients were re-evaluated a range of 6 to 9 months later (Riklan, Diller, & Weiner, 1960; Riklan, Levita, & Cooper, 1966a; Riklan & Levita, 1966b; Riklan & Levita, 1969). In like manner, studies of psychological functioning following unilateral, and particularly bilateral temporal lobe surgery for epilepsy (with or without hippocampal damage) generally report declines either in cognitive, learning, or perceptual functions as well as in visual and auditory memory during shorter range, and frequently during longer range testing (Milner, 1958, 1966, 1968; Kimura, 1961; Serafetinides & Falconer, 1962; Horowitz, 1970).

Not only did psychological tests fail to find postoperative declines in aspects of verbal or non-verbal intellectual functioning, but in contrast there were instances of apparent increases in performance, in some cases beyond that which might ordinarily be expected from practice effect, reduction in anti-convulsive medication, or from emotional-motivational factors. Such increases appeared to be more manifest in the seizure stimulation group where pre to shorter range and pre to longer range postoperative increases in full-scale IQ scores reached 20 points in some instances, increases not nearly approached by the seizure comparison group. Moreover, when such increases occurred, either in mean scores or individual cases, they tended to occur primarily in verbal sub-tests of intellectual functioning such as Information, Comprehension, Similarities, and Vocabulary. Paradoxically, this is somewhat in contrast to the usual test-retest finding for this type of adult intelligence scale, in which instance scores on performance sub-tests generally tend to increase more as a consequence of practice or familiarity effect than do the verbal sub-tests (Steisel, 1951a, b; Guertin, Frank, & Rabin, 1956; Wechsler, 1958; Coons & Peacock, 1959). Consequently, the increases in verbal performance seem especially salient as indicative of gains made by the seizure stimulation patients, as do the occasional decreases in certain performance sub-tests, warrant special notice.

Since in only a few instances were statistically significant differences found, and since some differences in verbal scores between the seizure stimulation and hypertonic stimulation group were also noted, one must be cautious in attempting to interpret the increments in verbal output shown by the stimulation patients in general. In this respect, also, one hesitates to attribute these gains to any "real" improvement in basic intellectual functions, and to seek other possible sources of explanation. Since the concept of general intelligence includes the end result of a wide scope of sensory, perceptual, motor, emotional, motivational, and activational processes, many alternate explanations become available. In the ensuing discussion we shall hypothesize that the behavioral alterations are at least, in part, a function of mechanisms initiated by cerebellar stimulation. We recognize, however, that such variables as medication, symptomatic relief, practice effects and motivational-emotional factors may also play some role. Furthermore, since much current thinking concerning efferents from the cerebellar cortex concerns the role of the Purkinje cells as inhibitory (Eccles, Ito, & Sentagothai, 1967), and the consequences of this inhibition upon the cerebellar nuclear masses and other ascending and descending pathways, it may be well to view the intellectual changes and other findings later to be considered, from the viewpoint of inhibition (and facilitation) within the nervous system, with possible implications for behavior. In this respect it might be reiterated that while initial Purkinje cell action is inhibitory and is exerted upon the deep cerebellar nuclei, nevertheless the output of the deep cerebellar nuclei tend to be excitatory, indicating that both excitatory and inhibitory impulses somehow reach these nuclei. Finally, since cerebellar influences upon other parts of the nervous system, and eventually upon behavior, are mediated by numerous relay nuclei at all levels of the brain stem as well as in various other ascending and descending efferent tracts, numerous potentials are available for various combinations of inhibitory and facilitatory impulses to occur.

In this context, the tendency of the stimulation groups to increase in verbal IQ scores might be interpreted as a form of verbal-motor facilitation. This facilitation may be further delineated as an improvement in the type of verbal fluency and articulation and output required to respond to verbally presented material concerning such functions as information,

comprehension, and word definition. This type of verbal-motor facilitation is also suggested by the tendency for Memory Quotient scores to increase somewhat more in the stimulation groups than in their comparison
groups. It is also of some interest to note that the Memory Quotient
sub-test of Associate Learning, concerned primarily with verbal association
and memory, shows the greatest increase. These increments in verbal output are maintained during both shorter and longer range testing, at least
for the seizure group for which data are available. There exists some
experimental evidence concerning the effects of cerebellar stimulation on
the excitability of the motor area of the cerebral cortex. Rossi's discovery (1912) that stimulation of the cerebellum increases the excitability of
the motor cortex has repeatedly been confirmed (Bremer, 1935; Dusser de
Barenne, 1937), and is generally regarded (Bremer, 1935; Holmes, 1939)
as direct evidence of a facilitatory influence exerted by the cerebellum
on the cerebrum. Moreover, since a generalized EEG arousal may be
elicited by stimulating the cerebellar cortex of the anterior lobe (Mollica,
Moruzzi, & Naquet, 1953) or the festigial nuclei (Moruzzi & Magoun,
1949), Dow and Moruzzi (1958) had previously raised the question as to
whether the ascending reticular system may be impinged upon by cerebellifugal impulses (cf Snider, 1967). According to Dow and Moruzzi there
is anatomical evidence supporting an affirmative answer since cerebellifugal
fibers do reach those areas of the reticular formation in which the long
ascending fibers have their origin (Brodal & Rossi, 1955). Physiologically
this hypothesis is supported by the results of various stimulation experiments
and by the observation that units located in the pontine areas of the reticular formation that give rise to the long ascending fibers may be influenced by cerebellar stimulations (Palastini, Rossi, & Zanchetti, 1957).
Consequently, reticular systems may play a significant role in the observed
verbal-motor output.

     At this point we might tentatively suggest that other candidates for
the verbal-motor facilitation observed may involve ascending cerebellar
influences which may somehow eventually facilitate (perhaps modulate)
motor cortex, through their pathways via red nucleus and perhaps non-
specific thalamus, or may involve cerebellar-motor cortex feedback systems
initiated by cerebellar cortex stimulation. The slight tendency for some
seizure patients to improve in memory test scores may in turn be related
to hippocampal stimulation resulting from efferent cerebellar influences
(cf Iwata & Snider, 1959; Babb & Crandall, this Symposium). In contrast,
lesions involving the hippocampal complex in man result in various forms
of memory impairment (Victor, Angouine, Mancall, & Fisher, 1961;
Drachman & Arbit, 1966).

2. Visual Perception

The choice of visual perception as an area of investigative interest was suggested, in part, by current concepts that the cerebellum may influence (and be influenced by) sensory as well as motor phenomena. Numerous studies have confirmed Snider's (1950) earlier views in this respect and it is now generally accepted that stimulation of the so-called cerebellar "audiovisual area" (simple lobule and tuber) evokes responses in the cortical auditory area and in parts of the cortical visual area. In turn, auditory and visual areas of the cerebral cortex project to similar regions of the cerebellar cortex. Earlier, mention was made of the finding that cerebellar cortex stimulation results in lesser increases, and in some instances decreases, in test-retest scores on certain performance tasks of the intelligence scale. Such performance sub-tests generally involve visual perception, visual alertness, and the coordination of visual perception with motor functions. In most of these functions the stimulation patients failed to increase in scores to a degree greater than would ordinarily be expected from practice effects. Furthermore, for both the seizure and hypertonic stimulation groups, postoperative increases are less than those shown by their comparison groups, suggesting the possibility of actual decreases. These data provided a first clue that in contrast to increases in verbal-motor output, the possibility exists of decrements in tasks involving spatial and visual perception functions. And, for the hypertonic stimulation group the Picture Arrangement and Object Assembly sub-tests actually decreased in score during the shorter range postoperative testing, a clearcut suggestion of some loss in functions related to visual-spatial integration.

The main body of evidence, however, with respect to visual-spatial perception was derived from response time scores on the Tachistoscope presentation of single and combined words and symbols. To recapitulate, it was noted that such scores (i.e., number of seconds to respond correctly) for the seizure stimulation group tended to increase during the shorter range postoperative period, relative to its comparison group which tended to improve somewhat in this function. In partial contrast, the hypertonic stimulation group tended to improve slightly, overall, relative to its comparison group. This difference was further amplified when the two stimulation groups were compared with each other, in which instance the seizure stimulation group worsened overall whereas the hypertonic stimulation group improved somewhat although these differences did not achieve statistical significance.

Closer analysis of the particular stimulus cards in which the seizure group performance worsened indicated the higher decrements in stimuli which involved double figures, specifically word-word, word-figure, and figure-word. Furthermore, the two highest decrements, word-word and figure-word, occurred in which the word was in the right half of the field of vision. In essence, the seizure stimulation group tended to worsen in identifying words of double stimulus cards, shorter range postoperatively, when the word appeared on the right field of vision. This is in contrast to both comparison groups, and to the hypertonic stimulation group whose greatest mean improvement was in the figure-word stimulus card, where the word appeared on the right half of the visual field.

The increased time required by the seizure group for accurate word identification may be described as an inhibition of some aspect of visual-perception. It should be noted here that in longer range testing these decrements no longer obtain, whether due to continuing practice effects, or to some rebalancing or redistribution of such functions in the central nervous system. Moreover, as previously noted, CFF scores, which represent another form of "perceptual efficiency", but not lateralized, tended to increase during both the shorter and longer range postoperative testing. Nevertheless, we are encountering somehow a reduction in the efficiency of exteroceptive input, an example perhaps, of CNS efferent control of its own input (cf Pribram, 1971). This control, ultimately, may be modulated by cerebral cortical sensory zones. As a working hypothesis, this process of inhibition may be related to ascending influences initiated from (right) cerebellar cortical stimulation which somehow alters sensory-perceptual areas of the (left) cerebral cortex, and vice versa. This hypothesis is compatible with the findings of Dow, Fernandez-Guardiola, and Manni (1962) who reported that cerebellar stimulation both inhibited cobalt produced epileptic waves and depressed sensory responses in the cerebral cortex. It also closely relates to the concept of Snider and his associates concerning cerebellar cortex modulation of cerebral sensory areas (Snider, Sato, & Mizuno, 1964; Snider, 1967; Snider, Mitra, & Sudilovsky, 1970). Alternately, and concomitantly, some ascending fibers from the superior cerebellar peduncle may pass through intralaminar thalamic nuclei and in turn might inhibit cells of the diffuse thalamocortical projection system, which in turn may be related to the decreased visual efficiency.

Many experimental data relate exteroceptive sensory functions to cerebellar action. Among the earliest reports concerning visual and auditory projections to the cerebellar cortex was that of Snider and Stowell (1944), a finding also related to the fact that a variety of visual and visual-motor responses would appear to be very much involved in patterns of coordination of movements. In turn, a study concerning responses of the cerebral cortex to cerebellar stimulation was undertaken by Henneman,

Cooke, and Snider (1952), in which instance the authors noted that stimulation of the anterior lobe and the lobulus simplex elicited responses in
the somatic sensory and motor areas of the contralateral cortex. Stimulation of the visual and auditory areas of the cerebellum yielded a response
in both auditory areas 1, although no clearcut effects were observed in
the visual cortex of the cerebrum.

In summarizing their concepts on the functions of the cerebellum
Dow and Moruzzi (1958) emphasized that the cerebellum is impinged upon
not only by proprioceptive volleys, but also by tactile, visual, auditory,
and even by visceral impulses. Moreover, cerebellifugal volleys reach
not only the postural centers of the brain stem and motor cortex, but also
project upon cerebral cortical areas not strictly related to motor functions
as well as upon several somatic and autonomic structures of the diencephalon and brain stem. Finally, even the spindle receptors and possibly
many sensory neurons may be influenced by the cerebellum. A control
thus may be exerted by the cerebellum in the sensory sphere and on autonomic functions. On this basis, an alternate hypothesis for the "inhibition"
of certain aspects of visual perception might concern the effects of cerebellar stimulation on sensory receptors, primary sensory neurons, and post-
primary sensory neurons. In effect, the inhibition, rather than directly
involving the sensory areas of the cerebral cortex may, through feedback
processes actually induce an inhibition of the sensory receptors or their
immediate neurons.

There are some more recent experimental data with respect to visual
learning and the cerebellum. In rats, Buchtel (1970) noted that visually
evoked responses come to the cerebellum by two routes, the first from the
optic nerve via tectal and pontine relays, and the second from primary
visual cortex of the cerebrum (Fadiga & Pupilli, 1964). Damage to the
rat cerebellum causes a deficiency in learning certain visual cues under
conditions of high motivation. In some animals, however, the learning
of certain stimuli was normal. The cerebellar damage evidently hindered
"learning" but not "performance" under conditions of high motivation.
Both placement and size of the lesion affected learning speed. The deficits were greatest with small lesions in lobule V (culmen) and small lesions in lobule VI (simplex) except when in the latter case they involve
medial cortex alone. The author suggests that there appears to be an
interaction between cerebellar damage and level of motivation, with the
cerebellum acting to reduce disruption of learning during periods of high
motivation by preventing overfacilitation of motor responses, especially in
tasks where inappropriate responses already have a high probability of
expression.

In dogs, ablation of the posterior cerebellum and lingula lead to deficiencies in spatial perception in which labyrinthine cues are necessary (Beritoff, 1965). Ablation of the entire cerebellum also results in losses of "vestibular" type of orientation in space. Such findings led Beritoff to postulate that the cerebellum contributes to the spatial function of the cerebral cortex, i.e., its capacity for projecting perceived objects into space and generating orienting movements toward these objects. Although only eye movements seem to be involved in the Tachistoscope alterations we noted, anterior (and posterior) cerebellar cortex may play some role in this type of visual-motor orientation inhibition, since functional movements of eye and body would seem to relate to much visual perception.

3. Emotional Functions (Depression, Anxiety, Tension, and Arousal)

The primary data concerning intellectual and visual-perceptual functions were derived from standardized tests in contrast to data with respect to the "emotional" functions now under consideration which were derived largely from observation of patients and interviews undertaken with them and their families at specifically stated times postoperatively. As previously indicated, almost invariably seizure stimulation patients reported alterations in these areas, primarily improvements, as did a portion of the hypertonic stimulation group. The general pattern was for patients to report varying degrees of reduction of preoperative depression, alleviation of tension and anxiety, and generally an increased feeling of well-being and optimism. Clearly, such "subjective" data must be interpreted with great caution, since many questions of reliability and validity of the data naturally arise, and furthermore there exists a wide variety of possible interpretations of these observations. Among the possible explanations, as previously noted, include the simple fact that generally seizure activity and spasticity were reduced in most instances during cerebellar stimulation, and that patients tended to be more optimistic with concomitant reduction in depression and anxiety and increased feelings of self-esteem. However, these impressions must be qualified to some degree. For example, in one instance (R.S.) very little in the way of actual seizure reduction was noted during the first two months following cerebellar cortex stimulation. Yet this patient reported "improved thinking", "increased relaxation", and a reduction in "anxiety and tension". In contrast, the one seizure stimulation patient who failed to describe any changes of this nature (M.B.) was observed by nurses and professional staff to have had significant improvement in seizure activity, and progress notes at various times postoperatively indicated that she appeared to be more relaxed, more calm, and less anxious than preoperatively.

One other behavioral variable, aggression, was particularly monitored by patients, their families, and the professional staff. Specifically,
this relates to episodes of aggression, hostile behavior, and loss of self-
control documented in the history of three seizure patients (W.B., M.C.,
and S.H.), behaviors which occurred most frequently during actual seizures, but in some instances as a behavior pattern even between seizures.
One other patient (B.M.) with a diagnosis of basilar artery thrombosis,
was observed preoperatively to have "extremely poor emotional control"
with frequent and inappropriate giggling and laughing. In each of these
instances, following several weeks of stimulation, there was observed by
the patient, his family, and the professional staff, a clearly defined
reduction in aggressive, violent, and uncontrolled behavior. In the case
of the three seizure patients, improved behavioral control correlated with
the decrease in the number and frequency of seizures, and might be interpreted, in part, simply within a pattern of seizure reduction and concomitant reduction of ictal phenomena. However, in two instances, observations and reports from the patient's family indicated a commensurate decrease of aggressive and acting out behavior even during times between
seizures. Furthermore, in the case of one non-seizure patient, reduction
in inappropriate laughter and poor self-control was noted after several
weeks of stimulation, despite the fact that rather minimal improvement
had occurred in his hypertonicity.

Three behavioral functions, perhaps related, must be considered at
this point. The first may be described as aggression and its correlates;
the second as anxiety and its concomitants; and the third as depression.
The notable reduction in aggression just described may clearly be described
as an instance of behavioral inhibition. It is quite probable that this behavioral inhibition is related to the same type of mechanism as the seizure
inhibition, representing ascending pathways of physiological inhibition from
the cerebellar cortex to other subcortical and cortical areas from which
seizure activity may originate in the individual instances. The possible
physiology of these mechanisms have been described in a number of experimental studies (Cooke & Snider, 1955; Dow & Moruzzi, 1958; Dow,
Fernandez-Guardiola, & Manni, 1962; Hutton, Frost & Foster, 1972) and
will not be repeated here. A specific thalamic role may be present.
Williams (1965), for example, has postulated that focal epileptic attacks
leading to a general convulsion abnormally activate thalamic reticular
structures which are essential to the development and spread of the general discharge. It is also possible that paleocerebellar cortex stimulation
may influence (inhibit) certain limbic structures, amygdala and hippocampus, for example, and result in seizure-aggressive reduction (Iwata &
Snider, 1959; Narabayashi, Nagao, Saito, Yoshida, & Nagahata, 1963;

Mark & Ervin, 1970).   Finally, there is some evidence that posteromedial hypothalamectomy may reduce aggressive behavior in some instances (Sano, Yoshioka, Ogashima, Ishijama, & Ohye, 1966).   This report, along with earlier experimental evidence that stimulation of the anterior cerebellar lobe may modify electrical activity of certain hypothalamic nuclei (e.g., ventromedial)(Ban, Inove, Ozaki & Korotsu, 1956; Zanchetti & Zoccolini, 1954) lends credence to a certain cerebello-hypothalamic factor in aggression reduction in those seizure stimulation patients.

The other behavioral alterations, notably anxiety and depression reduction, while in part related to seizure reduction and related physiological mechanisms, as well as to numerous psychological factors, might also be amenable to alternate explanations, in which cerebellar influences may participate.   In this respect, the inhibition-facilitation continuum may again be invoked.   According to Worden and Livingston (1961) there is anatomical evidence of reciprocal connections between the reticular formation and the cerebellum (Snider, 1950; Brodal, 1953; Cajal, 1955). Mollica, Moruzzi, and Naquet (1953), von Baumgarten (1954), Combs (1954), and others have shown that the reticular formation is capable of firing the cerebellum and that the cerebellum in turn is capable of firing the reticular formation.   It appears that the entire cerebellar mantle is aroused by reticular-formation stimulation very much in the same way as the cortex of the major cerebral hemisphere.   Moreover, among the feedback systems of the cerebellum are included fibers from the superior cerebellar peduncle which descend in the brain stem, terminating upon reticular nuclei, and then project back to the cerebellum.   Clearly, cerebellar-reticular systems may be activated as a result of paleo- and neocerebellar cortex stimulation.   These systems, in turn, play a significant role in the modulation of muscle "tone".   While the relationship of skeleto-muscular tone to anxiety or tension has been little explored, one may argue that considered as a continuum for any one individual, increased skeleto-muscular tone might lead to (i.e., be interpreted subjectively as) anxiety or tension, while reduction in such tone might in turn be regarded as anxiety or tension alleviation.   As Pribram (1971) noted tone is not merely the amount of spasticity of flaccidity of contractile tissue, "it is the state of readiness of the entire neuromuscular apparatus - the precondition for action (p. 226)".   This readiness, this precondition may, in subjective terms, be very much related to the muscular equivalent of felt anxiety.   Thus, it is conceivable that through modulation of cerebellar-reticular systems, yet to be fully delineated, a "tone-anxiety-tension" reduction may occur.   Furthermore, reticular and other descending cerebellar influences may in turn affect the activity of autonomic centers which involve visceral organs and hormone processes also related to somatic aspects of tension and anxiety.

There is much experimental evidence to suggest cerebellar relationships to such vegetative functions as circulation, respiration, digestion,
and to the endocrine glands (Dow & Moruzzi, 1958, pp. 290-309).
Recently, the effects of stimulation of the cerebellar vermis on some
vegetative functions and the electrical activity of limbic and other regions
of the brain were studied by Rasheed, Manchanda, and Anand (1970).
Lobules located more anteriorly in the vermis were more responsive than
those located posteriorly.   In anesthetized preparations the preponderance
was that of depressor responses and respiratory inhibition, whereas in
unanesthetized preparations mostly pressor responses were obtained on
stimulation of the vermian cortex.   Similarly in the anesthetized animals,
pupillary changes or intravesical pressure changes were not conspicuous.
On the other hand, marked but variable effects on the intravesical pressures and the pupillary changes were obtained on stimulation of the vermian cortex in the unanesthetized preparations.   Results do not permit the
parcellation of the cerebellar vermis into anterior sympathicotonic or posterior parasympathicotonic regions, but it was suggested that the fiber
pathways involved in producing these responses of cerebellar stimulation
can be more fruitfully analyzed by correlating the neuroaxial hierarchy
with the complexity or type of autonomic activity pattern.   Stimulation of
the cerebellum also produces other autonomic responses.   Excitation of the
anterior lobe inhibits vasoconstrictor and respiratory mechanisms, and stimulation of the median lobule produces parasympathomimetic effects on pup-
illory responses (Grossman, 1967).

If a pattern of inhibition in skeleto-muscular tone, vegetative functions, and hormonal output occurs, then one may conceive of a resulting
reduction in subjectively felt anxiety or tension.   One also may argue
that even facilitation of certain descending fibers may also reduce skeleto-
muscular tone in some instances and consequently relate to anxiety and
tension reduction.   The feelings of depression described preoperatively by
some patients, and seemingly alleviated by cerebellar stimulation, may
represent an epiphenomenon of the anxiety and tension, a psychodynamic
factor related to the patient's overall condition, an alteration in patterns
of biogenic amines, or some combination of these and perhaps other factors.   Further investigation is warranted in this area.

4. Role of Side, Site, and Frequency of Cerebellar Stimulation

In the earlier discussions of intellectual functions, visual-perception,
and emotional functions, brief implications were drawn with respect to the
possible role of side and site of the cerebellar stimulation, and there also

exists experimental evidence that frequency of stimulation may be an important variable. It is our present purpose to consider in further detail
some aspects of side, site, and frequency. However, the relatively small
number of patients which fall into each of the specific sub-categories involved does not allow for useful statistical assessment and much of the
following discussion is based upon small numbers, observation of data, and
mean scores, and must be considered suggestive rather than definitive.

The area involving the strongest possibility for reliable interpretation
concerns the side of cerebellar stimulation. In this instance, it will be
recalled that right-sided cerebellar stimulation, which included all the
seizure stimulation patients, resulted in decrements in visual-perception
for words in the right field of vision in contrast to no reduction, and even
increases for the hypertonic group, one of whom had right and two others
of whom had left-sided stimulation (three hypertonic patients were untest-
able on the Tachistoscope). In contrast, the two hypertonic patients with
left cerebellar cortical stimulation showed decrements to stimuli on the left
field of vision whether for a word or a figure. This finding, while not
submitted to statistical assessment because of the small numbers involved,
tends to extend previous concepts of cortical (Reitan, 1954, ·1955; Bauer,
1957; McFie & Zangwill, 1960; Piercy, Hecaen, & Ajuriaguerra, 1960;
Piercy & Smyth, 1962; Piercy, 1964), and subcortical (Allan, Turner, &
Gadea-Ciria, 1966; Riklan & Levita, 1968; Bell, 1969) lateralization to
the cerebellum. In essence, verbal-symbolic perceptual functions appear
to be inhibited by right cerebellar stimulation, whereas spatial-symbolic
perception is altered by left cerebellar stimulation. The decussation of
ascending cerebellar pathways would seem to provide a suitable anatomic
basis for such a finding. With respect to verbal-motor output, stimulation
of either cerebellar hemisphere seems to have a facilitating effect. Further studies are required in this area to determine the possible role of
occipital lobe manipulation during surgery.

Interpretation of the role of site and frequency of stimulation becomes
somewhat confounded by the fact that in most instances side, site, and
frequency were similar or identical for the seizure group on the one hand,
whereas sides differed for the hypertonic group, but site and frequency were
similar. Nevertheless, some comparisons were possible. In the first instance a statistical comparison to 2 seizure patients with anterior and posterior sites, with respect to VIQ, PIQ, Memory Quotient, and the Tachistoscope presentations. On the basis of two-tailed tests no significant or
near significant differences were found in performance, with the exception
of the single figure of the Tachistoscope in which p = .27, two-tailed,
was found, suggesting a slight tendency for the patients with combined
anterior and posterior stimulation to improve in performance pre to shorter

range, whereas the anterior stimulation group tended to worsen. This slight trend, combined with previous data, might suggest that the decrement of response to spatial-visual stimuli might conceivably be related more to anterior than posterior placement, although the data are highly tenuous in this respect.

With respect to frequency of stimulation, a similar data analysis problem exists as did with respect to anterior and posterior placement. That is to say, the general pattern was for the seizure disorder group to have frequencies of 10 cycles per second and for the hypertonic group to have frequencies of 200 cycles per second. Since the frequency data correlated both with the site and side, it was not possible, statistically or clinically, to separate the alterations or effects of stimulation frequency and placement from that of side of lesion. Further data are required in this area, and are now in the process of being collected.

SUMMARY

In summary, 13 patients undergoing chronic cerebellar lobe stimulation primarily for the relief of seizure disorders or hypertonicity underwent extensive psychological testing and interviewing before surgery and during the shorter and longer range stages of chronic cerebellar stimulation. Included among the group were 7 seizure patients and 6 hypertonic patients (with the exception of 1 individual with intention myoclonus) and 2 groups of comparison, unoperated subjects.

The pattern of findings indicated a form of verbal-motor facilitation for the stimulation groups, in contrast to decrements in visual-spatial perception. The verbal-motor facilitation held for chronic stimulation whether of seizure or hypertonic patients, of left or right side, of the anterior or paleo-cerebellar cortex, and for high or low frequency stimulation. Decrements in visual-spatial function tended to be more closely associated with the seizure stimulation group where placements were primarily in the right cerebellar lobe, and in which all individuals had anterior placements (3 had posterior placements as well), and the frequency of stimulation was within the lower area. In this respect, a lateralization effect also obtained in which visual-perceptual functions showed greater decrements on the right field of vision, particularly for words, for individuals with right cerebellar lobe stimulation. In contrast, left cerebellar lobe stimulation tended to reduce efficiency on the left field of vision, both for words and figures. In most patients reduction of anxiety, tension, and depression were reported, for both the seizure and hypertonic stimulation groups.

Better control of aggression and emotion in general was observed following chronic stimulation, particularly in three patients with histories of aggressive and assaultive behavior associated with seizures but also occurring between seizures.

Hypotheses were offered for the behavioral alterations in terms of neural systems inhibited or facilitated by cerebellar stimulation, although alternate possibilities were noted also. With respect to the cerebellar hypotheses it was suggested that as a result of cerebellar cortex stimulation a facilitation of verbal-motor output occurs in contrast to a decrement in visual-perceptual input, and that the latter tends to be lateralized in a manner similar to the lateralization frequently reported for cortical and thalamic areas. The intimate relationship between sensory, vestibular and motor functions was emphasized. Reduction in anxiety, tension, and aggression was related to possible mechanisms in which the cerebellum influences reticular systems and their secondary effects through ascending and descending pathways which modulate cortical function as well as somato-muscular and visceral-hormonal mechanisms. The preliminary nature of these findings, and particularly of the interpretations, was emphasized, and clearly more extensive studies are indicated in this area.

REFERENCES

ALLAN, C.M., TURNER, J.W., & GADEA-CIRIA, M. Investigations into speech disturbances following stereotaxic surgery for parkinsonism. Brit. J. Dis. Commun. 1:55-59, 1966.

BAN, T., INOUE, K., OZAKI, S., & KUROTSU, T. Interrelation between anterior lobe of cerebellum and hypothalamus in rabbit. Med. J. Osaka Univ. 7:101-115, 1956.

BAUER, R.W. & WEPMAN, J.M. Lateralization of cerebral functions. J. Speech Hear. Dis. 20:171-177, 1955.

BAUMGARTEN von, R., MOLLICA, A., & MORUZZI, G. Modulierung der Entladungsfrequenzeinzelner Zellen der Substantia reticularis durch corticofugale und cerebellare Impulse. Pflug. Arch. ges. Physiol. 259:56-78, 1954.

BELL, D.S. Speech functions of the thalamus inferred from the effects of thalamotomy. Brain, 91:619-638, 1969.

BENDER, L. "A Visual-Motor Gestalt Test and Its Clinical Use." American Orthopsychiatric Association Research Monograph, No. 3, 1938.

BERITOFF, J.S. "Neural Mechanisms of Higher Vertebrate Behavior". Boston: Little, Brown, 1965.

BREMER, F. Le cervelet. In Roger, G.H. & Binet, L. (Eds.) "Traité
de Physiologie Normale et Pathologique", Vol. 10, pt. 1-2.
Paris: Masson, 1935.

BRODAL, A. Reticulo-cerebellar connections in the cat. An experimental study. J. Comp. Neurol. 98:113-153, 1953.

BRODAL, A. & ROSSI, G.F. Ascending fibers in brain stem reticular
formation of cat. Arch. Neurol. Psychiat. 74:68-87, 1955.

BROOKHART, J.M. The cerebellum. In Field, J. (Ed.) "Handbook
of Physiology". Section 1, Neurophysiology II. Washington:
American Physiological Society, 1960, pp. 1240-1280.

BUCHTAL, H.A. Visual-learning deficits following cerebellar damage in
rats. J. Comp. Physiol. Psychol. 72:296-305, 1970.

CAJAL, S. Ramon y. "Histologie du système nerveux de l'homme et des
vértébrés." Translated from the Spanish by L. Azoulay (1909-11).
Madrid: Instituto Ramon y Cajal. Vol. 1, 1952, Vol. II, 1955.

CHAMBERS, W.W. & SPRAGUE, J.M. Functional localization in the
cerebellum. II. Somatotopic organization in cortex and nuclei.
Arch. Neurol. Psychiat. 74:653-680, 1955.

COOKE, T.M. & SNIDER, R.S. Some cerebellar influences on electrically induced cerebral seizures. Epilepsia, Series III, 4:19-28, 1955.

COONS, W.H. & PEACOCK, E.P. Inter-examiner reliability of the
WAIS with mental hospital patients. OPA Quart. July 1959.

COMBS, C.M. Electro-anatomical study of cerebellar localization:
Stimulation of various afferents. J. Neurophysiol. 17:123-142,
1954.

COOPER, I.S., CRIGHEL, E., & AMIN, I. Clinical and physiological
effects of stimulation of the paelocerebellum in humans. J. Amer.
Geriatr. Soc. 21:40-43, 1973a.

COOPER, I.S., CRIGHEL, E., & AMIN, I. Effect of chronic stimulation of cortex of paleocerebellum and neocerebellum upon muscular
hypertonus and EEG of neocortex of man. 25th Annual Meeting
American Academy of Neurology, Boston, Mass. April 1973b.

COOPER, I.S. & GILMAN, S. Effect of chronic cerebellar stimulation
upon epilepsy in man. 98th Annual Meeting, American Neurological Assn., July 11-13, 1973c, Montreal.

CROSBY, E.C., HUMPHREY, T., & LAUER, E.W. "Correlative Anatomy
of the Nervous System". New York: The MacMillan Co., 1962.

DOW, R.S., FERNÁNDEZ-GUARDIOLA, A., & MANNI, E. The
influence of the cerebellum on experimental epilepsy. Electroenceph. Clin. Neurophysiol. 14:383-398, 1962.

DOW, R.S. & MORUZZI, G. "The Physiology and Pathology of the
Cerebellum". Minneapolis: University of Minnesota Press, 1958.

DEUTCH, J.A. & DEUTCH, D.   "Physiological Psychology".   Homewood,
    Ill.: Dorsey, 1966.
DRACHMAN, D.A. & ARBIT, J.   Memory and the hippocampal complex.
    II. Is memory a multiple process?   Arch. Neurol. 15:52-61, 1966.
DUSSER de BARENNE, J.G.   Experimentelle Physiologie des Kleinhirns.
    In Bumke, O. & Foerster, O. (Eds.) "Handbuch der Neurologie"
    Vol. 2.   Berlin: J. Springer, 1937, pp. 235-267.
ECCLES, J.C., ITO, M., & SZENTAGOTHAI, J.   "The Cerebellum as
    a Neuronal Machine".   New York: Springer-Verlag, 1967.
FADIGA, E. & PUPILLI, G.C.   Teleceptive components of the cerebel-
    lar function.   Physiol. Rev. 44:432-486, 1970.
FOX, C.A. & SNIDER, R.S. (Eds).   "The Cerebellum.   Progress in
    Brain Research".   Vol. 25.   Amsterdam: Elsevier, 1967.
GRIMM, R.J., FRAZEE, J.G., BELL, C.C., KAWASAKI, T., & DOW,
    R.S.   Quantitative studies in cobalt model epilepsy: The effect
    of cerebellar stimulation.   Int. J. Neurol. 7:126-140, 1970.
GROSSMAN, S.P.   "A Textbook of Physiological Psychology".   New
    York: Wiley, 1967.
GUERTIN, W.H., FRANK, G.H., & RAVIN, A.I.   Research with the
    Wechsler-Bellevue Intelligence Scale.   Psychol. Bull. 53:235-257,
    1956.
HENNEMAN, E., COOKE, P.M., & SNIDER, R.S.   Cerebellar projec-
    tion to the cerebral cortex.   Assn. Res. Nerv. Ment. Dis. Proc.
    30:317-333, 1952.
HOLMES, G.   The cerebellum of man (Hughlings Jackson memorial
    lecture).   Brain, 62:1-30, 1939.
HONIGFELD, G.   Neurological efficiency, perception and personality.
    Perc. Mot. Skills, 15:531-553, 1962.
HUTTON, J.T., FROST, J.D., Jr., & FOSTER, J.   The influence of
    the cerebellum in cat penicillin epilepsy.   Epilepsia, 13:401-408,
    1972.
HOROWITZ, H.J.   "Psychosocial Function in Epilepsy".   Springfield:
    Charles C. Thomas, 1970.
IWATA, K. & SNIDER, R.S.   Cerebello-hippocampal influences on the
    electroencephalogram.   Electroenceph. Clin. Neurophysiol. 11:
    439-446, 1959.
KIMURA, D.   Some effects of temporal-lobe damage on auditory
    perception.   Canad. J. Psychol. 15:156-165, 1961.
KREINDLER, A.   Active arrest mechanisms of epileptic seizures.
    Epilepsia, 3:329-337, 1962.
LARSELL, O. & JANSEN, J.   "The Comparative Anatomy and Histology
    of the Cerebellum. The Human Cerebellum, Cerebellar Connections,
    and Cerebellar Cortex".   Minneapolis: University of Minnesota
    Press, 1972.

MARK, V.H. & ERVIN, F. "Violence and the Brain". New York: Harper & Row, 1970.

MARR, D. A theory of cerebellar cortex. J. Physiol. 202:437-470, 1969.

McFIE, J. & ZANGWILL, O.L. Visual constructive disabilities associated with lesions of the right cerebral hemisphere. Brain, 83:243-260, 1960.

MILNER, B. Psychological defects produced by temporal lobe excision. In "The Brain and Human Behavior." Research Publications of the Association for Research on Nervous and Mental Disease. Baltimore: Williams & Wilkins, 1958, pp. 244-257.

MILNER, B. Amnesia following operation on the temporal lobes. In Whitty, C.W.M. & Zangwill, O.L. (Eds.) "Amnesia". London: Butterworth, 1966, pp. 109-133.

MILNER, B. Brain mechanisms suggested by studies of temporal lobes. In Darley, F.L. (Ed.) "Brain Mechanisms Underlying Speech and Language". New York: Grune & Stratton, 1967, pp. 122-145.

MISIAK, H. The Flicker-Fusion test and its applications. Trans. N.Y. Acad. Sci. 29:616-622, 1967.

MOLLICA, A., MORUZZI, G., & NAQUET, R. Decharges reticulaires induites par la polarisation du cerevelet; leurs rapports le tonus postural et la reaction d'eveil. Electroenceph. Clin. Neurophysiol. 5:571-584, 1953.

MORUZZI, G. "Problems in Cerebellar Physiology". Springfield: Charles C. Thomas, 1950.

MORUZZI, G. & MAGOUN, H.W. Brain stem reticular formation and activation of the EEG. Electroenceph. Clin. Neurophysiol. 1: 455-473, 1949.

NARABAYASHI, H., NAGAO, T., SAITO, Y., YOSHIDA, M. & NAGAHATA, M. Stereotaxic amygdalotomy for behavior disorders. Arch. Neurol. 9:11-26, 1963.

NASHOLD, B.S., Jr. & SLAUGHTER, D.G. Effects of stimulating or destroying the deep cerebellar regions in man. J. Neurosurg. 31: 172-186, 1969.

PALESTINI, M., ROSSI, G.F., & ZANCHETTI, A. An electrophysiological analysis of pontine reticular regions showing different anatomical organization. Arch. Ital. de Biol. 95:97-109, 1957.

PIERCY, M. The effects of cerebral lesions on intellectual functions: A review of current research trends. Brit. J. Psychol. 110:310-352, 1964.

PIERCY, M., HECAEN, H., & AJURIAGUERRA, J. de. Constructional apraxia associated with unilateral cerebral lesions - left and right-sided cases compared. Brain, 85:775-790, 1962.

PIERCY, M. & SMYTH, V.   Right hemisphere dominance for certain
    non-verbal intellectual skills.   Brain, 85:775-790, 1962.
PRIBRAM, K.H.   "Languages of the Brain".   Englewood Cliffs, N.J.:
    Prentice Hall, 1971.
RASHEED, B.M.A., MANCHANDA, S.K., & ANAND, B.K.   Effects
    of the stimulation of paleocerebellum on certain vegetative functions
    in the cat.   Brain Research, 20:293-308, 1970.
REITAN, R.M.   Intelligence and language functions in dysphasic patients.
    Dis. Nerv. Syst. 15:131-137, 1954.
REITAN, R.M.   Certain differential effects of left and right cerebral
    lesions in human adults.   J. Comp. Physiol. Psychol. 48:474-477,
    1955.
RIKLAN, M., DILLER, L., WEINER, H., & COOPER, I.S.   Psycholog-
    ical studies on effects of chemosurgery of the basla ganglia in
    parkinsonism.   I. Intellectual functioning.   Arch. Gen. Psychiat.
    2:22-31, 1960.
RIKLAN, M., LEVITA, E., & COOPER, I.S.   Psychological effects of
    bilateral subcortical surgery for Parkinson's Disease.   J. Nerv.
    Ment. Dis. 141:403-409, 1966.
RIKLAN, M. & LEVITA, E.   "Subcortical Correlates of Human Behavior".
    Baltimore: Williams & Wilkins, 1969.
ROSSI, G.   Sugli Effeti conseguenti alla stimolazione contemporanea
    della corteccia cerebrale e du qyekka cervekkare.   Arch. Fisiol.
    10:389-399, 1912.
SANO, K., YOSHIOKA, M., OGASHIWA, M., ISHIJIMA, B., &
    OHYE, C.   Posteromedial hypothalamectomy in the treatment of
    aggressive behavior.   Confin. Neurol. 27:164-167, 1966.
SERAFETINIDES, E.A. & FALCONER, M.A.   Some observations on
    memory impairment after temporal lobectomy for epilepsy.   J.
    Neurol. Neurosurg. Psychiat. 25:251-255, 1962.
SNIDER, R.S.   Recent contributions to the anatomy and physiology of
    the cerebellum.   Arch. Neurol. Psychiat. 64:196-219, 1950.
SNIDER, R.S.   Interrelations of cerebellum and brain stem.   Res. Publ.
    Assn. Nerv. Ment. Dis. 30:267-281, 1950.
SNIDER, R.S.   Functional alterations of cerebral sensory areas by the
    cerebellum.   The Cerebellum.   In Fox, C.A. & Snider, R.S. (Eds.)
    "Progress in Brain Research", V. 25.   Amsterdam: Elsevier, 1967,
    pp. 322-332.
SNIDER, R.S., MITRA, J., & SUDILOVSKY, A.   Cerebellar effects on
    the cerebrum.   A microelectrical analysis of somatosensory cortex.
    Int. J. Neurol. 7:141-151, 1970.
SNIDER, R.S., SATO, K., & MIZUNO, S.   Cerebellar influences on
    evoked cerebral responses.   J. Neurol. Sci. 1:325-339, 1964.

SNIDER, R.S. & SINIS, S.   Cerebellar influences on sensory relay
    nuclei of thalamus.   Int. J. Neurol. 8:230-237, 1971.

SNIDER, R.S. & STOWELL, A.   Receiving areas of the tactile, auditory
    and visual systems in the cerebellum.   J. Neurophysiol. 7:331-
    357, 1944.

SNIDER, R.S. & WETZEL, N.   Electroencephalographic changes induced
    by stimulation of the cerebellum in man.   Electroenceph. Clin.
    Neurophysiol. 18:175-183, 1965.

STEISEL, I.M.   The relationship between test and retest scores on the
    W-B Scale Form I for selected college students.   J. Genet.
    Psychol. 79-155-162, 1951a.

STEISEL, I.M.   Retest changes in W-B scores as a function of the time
    interval between examinations.   J. Genet. Psychol. 79:199-203,
    1951b.

STERIADE, M. & STOUPEL, N.   Contribution a l'etude des relations
    entre l'aire auditive du cervelet et l'ecore cerebrale chez le chat.
    Electroenceph. Clin. Neurophysiol. 12:119-136, 1960.

TRUEX, R.C. & CARPENTER, M.D.   "Human Neuroanatomy".   6th Ed.
    Baltimore: Williams & Wilkins, 1969.

VICTOR, M., ANGEVINE, J.B., MANCALL, E.L., & FISHER, C.M.
    Memory loss with lesions of hippocampal formation.   Arch. Neurol.
    5:26-45, 1961.

WECHSLER, D.   "The Measurement and Appraisal of Adult Intelligence".
    4th Ed.   Baltimore: Williams & Wilkins, 1958.

WECHSLER, D.   A standardized memory scale for clinical use.   J.
    Psychol. 19:87-95, 1945.

WECHSLER, D. & STONE, C.P.   "Wechsler Memory Scale Manual".
    New York: The Psychological Corp., 1959.

WHITESIDE, J.A. & SNIDER, R.S.   Relation of cerebellum to upper
    brain stem.   J. Neurophysiol. 16:397, 1953.

WILLIAMS, D.   The thalamus and epilepsy.   Brain, 88:539-556, 1965.

WORDEN, F.G. & LIVINGSTON, R.B.   Brain stem reticular formation.
    In Sheer, D.E.C. (Ed)   "Electrical Stimulation of the Brain".
    Austin: University of Texas Press, 1961, pp. 263-276.

ZANCHETTI, A. & ZOCCOLINI, A.   Autonomic hypothalamic outbursts
    elicited by cerebellar stimulation.   J. Neurophysiol. 17:475-483,
    1954.

SOME ETHICAL CONSIDERATIONS OF CEREBELLAR STIMULATION AS AN INNOVATIVE THERAPY IN HUMANS

Harmon C. Smith

The Divinity School
Duke University
Durham, North Carolina

Since words like "ethics" and "morals" are heir to many variant interpretations and meanings, I want to begin with a kind of apologia pro vita sua which will at least indicate what I understand myself to be doing in this paper.

Moral philosophy or ethics is typically characterized by a spirit of radical inquiry; it does not attempt to supply solutions for moral dilemmas, but it does undertake to provide a rational framework for comprehending the complexities of moral judgment. Historically, therefore, ethics has been distinguished from morals in that ethics is the formal study and analysis of the values which inform behavior; while morals is the word for those phenomena (particularly actions, behaviors, codes of rules, etc.) which are studied by ethics.

Ethics, then, has no immediate concern for furnishing any form of specific moral guidance, such as rules for right behavior; that is the purpose and function of particular systems of morality (e.g., the Ten Commandments, the Hippocratic Oath, or the "code of ethics on human experimentation" called the Declaration of Helsinki). On the other hand, ethics impinges on morals at the point of assessing coherence and comprehensiveness between categories like character and conduct, belief and behavior, affirmation and action. Moral codes call for conformity; ethics requires reflection.

In the history of medicine, phrases like "respect for life", "relief of suffering", and "service to mankind" provide the ethical context for

343

the practice of medicine. Physicians are expected to honor these formal
and generalized maxims; and I have yet, in my personal experience, to
meet a physician who would (if allowed to say what he means by these
phrases!) refuse to affirm them. But it is precisely in this "saying what
he means" -- whether in his day-to-day practice or in some more formal
attempt to articulate his understanding -- that the physician more or less
systematically and critically reflects upon these terms and their implica-
tion(s) for his personal and professional conduct and choice-making.
Socrates is reported, in the Apology, to have said, "the unexamined life
is not worth living". To examine life, in terms of the values which support and inform it, is to practice ethics.

Within the scope of this definition, physicians are of course daily engaged (in either implicit or explicit ways) in practicing ethics; and it
might appear redundant, therefore, to solicit the opinion of non-medical
persons on medical practices. Probably the clearest and most succint
reasons for the "external examiner" in these settings are that different
interests and competences are at stake in patient care -- a fact already
acknowledged by many disciplinary sub-specialties within medicine itself--
and that one of the obvious ways by which comprehensive evaluation is
achieved is to invite a "consultant" whose special interest and knowledge
will hopefully complement and enlarge awareness and perspective.

I do not intend, however, to emphasize this difference out of pro-
portion. There is surely an important and profound sense in which medical and non-medical professionals share a common interest -- which we
could perhaps call "health" or "well-being" or "patient care" -- and we
ought to affirm and celebrate this, since without it there would be no
serious reason for dialogue between us. But as important to purposive
and meaningful conversation as commonality is, we should neither ignore
nor disparage our differences which are sometimes competing or conflicting. Because this paper represents "clinical investigation" by an ethicist,
and because some of my questions may seem to be provincial to my own
discipline, it is appropriate to state these working assumptions from the
beginning. Of course, none of this would be either needed or fitting
except for the uncommon opportunity afforded me to undertake this study;
and I want here to acknowledge my thanks for that.

The introduction of a new method of treatment -- in this case, electrical stimulation of the cerebellum for relief of physiologic motor disorder -- is particularly well-suited to ethical examination at several points;
and four areas of ethical inquiry appear to be specifically relevant to this
procedure: 1) the suitability of the procedure for human trials; 2) the

adequacy of consents; 3) the efficacy of the treatment; and 4) certain implications of the operation for mind and mood manipulation, or behavior modification. These areas do not exhaust the ethical significance of cerebellar stimulation, but they are arguably among the obvious and urgent considerations for ethical examination.

1. Human experimentation is inevitable, most of us would agree, with any innovative technique irrespective of that technique's prior theoretical reliability and its successful laboratory bench and animal studies. Indeed, it is not only generally accepted now that human experimentation is necessary in order to develop valid conclusions; but, given the operational values of modern society in general and scientific medicine in particular, human trials are generally acknowledged to be highly desirable in order to push back further the frontiers of human knowledge and thereby increase (hopefully) the human capacity for exercising deliberate and discriminating control over human health and life, and disease and death. But the need for scientific inquiry in order to advance scientific knowledge must be reconciled with the inviolability which our society accords to persons, their minds and bodies. In this society it is axiomatic that the right to personal inviolability forbids medical or scientific violation of that right without competent, knowing, and voluntary consent.

Therefore it is important to keep in mind also that human experimentation is not limited to trials of innovative therapies with the intention of improving a specific condition in a particular patient or population. More precisely, human investigation affects human subjects in three distinct (but not always separable) ways: a) as a direct benefit (e.g., by applying a new drug or surgical technique which is thought to be immediately pertinent to the primary patient's physiologic disease); or b) as an indirect benefit (e.g., by acquiring information or data that is uncertainly related to the subject's immediate distress); or c) of no benefit (e.g., by studying physiologic processes, drug effect, etc., which have no known or suspected relevance for the subject). The first two types almost always occur in the context of clinical care; the third type occurs (almost always) outside clinical care because normal volunteers are used as either experimental subjects or controls.

In view of the present widespread public and professional interest in human experimentation, it is important to delineate these types precisely in order to assess particular experimental therapeutics accurately. Moreover, because electrical stimulation of the cerebellum has been and is being employed in the treatment of patients with physiologic motor disorders, this procedure is accountable as one which combines professional care with clinical research, i.e., type (a) above. Among several professional "codes of ethics" which bear upon human experimentation, the World Medical Association's 1964 "Declaration of Helsinki" provides tests for the ethical acceptability of a procedure like cerebellar stimulation. Section II of that declaration, on "Clinical Research Combined with Professional Care, "states:

"1. In the treatment of the sick person the doctor must be free to use a new therapeutic measure if in his judgment it offers hope of saving life, re-establishing health, or alleviating suffering.

If at all possible, consistent with patient psychology, the doctor should obtain the patient's freely given consent after the patient has been given a full explanation. In case of legal incapacity consent should also be procured from the legal guardian; in case of physical incapacity the permission of the legal guardian replaces that of the patient.

2. The doctor can combine clinical research with professional care, the objective being the acquisition of new medical knowledge, only to the extent that clinical research is justified by its therapeutic value for the patient."

The ethical question here, quite directly, is: how does electrical stimulation of the cerebellum for treatment of physiologic motor disorder fulfill, or fail to fulfill, these criteria for acceptable human investigation when combined with clinical care?

The theoretical bases for controlling spasticity by stimulating the cerebellum have long been known; and successful experimentation with animals (cats and rats) was demonstrated many years ago. Dr. Cooper's paper, in this volume, has described the scientific history and development of cerebellar stimulation. Now, in view of these achievements, one must ask: If it is theoretically sound and laboratory demonstrated that spasticity and/or convulsive seizures can be relieved by chronic cerebellar stimulation, if the surgical and neuroanatomy problems could be resolved, and if the procedure could be done with reasonable knowledge of safety and absence of inordinate risk, would installation of stimulating electrodes on the cerebellum offer "hope of saving life, re-establishing health, or alleviating suffering" in selected spastic or epileptic patients?

These patients are not in immediate threat of death, and therefore the way(s) in which this procedure would offer hope of saving life must be more broadly conceived than as avoiding or deferring imminent death. The procedure, if effective, would surely tend toward re-establishing health in the measure to which patients developed seizure control and/or realized relief of spasticity and hopefully regained use of limbs and movement. Experience with 32 patients to date, whose conditions include cerebral palsy, stroke, spastic hemiplegia, amyotrophic lateral sclerosis, and intractable epilepsy, has been generally encouraging; and that assessment, together with the absence of any presently viable alternative therapy, would appear to support the judgment that this procedure meets the criteria of the Declaration of Helsinki. There was and is hope, now relatively well-founded, for "saving life" through relief of symptomatic distress (which I take to be one of the ways by which health is established) and relief of suffering.

In order to guarantee further the appropriateness of human investigations, it is now accepted procedure in many hospitals and medical centers (and in all those which receive government grants) that peer-review of experimental protocols be undertaken and approval given before inauguration of clinical trials. A "clinical research committee" exists in the institution where electrical stimulation of the cerebellum was inaugurated; but, owing to the general absence of clinical trials of innovative therapies in this institution, the committee is largely dysfunctional unless an application for a grant is involved. When it has acted, its role has been entirely advisory in this capacity. There is, then no peer committee per se which requires protocol review of clinical investigations which involve human subjects.

I do not suppose for an instant that decisions-by-committee are inherently or always better than those taken by an individual, nor am I unaware that the history of medicine is replete with incidents of pioneering investigators who have heroically swum against the stream of conventional wisdom. Nevertheless, it is not inconsequential to consider the advantages and disadvantages of a decision-making process which allocates to individuals adjudication of the large range of issues ineluctably at stake in innovative therapies. I do not intend this retrospective raising of that question to be pedantic, but only to indicate again the spirit of radical inquiry which characterizes moral philosophy.

As an ethicist, I do not of course claim competence to judge the scientific and technical merit of a proposal for innovative therapy except as any well-informed layman might be. Nor can we probably venture a meaningful judgment, from the present retrospective viewpoint, as to the technical or ethical propriety of the initial protocol for the cerebellar stimulation procedure, even though clinical experience is preliminarily supportive of the initial expectations from this new procedure. But it is precisely that need for expertise and competence at the outset, which the review committee ostensibly represents, which raises questions about the inauguration of an investigative therapeutic without appropriate peer review and sanction.

To my first question, then -- i.e., whether this procedure was, in its conception and inauguration, suitable for human trials -- I have not come to a clear and precise answer. All of us, as the cliche goes, have 20/20 hindsight, and in retrospect the procedure appears to have offered some patients a new hope without exposing them to inordinate risk; indeed, some of the patients have received demonstrable benefit from the procedure. The matter of initial review, however, remains a lacuna.

2. The second principal area of ethical inquiry has to do with the adequacy of patient consent to surgery. Here I want to draw rather extensively upon interviews with patients and their families, both pre- and postoperatively. I have chosen this method for two pre-eminent reasons: first, the formal validity of the consent mechanism ultimately lies in the patient's own voluntary and understanding "yes" to the physician's proposal; and, secondly, I have participated in and observed enough consent-getting to know that both physicians and third-party observers like myself may be prematurely satisfied with the adequacy of the consent given.

Owing to the limited time during which these studies were undertaken, and the absence of a control group against which these responses could be measured, it might be argued that these findings are serendipitous and not representative of all (or even a majority of) patients undergoing the procedure for cerebellar stimulation. Nevertheless, the six patients studied, together with their families, constitute 25% of those who have received this therapy; and extensive interviews with them, while not definitive, may yet be instructive at several points in the consent situation.

Preoperative understanding by patients varied considerably with respect to both general awareness and specific detail. Three of the patients studied were, by reason of age, legally incompetent to give valid consent; and in these cases it is interesting to compare patient perceptions with parental comprehensions.

The youngest patient, a 14-year old boy, knew that he was admitted "for the other operation...last time they did the cryo operation and it

TABLE 1

Personal and Medical Profile of Patients Interviewed

Patient	Age/Sex	Previous Surgical Procedures for Present Complaint	Diagnosis	Surgical Procedure
R.L.	14/M	1 – Performed at St. Barnabas Hospital for opposite side; successful	Cerebral Palsy with choreoathetosis	Left suboccipital craniectomy, anterior and posterior; cerebellar stimulator installed unilaterally
D.P.	16/M	None	Cerebral Palsy with involuntary movements in all limbs and quadriparetic condition	Suboccipital craniectomy, anterior and posterior; cerebellar stimulator installed unilaterally
R.K.	17/M	3 – Performed at St. Barnabas Hospital, for same side; relieved involuntary movements but not spasticity	Cerebral Palsy with hemi–athetosis and left spasticity	Suboccipital craniectomy, anterior and posterior; cerebellar stimulator installed
W.B.	24/M	7 – All performed elsewhere	Epilepsy; right temporal and right frontal lobe seizure disorders	Left suboccipital craniectomy, anterior and posterior; cerebellar stimulator installed unilaterally
B.M.	26/M	None	Thrombosis of the basilar artery with partial quadriparesis, 10 years' duration	Suboccipital craniectomy, anterior and posterior; cerebellar stimulator installed, left cerebellum
D.C.	39/F	None	Intention Myoclonus	Suboccipital craniectomy, cerebellar stimulator installed left and right cerebellum

stopped my right side from shaking....I'm glad they won't use the head-
clamp tomorrow because they used that before and it hurt". He could not
explain in any detail what awaited him in the OR; nevertheless, he rather
looked forward to surgery and expressed no anxiety about it.

An extended conversation with the boy's father, who signed the consent, disclosed that he had not discussed the surgical procedure except
during an initial conversation when his son was admitted. At that time
Mr. L. expressed the hope that "something could be done" for his son.
The mother sometime later discussed the procedure "with one of the doctors" by telephone, and that information was also relayed to the father.
Mr. L. was not certain when he had signed the consent form, but thought
that it was probably done at the time of his son's admission. The consent
form is illustrated in Figure 3. He expressed no misgiving about his con-
sent-giving, and gave as his reason a profound trust and confidence in the
doctors: "I would never go back on the doctors", he said. "If my son
goes through this and has no improvement, the operation was worth it....
there is nowhere else I know that can help these kids so much...no matter
how things work out, it's the Lord's will". It may be worthy of noting
here that in this case the father's sense of trust and confidence in the surgeons was probably due to the successful alleviation of his son's cerebral
palsy tremor of his right extremities, which was accomplished by the first
operation a year earlier.

Another patient, D.P., is unable to speak due to his totally incapacitating spastic cerebral palsy, but his mother stated that both he and the
family were well informed regarding cerebellar stimulation. In addition
to the details about placing the receiver subcutaneously in the chest wall
and tunneling leads from the receiver to the posterior fossa, Mrs. P. understood (1) that the risk of surgical complication, largely due to general
anesthesia, was 1-2%; (2) that there was a 50/50 chance in favor of help-
ing her son, (3) that if cerebellar stimulation did not help, it would not
harm, and (4) that the procedure was an investigative therapy. She acknowledged that, in part, the family was precommitted by coming to the
hospital: "If the doctors think they can help D, the family is ready to
proceed". She added that she asked one of the physicians (not the operating surgeon) what he would recommend, and that he responded that he
would have the operation done if D.P. were his own son.

The parents of the third patient who is a legal minor volunteered
that they did not bother to read the entire operating consent because the
beginnings of the form itself contained the phrase,"...as explained by
Dr...." They did, however, sign the consent. They were aware

St. Barnabas Hospital
for Chronic Diseases
THIRD AVENUE, BETWEEN 181ST AND 183RD STREETS
BRONX, N. Y. 10457

295-2000

DATE _____

TIME _____ A.m.
                                  P.M.

AGE OF PATIENT _____

ADMISSION CONSENT FORM

1. I, the undersigned patient, request and authorize the above hospital, its physicians, agents, servants and employees to provide such hospital care and to administer such routine diagnostic, radiological and/or therapeutic procedures and treatment, including but not limited to the administration of pharmaceutical products, blood or blood derivatives and intravenous medication, as in the judgment of the physicians of the hospital as they deem necessary or advisable in my diagnosis, care or treatment.

2. I hereby authorize the above hospital to furnish such professional information, including the sending of a copy or abstract of my medical records, in accordance with the policy of the said hospital, as may be necessary for the processing and/or payment of any claim or right arising out of my hospitalization against any insurance carrier, any other third party payor, whether commercial or governmental, or for the purposes of any other treating, custodial, nursing, or health facility or treating physician, who may require same. I hereby release the above hospital from all legal liability that may arise from the release of the said information or records.

3. I certify that I have read and fully understand this consent for diagnostic and therapeutic procedures and treatment, and for release of medical information and records.

SIGNATURE OF PATIENT_____

OR (IF UNCONSCIOUS OR INCAPABLE OF SIGNING)

SIGNATURE OF PATIENT'S HUSBAND OR WIFE _____

When patient is a minor (under 21 years) or incompetent to give consent for any other reason, type in name of patient above and complete the following:

SIGNATURE OF PERSON AUTHORIZED TO CONSENT FOR PATIENT

_____

RELATIONSHIP TO PATIENT_____

WITNESS:

_____

_____

5M-8-72-B-81222

Fig. 1.   Admission Consent Form

St. Barnabas Hospital for Chronic Diseases
BRONX, N. Y. 10457

CONSENT FOR DIAGNOSTIC AND/OR THERAPEUTIC PROCEDURES

Date .... 19........

Time ....a.m.
                                          p.m.

I, the undersigned, hereby authorize Dr. ...., and whomever he may

designate as his associates or assistants, to administer or provide such medical, surgical, radiation or

other diagnostic or therapeutic services and anesthesia as they may consider necessary, upon

....
                               (NAME OF PATIENT OR "MYSELF")

to include the following..
                               (NATURE OF OPERATION, TREATMENT AND/OR PROCEDURE)

and/or such additional procedures, including the administration of blood and/or blood products, as are

considered necessary on the basis of findings during the course of said procedure or treatment, and I un-

derstand that no assurance of beneficial results has been promised or implied. I assume any possible

risks normally involved in this form of treatment or procedure. Any tissues or parts surgically removed

may be disposed of by the Hospital in accordance with accustomed practice.

I also consent to the taking and publication of any photographs in the course of this treatment or opera-

tion for the purpose of advancing medical education providing my identity is disguised.

I hereby certify that I have read and fully understand the above consent for diagnostic and therapeutic

procedures as explained to me by Dr. .... and any further explanation

that may appear on the reverse side of this form.

_____
SIGNATURE OF PATIENT

_____
SIGNATURE OF PARENT OR GUARDIAN

_____
SIGNATURE OF PATIENT'S HUSBAND IN CASE OF WIFE'S STERILIZATION PROCEDURE AND/OR
THERAPEUTIC ABORTION; OR SIGNATURE OF WIFE IN CASE OF HUSBAND'S STERILIZATION
PROCEDURE.

_____
WITNESS   5M-12-69-HIP-49900

Fig. 2.   Consent for Diagnostic and/or Therapeutic Procedures

ST. BARNABAS HOSPITAL FOR CHRONIC DISEASES
183rd Street and Third Avenue, Bronx, New York

Name of Patient_____ Date_____
          (Typed)
Chart and Reference No._____ Time_____ AM
                                                     PM

DESCRIPTIVE STATEMENT IN SUPPORT OF CONSENTS FOR:

        (1) PLACEMENT OF NEURO-STIMULATOR (DSC)
        (2) CRYOTHALAMECTOMY
        (3) CRYOPULVINECTOMY
        (4) CRYODENTATECTOMY

The following surgical procedures have been discussed with me by _____,M.D., a physician associated with the above hospital, and one or more of these procedures have been recommended in an effort to improve and/or control some of the symptoms of the condition of _____ for which (I) (The above patient) (is) (am) suffering. This condition is serious and incapacitating and has not responded favorably to other accepted forms of therapy. I understand that the sequence of these operations cannot be routinely established and that each procedure and the results from it will determine the next operation, if any. One procedure, a combination of several, or all four may be indicated. In some special circumstances reoperation may be necessary. I further understand that operative consent will be obtained prior to each operation.

(1) Placement of Neuro-Stimulator (DCS)

This involves first gaining access to the brain by an operation done under general anesthesia known as craniectomy or crainiotomy when the bone is replaced. In preparation for surgery, the entire head is shaved and the scalp is cleansed thoroughly with soap and water. A skin antiseptic is then applied, and all but the area to be operated upon, is covered with sterile drapes. The scalp is incised (cut), usually in a semicircular manner, and a number of holes are drilled in the underlying skull. In the case of a craniotomy, the holes are connected by means of a wire saw, thereby freeing a block of bone which is detached from the remainder of the skull. In the case of a crainectomy, the bone is removed by rongeur. Directly underneath the bone are the membranes overlying the brain. These are incised to reveal the dura mater (the outermost, toughest and most fibrous of the three meninges or membranes of the brain), but in this procedure no brain tissue is destroyed. Electrode devices are placed over or in a specific area of the central nervous system occasionally requiring more than one and they are connected to a small receiver, all of which is placed beneath the skin in an inconspicuous place. A small transmitter is used to activate the receiver. This procedure carries with it a surgical risk, including those involved in general anesthesia and the exposure of the central nervous system. Occasionally, the apparatus may have to be removed because of undesirable effects of the stimulator or mechanical failure. Although recovery from this procedure is the same as with most major operations, hospitalization may be prolonged because the specific settings for the transmitter must be determined in each individual case.

Fig. 3. (see next page)

(2) Cryothalamectomy

This procedure is done under local anesthesia with a patient awake, the head being placed in a holder to prevent movement. A small incision is made in the scalp and a hole about the size of a dime is drilled in the skull. Air is introduced into the ventricle (one of the several cavities of the brain) to localize the target. A tiny probe is introduced into the brain tissue, which is pushed aside, until the probe reaches the desired area as confirmed by x-rays. A small lesion (a change in tissue structure) is made by freezing the tissue with the probe. Throughout the procedure the cooperation of the patient is necessary in order that the size of the lesion and the clinical results can be assayed. The procedure requires approximately one and one-half hours to complete and the physicians of this hospital have performed this procedure over 5,000 times. There are certain risks, discomforts, complications and consequences associated with the procedure which the patient must understand and assume. These include a mortality (death) risk of   percent; a risk of permanent weakness or paralysis of   percent; a risk of speech problems of   percent which are usually temporary and responds well to speech therapy; a risk of balance difficulty of   percent, which difficulty is usually temporary and responds well to physical therapy; a risk of mental confusion of   percent which may occur immediately following the surgery or possibly three to five days after surgery, which condition is usually temporary but can last for several weeks.

(3) Cryopulvinectomy

This procedure is done exactly like the cryothalamectomy but the placement of the lesion is slightly different. The complication percentages with this procedure are the same as cryothalamectomies.

(4) Cryodentatectomy

This procedure is carried out with the patient asleep under general anesthesia. An incision is made at the back of the head and neck and a small amount of bone is removed by craniectomy or craniotomy as described in procedure (1) and the dura mater is exposed. Air and/or a radio-opaque material is introduced into the ventricular (brain cavity) system for localization purposes. A special cryogenic (low temperature) probe is then placed into the cerebellum (not the main portion of the brain) and the dentate nucleus (a large and rather dense spheroid body embedded within the hemisphere of the cerebellum from which certain fibers arise) is destroyed by freezing and removed. Complications may occur from the general anesthetic as with any operation. Postoperatively, swelling of the cerebellum can occur which may temporarily cause balance or coordination problems. Although it has not occurred in the series performed in this hospital, we feel that there does exist the possibility of postoperative hemorrhage or infarction which could cause a permanent cerebellar or other brain dysfunction (disturbance or impairment) such as hemiplegia or even death.

                                        (Signed)_____
                                                            (Patient)

Note: If patient is a minor under 18, or incompetent, or unable for any reason to give consent, complete the following:

        The above patient is (a minor under 18) (unable to consent because):_____

_____

Witness:

                                        _____
                                                      (Signature)

_____   _____
          (Signature)   (Indicate whether parent, legal
_____   guardian, responsible next of kin, etc.)
          (Address)

Fig. 3. Descriptive statement in support of consents for: 1) placement of neuro-stimulator (DSC); 2) cryothalamectomy; 3) cryopulvinectomy; 4) cryodentatectomy.

beforehand, they said, of the subcutaneous receiver placement, the tunneled leads, and the power-pack transmitter. In addition, they understood that about 65% of patients had experienced "good results" from the operation, that the operation is "not dangerous because no tissue is destroyed" but that there is "always a risk with general anesthetic", and that "if it works, R.K. will have improved use of his left arm, hand, and leg". The patient himself knew that he was admitted for cerebellar stimulation in order to "correct my left arm and leg", and he indicated familiarity with the technical aspects of the procedure. As with every other patient I talked with, R.K. professed to have learned a good deal about what was imminent for himself through conversations with patients who had already been operated.

Leaving aside just now the case of D.P., who cannot speak and whose understanding we therefore cannot compare with that of his mother, some interesting complementarities are evident in the other cases. Most apparent is that patient and parent tend to share similar kinds and quantities of information -- in one case probably not enough to provide "informed consent" but in the other a quite adequate understanding of the procedure, even though neither apparently bothered to read the formal consent instrument very thoroughly. What accounts for this differential would be largely conjectural without more evidence, but I suspect that a basic familial attitude toward knowing and accepting is indicated here. Both patients and both families professed unqualified confidence in the surgeons; but one set, I think, knew and understood better (i.e., more thoroughly and comprehensively) than the other, even though both were presumably offered the same information.

As might be expected, the quality of consent appeared more consistent among the adult patients whom I studied. One seemed to speak for the rest when she said, "Most of us are grasping for straws". (See case W.B., Cooper et al., in this volume). Another stated: "I came in as a test patient....amd I'm game for tests....if they don't help me, maybe they can help somebody else". This was the second cerebellar electrode installation for the third patient in this group who said that while he was "a little disappointed in the first operation because I was reaching for the moon" he agreed again because "I want to find out if the second one will help". All three of these patients appear to have been well informed and knowledgable prior to surgery.

But the criteria for valid consent are not exhausted by information necessary to understanding and legal competency to consent; and while I discovered some disparity with respect to "informed" consent there seemed

to be a profoundly univocal attitude among these patients toward the
"voluntary" aspect. Although some patients who had been offered surgery
declined or deferred it, none of these patients interviewed, or their families, felt free to refuse the hope offered by this innovative therapy. "I
want everything I can get (to help my condition)....I'm a very greedy
person", was one patient's way of putting it. Another said, "I wasn't
free to refuse at all....it was a foregone conclusion....the possible benefits are so significant that I just couldn't refuse". And one set of parents seemed to speak for the others: "How can we possibly deny our son
any chance....we are not at all free....we don't have that choice."

That this sentiment should be so strongly and pervasively felt is not
surprising in view of the protracted illness, unremitted pain, and severe
physical disability of these patients. And what comes through clearly in
extended conversation with them and their families, sometimes more emo-
tive than articulate, is that they somehow find the will to exceed the
apparent limit of their endurance. So one parent confessed that they
"grasp for straws" while simultaneously acknowledging that "I don't know
how many more operations we can endure....my husband and I are only
human, and we're both very tired."

A more pragmatic, although still provisional, measure of ethics in
the consent situation is to compare whether postoperative experience confirmed preoperative expectations and whether, in view of that, the patients would make the same decision again. Although the patients recognized that more time was needed for full evaluation, in one case the
answer was a definite "no"; in another, agnosticism; but in the others,
both patients and families affirmed that knowing what they know now,
they would make the same decision. Perhaps I should add that in this
latter group the enthusiasm for saying "yes" to that question was variable!
Still, there was no doubt that, with whatever equivocation, this was their
answer.

Anybody who has considered seriously the voluntary aspects of the
consent situation knows that "freedom" in this setting is a very elusive
and fragile concept. Indeed, the predicament which the physician faces
here is not substantially different from gaining "informed" consent. I
have observed consents in a variety of settings which, to the satisfaction
of both the physician and myself, were exemplary models of unhurried and
clear information which was repeated several times. Still it was abun-
dantly clear to both of us that the patient, for whatever reason(s) was not
comprehending what was being said. Undoubtedly those reasons are complex, and probably vary from patient to patient. Nevertheless, the result

is very similar: the patient appears to be either unable or unwilling to grasp what is being said.

Something like that also happens with the voluntary aspect of the consent situation. It is clear that freedom, like knowledge, is contingent and hedged by many forces over which we exercise only more or less control. This is dramatically the case with victims of chronic disease, who have either never been free from the limitations imposed upon them by their disease or who, even remembering a time when they were not shackled by this disability, know themselves now to be controlled by it. They are significantly "un-free" and they know this about themselves - and they seem compelled, therefore, to embrace anything that offers the slightest hope for release from this bondage. So their captivity is complete; and they appear to be no more free to refuse a hoped-for escape through symptomatic relief than they are free to deny the reality of their subjection to a chronic disease.

This suggests that in fulfilling the criteria for valid consent, sensitivity for the minimalization of "free" consent should be complemented by heightened concern for full and complete disclosure of information to the patient's understanding. I know, of course, that this objective will sometimes be very difficult to achieve. Even in pre-admission patient consultations, it is quite clear that many patients and their families present themselves as already prepared to accept gladly whatever is offered to them; and it is the exceptional patient (in my experience) who fails to say, or refuses to say, "whatever you think is best, doctor." Why is this so pervasively the case? Are there demonstrable differences in attitude and acceptance between these patients with chronic physiologic brain disease and their fellow patients on other services? Does protracted disability and pain naturally give rise to a vigorous determination to gain symptomatic relief? Why do these patients, many of them with diseases and disorders of unknown etiology and uncertain prognosis, display a kind of stoicism which is at once profound and casual? All of us are likely to have intuitive answers - predicated on more or less clinical experience - to these questions; but they are worthy of serious and sustained study, particularly with a patient population whose physiologic disorder is so closely related to their psychological temperament.

I stated at the outset that the data from these consent studies, while perhaps not definitive, might nevertheless be instructive; and I have suggested some of the ways in which I think this to be the case. With respect to the principal inquiry of this part of the paper, viz., the adequacy of the consent situation, I tend to think that the special circumstance of these patients, together with the innovative procedure offered them, poses subtle issues in consent-getting; and this, in turn, places a greater-than-usual responsibility upon the physician in requesting and accepting the patient's consent. Notwithstanding the obvious value of legal codes and ethical considerations of "valid consent", I do not know of any formal mechanism which will guarantee the result that is wanted here; and our best hope probably lies, therefore, in compassionate and conscientious physicians who are committed to the spirit as well as the letter of the law of valid consent, and who are open to sympathetic review of the nuances in the consent situation.

Although writing with a somewhat different emphasis, Dr. Ingelfinger's observation is not inapposite here:

"Incapacitated and hospitalized because of illness, frightened by strange and impersonal routines, and fearful for his health and perhaps life, he (the patient) is far from exercising a free power of choice when the person to whom he anchors all his hopes asks, 'Say, you wouldn't mind, would you, if you joined some of the other patients on this floor and helped us to carry out some very important research we are doing?'....the process of obtaining 'informed consent', with all its regulations and conditions, is no more than an elaborate ritual, a device that, when the subject is uneducated and uncomprehending, confers no more than the semblance of propriety on human experimentation. The subject's only real protection, the public as well as the medical profession must recognize, depends on the conscience and compassion of the investigator and his peers." (Ingelfinger, 1972).

3. A third area of ethical interest has to do with the efficacy of this operation. Maurice Strauss (1973) has recently argued that "no experimental method of treatment may be ethically employed except under such conditions that valid conclusions may be drawn." Dr. Strauss' concern is that new forms of therapy be objectively and prospectively evaluated in controlled clinical trials before they are introduced and accepted by physicians at large; and he quotes approvingly Lord Cohen's aphorism: "The feasibility of an operation is not the best indication for its performance." I agree with Dr. Strauss' principal point, and want here only to extend (what I take to be) his scientific and technical evaluation to the humanistic dimensions of patient response. I should also indicate that provision for scientific and technical evaluation of chronic cerebellar stimulation in humans has attended this procedure since its inauguration;

and that, in addition to these aspects, independent clinical and psychological evaluations of each case are conducted by a non-surgical neurologist and a clinical psychologist.

In any innovative therapy precise diagnosis for applicability is frequently the key to success. This appears also to be the case with cerebellar stimulation. And although I disclaim competence to judge the
scientific or technical achievement of this new procedure, there is evidence
which the informed lay eye and ear can perceive and evaluate. Thus,
among the patients I have studied, the most conspicuous and encouraging
preliminary results appear to have been achieved with diagnoses of epilepsy
and intention myoclonus. These patients show marked improvement in motor
control together with absence, or significant diminution, of involuntary
movement and seizure. In addition, they tell me (despite a somewhat more
cautious assessment by their physicians!) that they are entirely convinced
of the efficacy of the procedure because they feel that they have been
given a "new lease on life" with their newfound control and mobility.
They are eager for discharge from the hospital, and even enthusiastic
about the prospect of extended physical therapy! The external hardware
which they must carry - battery-pack, leads, and transmitter antennae -
is only a casual annoyance to them, and even the requirement to regulate
their stimulation periodically does not dampen their optimism.

The prognosis for patients diagnosed with cerebral palsy must, however, be even more open because it is simply too early to draw firm conclusions. Moreover, the time of onset, together with additional complications, appears to be significant in these patients.

There is need to develop diagnostic precision for the applicability
of innovative therapies, just as there is the need for technical and scientific excellence in the design of the therapy. And a crucial part of what
is learned in early human trials is the disease or disorder for which the
therapy is best suited. Those human trials which have treated indiscrim-
inately the application of an innovative therapy have been most disastrous.
The use, for example, of a special high protein diet in the treatment of
liver disease seemed to have a sound theoretical basis and to be adminis-
tratively innocuous; but lacking demonstration of the benefit of this regimen,
a decade has passed before it became apparent that many patients were
dying in hepatic coma as a result of this diet. That kind of risk is inherent in any experimental therapeutic; but the risk need not be made inordinate by supposing it an unqualified success before adequate evidence is
in. On the other hand, some procedures must, in the nature of the case,
be accepted largely on an empirical basis because the number of subjects

required for conclusive demonstration would be unrealistic. Cerebellar
stimulation probably falls into this latter category, and its demonstrated
efficacy will likely depend upon its restricted application to precisely
diagnosed patients.

4. To this point, we have considered cerebellar stimulation as an
innovative therapy for physiologic motor disorder and we have presumed
that the sole intention and function of the procedure, insofar as it affects
recipient patients, is relief of seizure and spasticity. But there may be
other sequelae, which are psychological, that also accompany (in some
cases) electrical stimulation of the cerebellum. Dr. Riklan (this volume)
has described these psychological alterations in his paper as a further
instance of the linkage between clinical care and research. Certain
implications of cerebellar stimulation for behavior modification or mind
and mood manipulation are therefore already before us.

It deserves stating at the outset that this operation is quite different
in both method and intention from what is conventionally referred to as
psychosurgery. The principal methodological difference lies in the fact
that cerebellar stimulation entails no destruction of brain cells and is, for
that reason, reversible. The significant intentional distinction is that
cerebellar stimulation is undertaken to treat a physiologic motor disorder.
In no customary or common-sense use of language, therefore, can this operation be called psychosurgery.

That there are psychological sequelae, more or less detectable, to
virtually every surgical procedure is not unexpected; but that behavior
modification or some other psychological alteration should be the primary
focus of irreversible surgery raises some vital questions with respect to the
recipients of these procedures. At least until the advent of psychiatry,
the pre-eminent concern of a physician was supposed to be the treatment
of his primary patient. Family wishes (unless the patient were a minor),
advancement of scientific knowledge through human experimentation, political interests of the state, and the like have not been ordinarily allowed
to infringe or compromise the well-being of the primary patient. To suggest that absolutely no one else benefited from the medically-derived well-
being of the primary patient would, of course, be myopic and absurd. But
the priorities are important, and the point, withal, is that if other persons
benefited they did so tangentially and indirectly and not as a function of
some primary intention for social benefit which the treatment of a primary
patient would achieve. The "principle of totality" - which argues that
a patient may submit to mutilation of a part of his body when the whole
body benefits thereby - has been an operational rubric for centuries of
medical practice.

The advent of organ transplantation raised, in its early days, the question of the applicability of the principle of totality to living donors who, it could be argued, subjected themselves to mutilation for the benefit of another. That argument continues, but principally with reference to the use of legally certified minors and incompetents as organ donors. Courts in Massachusetts and Kentucky have held, respectively, that the psychological well-being of minors and an inmate in a state mental institution would be served by, and was sufficient warrant for, an order permitting these persons to be organ (kidney) donors. These decisions, in response to petitions by hospitals and physicians, have not gone unnoticed by persons who are concerned for the moral health of medicine in the wake of unprecedented scientific and technological innovation; and they are important to note here as another instance of the thin edge of the wedge that tends to jeopardize honored professional and humane values in the interest of technocratic novelty. We claim to be, as the Watergate hearings are desperately trying to show, a people governed by laws rather than men; and the preferential benefit of some citizens at the expense of others, in instances like this, challenges our best instincts and conventions for guaranteeing human dignity and social justice.

It was recently suggested to me that hemorrhoidectomy, because its results include a modification of patient behavior and attitude, could be called psychosurgery; and I acknowledged that while in some sense excision of hemorrhoids probably could be called psychosurgery, we should be aware that engaging in that kind of extension of meaning logically impels us to a nonsensical vocabulary. Bills are now before both houses of the Congress to suspend Federal support of projects involving psychosurgery and to prohibit psychosurgery in federally connected health care facilities. In the House bill, psychosurgery is defined as

> ....those operations currently referred to as lobotomy,
> psychiatric surgery, and behavioral surgery and all other
> forms of brain surgery if the surgery is performed for the
> purpose of --
>   (A) modification or control of thoughts, feelings,
> actions, or behavior rather than the treatment of a known
> and diagnosed physical disease of the brain;
>   (B) modification of normal brain function or normal
> brain tissue in order to control thoughts, feelings, action,
> or behavior; or
>   (C) treatment of abnormal brain function or abnormal
> brain tissue in order to modify thoughts, feelings, actions,
> or behavior when the abnormality is not an established

cause for those thoughts, feelings, actions, or behavior.
Such term does not include electroshock treatment, the
electrical stimulation of the brain, or drug therapy,
except when substances are injected or inserted directly
into brain tissue.

                    H.R. 5371, p. 2, lines 7-24.

In the Senate bill, psychosurgery means

....brain surgery on (A) normal brain tissue of an
individual who does not suffer from any pathological disease, for the prupose of changing or controlling the
behavior or emotions of such individual, or (B) on dis-
eased brain tissue of an individual, if the sole object of
the performance of such surgery is to control, change, or
affect any behavioral or emotional disturbance of such
individual. Such term shall not include brain surgery
designed to cure, or ameliorate the effects of epilepsy;
nor shall such term be construed to include electric
shock treatments.

                    S.J. Res. 86, p. 3, lines 8-17.

On these definitions, electrical stimulation of the brain is explicitly
excluded from the term "psychosurgery" in the House bill; and it would
appear to be similarly excluded from the use of the term in the Senate
resolution.   Indeed, it is arguable that in the measure to which cerebellar
stimulation is therapy for physiologic motor disorder it is in principle not
different from medical or surgical interference with any other abnormal or
disordered physiologic process. That brain stimulation is involved may
suggest the need for greater care in the exercise of this surgery through
diagnostic precision in order to avoid the potential hazard posed by intervention in the brain.

What philosophers and theologians have for so long called "will" is
apparently what neurologists call "neuronal activity". In both cases, "will"
or "neuronal activity" is presumed to have some self-transcending capacity
for critical evaluation of self and development of a point of view. So
freedom from biomechanical successiveness and sentience - what we might
call the capacity for perennial and radical change - are ingredients of
human selfhood common to both philosophy and science; and they illustrate
in turn the reasons for our inability to define humanum in precise and
stable terms. Whatever we mean by "human" is always changing and to
define it is already to mis-identify it.

I tend to think, therefore, that in the interest of preserving at least those rudimentary ingredients of human selfhood we should be extremely cautious about elective surgeries for behavior and/or mood manipulation. Mark and Ervin (1973) make a strong case for anticipating violent behavior in certain individuals and proceeding then to curb that tendency by surgical means. Indeed, they are quite confident that Charles Whitman's killing of 17 people in Austin, and Richard Speck's murder of 8 nurses in Chicago, and Lee Harvey Oswald's assassination of President Kennedy could have been predicted by antecedent diagnosis and probably prevented by stereotactic electrode surgery. Perhaps so. But I wonder what social and political and personal price we would have to pay for this kind of prevention? And what philosophical anthropology underlies such an intention? Is all violent behavior "bad" and "abnormal" or is some violent behavior appropriate and desirable? And who is to say? What parties will have a voice, or the determinative voice, in decisions of this sort? These questions are arguably, certainly, in the first immediacy, not medical or technical but philosophical and ethical in character and substance. And where does one draw the line between abnormal behavior which is associated with brain disease and abnormal behavior which is not?

If one believes that "our past environment, once it is past, is no longer a sociological phenomenon" but that "it is imbedded in our brain and its use is dependent on the function or malfunction of the cerebral tissue" (Mark & Ervin, 1970), what is to prevent attributing any and every behavior, which we might want to describe as aberrant, to brain dysfunction? Could greed or avarice or compassion or gentleness qualify, depending on the circumstance, as a malfunction of cerebral tissue? Some physicians have suggested to me that all would be well if doctors would only affirm and practice the Golden Rule. Fine. Would there then be warrant for psychosurgery on all those physicians - presuming their consent! - who, for one or another reason, just could not naturally bring themselves to this affirmation and action? Are we at the point of resolving St. Paul's dilemma - the good that I would do, I do not; and the evil that I would not do, I do - by neurologic surgery? I am not myself ready for that; and not least because it represents the abdication of a moral struggle which has, in large measure, brought us to this alternative. The measure of our freedom is, in part, signified by our capacity to reject - as well as accept - technical innovation; and it is the surest sign of captivity to the technocratic mentality that we insist upon doing everything we are technically capable of doing.

I appreciate the distinction which Dr. Mark has himself drawn

between "advocating neurosurgical procedures for certain kinds of violent
behavior caused by organic brain disease or dysfunction" and advocacy of
these procedures "as general methods of behavior control (Mark, 1973).
But I am far from sanguine about either social and political restraints, or
the reluctance of physicians and surgeons to exceed appropriate limits in
accepting alleged therapies which are not yet objectively and prospectively evaluated.   Dr. Mark's own formulation of the principle seems to
me apt: "In my own practice, I and my group do not accept patients for
treatments who do not want therapy, and we do not believe that the
public good or public interest should intrude upon the personal medical
model in terms of protecting the public against violent individuals" (Mark,
1973).   It would appear that we are on safer therapeutic ground to restrict behavior modification to sequelae of neurologic surgery which is
itself directed toward the alleviation of precisely diagnosed physiologic
motor disorder; and, on these grounds, it is arguable that electrical stimulation of the cerebellum is not properly described as psychosurgery.

The preliminary conclusions of this paper, in summary, are:
1) inaugurating innovative therapies without extensive and intensive peer
review is very questionable practice, even though clinical experience thus
far with cerebellar stimulation is generally supportive of its initial expec-
ations and the hazards of the procedure appear to be minimal and not a
contraindication for clinical trials but commensurate with the hoped-for
benefit to patients;   2) the consent situation, probably owing largely to
the special circumstance of these patients, is complex and subtle and
therefore places an uncommon responsibility upon the physician to secure
a consent which is competent, knowing, and voluntary;   3) the clinical
efficacy of this procedure is yet largely unknown but appears to rest, in
some future assessment, upon restricted application to precisely diagnosed
physiologic diseases and/or disorders;   4) since electrical stimulation of
the cerebellum is directed toward the relief of symptomatic physiologic
disorder, is not undertaken to modify behavior, and is reversible, it is
not properly described as psychosurgery.

These observations, together with the questions I have raised, derive
from the spirit of radical inquiry which characterizes ethics and moral
philosophy.   One way, in summary, to state the general ethical problem
which faces us in innovative therapies is acknowledgment that we risk,
through our increasing scientific and technical sophistication, viewing our
species as merely the raw material for more and more manipulation, without attendant restraints.   We are on the threshold of mastering our life
but denying its mystery.   We are able to achieve brilliance without wisdom, and power without conscience; and ours can become a time of

technological giants and ethical infants. Our most urgent need is not to stop the world and get off, but to keep our priorities straight; and, in this case, I think that means remembering and understanding that, like the Sabbath, technics are made for man and not vice-versa.

REFERENCES

COOPER, I.S., AMIN, I., GILMAN, S., & WALTZ, J.M. The effect of chronic stimulation of cerebellar cortex on epilepsy in man. In Cooper, I.S. & Riklan, M. (Eds.) "The Cerebellum, Epilepsy and Behavior". New York: Plenum Press, 1973.

INGELFINGER, F.J. Informed (but uneducated) consent. N. Eng. J. Med. 287:466, 1972.

MARK, V.H. Brain surgery in aggressive epileptics. The Hastings Center Report, 3:1-5, 1973.

MARK, V.H. & ERVIN, F.R. "Violence and the Brain". New York: Harper & Row, 1970.

RIKLAN, M., MARISAK, K., & COOPER, I.S. Psychological studies of chronic cerebellar stimulation in man. In Cooper, I.S. & Riklan, M. (Eds.) "The Cerebellum, Epilepsy and Behavior". New York: Plenum Press, 1973.

STRAUSS, M.B. Ethics of experimental therapeutics. N. Eng. J. Med. 288:1183-1184, 1973.

PSYCHOSURGERY AND BRAIN STIMULATION:

THE LEGISLATIVE EXPERIENCE IN OREGON IN 1973

Robert S. Dow, Robert J. Grimm, and Donald S. Rushmer
Department of Neurology
Good Samaritan Hospital & Medical Center

Portland, Oregon

INTRODUCTION

This conference deals with the use of surgical and electrical techniques in the treatment of difficult disease states for which no fully satisfactory solutions are known. Historically, such problems have engendered experimental approaches to provide answers to such problems with the full recognition by physicians and patients that failure and dangerous consequences could follow. It is necessary that we focus on such problems having to do with brain dysfunction. In dealing with brain dysfunction, we find ourselves in a clinical area that extends far beyond the confines of the hospital or the technical rehabilitation of an impaired nervous system. When efforts are made to control or alter brain dysfunction, particularly when behavioral management is the goal, we enter a controversial area in which techniques, goals and attitudes of physicians are increasingly questioned.

We meet here to review new techniques which may be applied to the human cerebellum. As controversy mounts over surgical and electrical techniques designed to alter brain function, it is an opportune time to review ground rules for continuing to meet our obligations as physicians searching for better treatment methods. The vehicle for discussion will be the recent and pioneering legislative effort in Oregon to provide for the control of such techniques where modification of behavior is sought.

The past few years have seen the development of an awareness on the part of the public concerning operations on the brain and chronic

367

electrical brain stimulation (EBS) for purposes of controlling or modifying
behavior.   This is clear by considering just the volume of recent writings
on the subject in newspapers and periodicals (Mason, 1973; Salpukas,
1973; Hunt, 1973; Paradrini, 1973; Brody, 1973; Holden, 1973; Averback,
1973; Schmock, 1973; Aarous, 1973; Stokes, 1973; Leet, 1973; Dietz,
1972; Aarous, 1972; Opton & Stender, 1972; Mitford, 1972; Randel, 1972;
Breggin, 1972).   Apprehensions are expressed here and elsewhere that such
powerful behavior modifying techniques could and might be used to control
not only the mentally ill, but others for political purposes.   George Orwell
(1948, 1949) and Aldous Huxley (Brave New World, 1939) provided widely
discussed and chilling models of the consequences of this kind of state
control of behavior.   These have been augmented in our own time by
novels dealing explicitly with psychosurgery, e.g. One Flew Over the
Cuckoo's Nest (Ken Kesey, 1962), and electrical brain stimulation, e.g.
The Sirens of Titan (Kurt Vonnegut, Jr., 1959) and Terminal Man
(Michael Crichton, 1972).   Further, through the public writings of neuroscientists and clinicians (Delgado, J.   Physical Control of the Mind:
Toward a Psycho-Civilized Society; Skinner, G.F.   Beyond Freedom and
Dignity), Mark (1973), and Mark, V.J. and Ervin, F.R. (Violence and
and the Brain, 1972), considerable information is available to the public
on these subjects as to what some professionals are thinking about.   A
broad and real concern exists.

     Two general questions can be asked: First, are experimenters dev-
eloping the technology for "mind control" as might be used by the State
for its own ends?   Second, will the preliminary efforts to introduce these
techniques come via the authority and certification of medicine vis a vis
definition and management of the emotionally ill, or the touchier issue,
altering brain activity in prisoners or the violent?   That these are real
issues is clear.   They are raised by the charge that Soviet psychiatry was
employed to suppress political dissent in the Soviet Union in 1971, and
that some segments of U.S. psychiatry utilize treatment to maintain the
status quo and suppress behavior disapproved by the institution (see
Miller, 1973).

     What is the neuroscientists' role with regard to such public concern?
The key word is involvement and contribution of information.   It is our
view that our role should be characterized by candor, clear English, and
judgment based upon both data and sensitivity to the political issues at
stake.   Denials of bad intentions, supercilious responses in the authority
and jargon of science, or suggestion that the judgment of physicians shall
be final, we believe would foster concern and polarize issues along
irrational lines.   These things being so, how shall we proceed?

We begin with the view that public concern in this area is healthy and that neuroscientists must participate as knowledgeable citizens. When called upon, we have a real duty to respond. The response should be to provide full and explicit information to the public and to aid in drafting legislation if called upon. Let us provide the illustration of a response as it developed among our own laboratory group in the spring of 1973. As will be reviewed, we entered into this difficult public arena when concerns over brain control reached the legislative level. The result was the first legislation to be passed in the country on the subject of psychosurgical and EBS techniques.

Legislative Experience in Oregon in 1973

During the 1973 legislative sessions, an Orgeon State Senator (T. Hallock) introduced a bill to restrict the use of psychosurgery and electroconvulsive therapy (ECT) on patients in state institutions. The bill made it difficult to carry out either procedure without a specific medical review interposed between those requesting the procedure and the physician(s) carrying it out.

The Oregon branch of the American Civil Liberties Union, routinely surveying legislation dealing with informed consent, asked one of us (R. J. Grimm) to review the legislation for its medical and technical content as might pertain to questions of civil liberties. The matter was thereupon opened for discussion among colleagues and viewpoints on psychosurgery and EBS were solicited (in writing) from neurologists and psychiatrists attached to our department. A buildup of documentary information on psychosurgery and electrical brain stimulation was begun to provide an up-to-date review regarding the use of such methods in this country and throughout the world. As a result of this inquiry (Grimm, 1973), we decided that the initial bill needed a thorough revision. It was also felt that the ECT issue should be dropped since ECT is the treatment of choice in some psychiatric situations and its restricted use would not be supported by psychiatrists. It was felt, instead, that EBS, along with psychosurgery, should be examined for possible public control. These and other points pertaining to consent, civil liberties, and willingness of lab members to testify were background to the legislative effort.

Three members of our lab testified against the original bill in the Senate Human Resources Committee (D. S. Rushmer, C. C. Bell, and R. J. Grimm) resulting in a request from the committee's chairman that Donald Rushmer and Robert Grimm of our laboratory and H. Crawford of the Oregon Medical Association redraft it. A completely new bill was written and subsequently passed by the Oregon legislature in June 1973. This is the first legislation of its kind to be passed in the country dealing with psychosurgery and EBS. The bill in its entirety is provided in an appendix. What, then, was the philosophy which is expressed in this pioneer piece of legislation?

Psychosurgery and EBS Oregon Statute

The principle tenet of the legislation is that alteration of brain for the specific purpose of achieving behavioral goals is only to be carried out when two points have been satisfied. The first is that the proposed procedure must be known to provide the behavioral change sought; the second is that all other known therapies must have been tried and have failed, and that, therefore, such an approach, however, irreversible, is justified. Behind each of these points are a series of verifiable observations. The first is that scientific evidence exists that a proposed procedure on human brain will produce the desired results without catastrophic consequences. The questions here revolve around the assertions that specific, circumscribed brain sites are indeed of critical and unique importance in the pathophysiology of a behavioral disorder. Is there really a neural substrate with specific stereotaxic coordinates for violent behavior, anxiety, homosexuality, or a psychiatrically defined syndrome? If such brain loci do exist, the legislation implies that the procedure of stimulation at that site must be specific for a positive alteration of the function in question and will not damage other qualities. Secondly, it requires that other solutions, less drastic techniques--drastic meaning that brain tissue does not regenerate and any damage produced is irreversible-- be rigorously applied first to affect the desired change. A final and implicit part of the legislative philosophy is the view that the desired goal or change in behavior be known and recognizable in that individual.

In reflection, it is clear that all medical therapy requires that the physician make a calculated choice between the chances of benefit against the hazards of treatment. As the tools of medicine become more powerful, with a corresponding potential for harm, these choices become more difficult. As a result the necessity of informed consent has emerged in medical practice. At the present time this is generally held as an absolute necessity. The practitioner who fails to conform to this necessary procedure does so at his own ethical and legal peril.

The experiences which led to the Nuremburg Code (medical

experimentation, 1947), the Declaration of Helsinki (1964), American
Medical Association (1957), and numerous statements thereafter by medical
groups now impose stringent codes of conduct and demand a greater degree
of regulation when innovative and experimental methods of treatment are
contemplated.   As a result, most institutions today which engage in medical research on patients have established boards of inquiry consisting of
professional and lay people to approve and monitor such research.   This is
to insure that proposed experimental procedures are justified and will be
carried out with the motives of maximum protection of human rights.

The question then arose as to whether these internal safeguards are
adequate for psychosurgery and electrical brain stimulation which, as pointed out earlier, have become the object of general concern and contro-
versies.   Should the government itself, at a national or state level, impose some kind of review for the regulation of the use of these particular
techniques?   We felt that simple informed consent and a private physician's decision to employ psychosurgical or electrode implantation procedures for behavioral modification was not sufficient.   Further, as we reviewed the possibility of establishing such controls with physicians involved
in recommending or accomplishing these procedures, we found that they are
in the main uneasy about being the sole parties to making such decisions.
Rather, they welcomed a shifting of the responsibility involved to a group
empowered to make such judgments for them.   It appeared to us that stat-
utory guidelines for how such decisions are to be made and implemented
were indicated.

At the present, it is doubtful that any single physician in the country
can be in possession of the data bearing on the psychiatric, neurologic,
social, and legal aspects which attend the use of procedures such as
psychosurgery or electrode implantation for behavioral modification in
humans.   As these are the treatments of choice for no recognisable emotional illness, they are by definition experimental.   And as the use of
experimental techniques engenders a different set of criteria for decisions,
especially given the public concern already expressed concerning the use
of such tenchniques, it is proper that the agenda for decision should with-
stand a public test procedure regardless of the terminology and clinical
complexity of the issue.   Intelligent men everywhere are interested in the
question of what we are doing.   They rightfully insist on a role where
modifying behavior affecting their own social order is at stake.

The question then becomes one of federal vs local control.   It was
our view that federal control brings with it both inflexibility and inertia
ill equipped to foresee the future.   As an illustration of a federal agency

carrying out medical supervision the FDA can be cited. The FDA regulates the development and introduction of new drugs in the U.S.A. This agency has, in the opinion of some--its excellent supervisory work not withstanding--has slowed the introduction of drugs of proven value available in other medically advanced countries by the imposition of expensive and time consuming procedures. This has limited the number of new drugs available in the U.S.A. Therefore, it seemed to us that regulation at a state level where more flexibility and different approaches are possible would be more desirable. The federal government could then assume a role only if several states fail to act. This is already the case in the control of water and air pollution. This would provide for some diversity of action and with time and experience, a method of control might evolve which would permit the introduction of innovative treatment methods and at the same time permit a measure of control.

As will be seen on inspection of the bill, psychosurgery is defined as "any operation designed to irreversibly lesion or destroy brain tissue for the primary purpose of altering the thoughts, emotions or behavior of a human being". Psychosurgery does not include procedures which may irreversibly lesion or destroy brain tissues when undertaken to cure well defined disease states such as a brain tumor, epileptic foci or certain chronic pain syndromes. "Experimental" means a technique or a procedure about which there is not sufficient data to recommend it as a recognized treatment of choice, or to predict accurately the outcome of its performance. "Intracranial brain stimulation" means, as defined in this bill, the surgical implanting of electrodes within the brain for the purpose of directly stimulating specific brain structures to produce alteration of thoughts, emotions, or behavior in a human body. Intracranial brain stimulation excludes ECT. By inference, it would also exclude brain stimulation for the study or treatment of epilepsy or chronic pain syndromes.

A board made up of nine members will be appointed by the governor for a term of four years subject to his pleasure and reappointments are permitted. The board shall include one neurologist, two neurosurgeons, and two psychiatrists selected from three nominees for each physician position presented to the governor by the Oregon Medical Association. In addition to these five physicians, the governor shall also appoint a clinical psychologist, a neuroscientist actively engaged in research on the nervous system, and two members of the general public, one of whom shall be a member of the Oregon State Bar. No individual directly involved in psychosurgery or intracranial brain stimulation on human beings shall be a member of this review board. All decisions of the review board shall be made by the affirmative vote of not less than 6 members.

Once this board has been constituted, "any institution, hospital, or licensed physician intending to perform psychosurgery, or intracranial brain stimulation, for the primary purpose of altering the thoughts, emotions or behavior of a human being shall file a petition with the review board alleging that a patient is in need of such treatment, that the patient or his legal guardian, if any, has consented thereto and that the proposed operation has legitimate clinical value".

The remainder of the bill is taken up by defining the explicit terms of how the board proceeds to render a decision. As a first step, the board conducts a hearing to determine if informed voluntary consent has been given; the patient or his legal guardian may be provided with legal counsel if desired. Once this determination has been made, the review board then determines if, in their judgment, the proposed procedure has clinical merit and is appropriate for the particular patient in question. For this to be determined it must be shown that all conventional therapies have been attempted, the procedure offers hope of saving life, reestablishing health or attenuating suffering and all other viable alternative methods of treatment have been tried and have failed to produce satisfactory results. The review board may undertake specific diagnostic evaluation itself or by means of consultants of its choosing. It may subpoena witnesses if it chooses. Its decisions shall be rendered in writing and sent to the petitioner, the patient or the legal guardian, if any, and the patient or his legal guardian's counsel, if any. If, in the judgment of the review board, a legal guardian is necessary, they may request that this be provided.

On completion of the psychosurgery or intracranial brain stimulation operation, the petitioner shall render a written report to the board. All those involved in the review process or the operation are presumed to be acting in good faith and unless it is proven that their action violated the standard of reasonable professional care and judgment, they are immune from civil or criminal liability. Any one performing these operations without consent of the board shall be subject to civil liability and if a physician performs this without the approval of the board, his license to practice medicine may be suspended or revoked.

Having now briefly reviewed the provisions of this bill as it is now a part of the Oregon statues, we suggest that the members of this symposium discuss either positively or negatively our role as neuroscientists and clinicians in having helped prepare it and your thoughts concerning its specific provisions.

Included in the appendix is the statement of Dr. Donald Rushmer to the Oregon House Human Resources Committee reviewing the bill in its late stages before passage. It is illustrative of the nature and level of effective voice, in this case supporting local control, which neuroscientists can have.

In conclusion, the Oregon legislature has passed the first piece of legislation in the country to regulate the use of psychosurgery and electrical techniques for behavioral modification. The consequences of this legislation are yet unknown, the bill does provide the public with a clear message on the unique concern held for the brain and any procedures designed to alter it. It also provides the lay public with a voice in use of such procedures. For the clinician it establishes guidelines for the advocacy and use of such procedures, provides civil liability safeguards, and specifies that review of each candidate for such procedure undergo rigorous review. The decision of the board will determine whether or not such procedures are available, useful, and to be used. At this point we feel that we have established legislation which will provide the types of controls which are necessary without hampering the use of these procedures in well defined cases of "last resort". We consider this legislation to be an experiment to the extent that we have no real guides by which to measure its impact on the medical community nor do we know how effective it will be in meeting our intended goals. We plan to carefully study these points over the next two years with the aim of reexamining the issues and the statute when the legislature next convenes. It is also our view that such legislation, written elsewhere, may provide different and perhaps better approaches to the questions involved, and serve as models for evolving practical guidelines in future years.

REFERENCES

AAROUS, L.F. "Brain Surgery is Tested on Three California Convicts". Feb. 1972, The Washington Post.

AVERBACH, S. "Psychosurgery Assailed on Hill". Feb. 24, 1973, The Washington Post.

BREGGIN, P. "The Return of Lobotomy and Psychosurgery". Congress Rec. 118:E1602-E1612, 1972a.

BRODY, J.E. "Psychosurgery Will Face Key Test in Court Today". March 12, 1973, N. Y. Times.

CHRICHTON, M. "Terminal Man". New York: Bantam Books, 1972.

DECLARATION OF HELSINKI: Issued by World Health Association. In Ann. Int. Med. Supply, 7:74-75, 1964.

DELGADO, J., Jr. "Physical Control of the Mind: Toward a Psycho-Civilized Society". (Harper Calophon), 1969.

DIETZ, J. "Senate Urged to Kill "Brain" Study". Sept. 24, 1972, p. 38, Boston Sunday Globe.

GRIMM, R.J. Advocacy of psychosurgery and intracranial brain stimulation in the involuntarily committed: Medical, legal, and ethical objections. ACLU statement to Senate Human Resources Committee Hearing on SB-298, Oregon Legislature, March 20, 1973.

HOLDEN, C. Psychosurgery: Legitimate therapy or laundered lobotomy. Science, 179:1109-1112, 1973.

HUNT, J. "Two Boston Doctors Paid to Pacify the "Violent" by Cutting into the Brains". The Real Paper (Boston), May 30, 1973.

HUXLEY, A. "Brave New World". New York: Harper & Rose, 1932.

KESEY, K. "One Flew Over the Cuckoo's Nest". New York: Viking Press, 1962.

LEET, R. "Clergyman Asks Psychosurgery Halt". (Washington) Star and News, Feb. 5, 1973.

MARK, V.H. "Brain surgery in aggressive epileptics." Hastings Center Report, 3:1-7, 1973.

MARK, V.H. & ERVIN, F.R. "Violence and the Brain". New York: Harper & Row, 1970.

MASON, B.J. "Brain surgery to control behavior." Ebony, Feb. 1973.

MILLER, J. APA: Psychiatrists reluctant to analyze themselves. Science, 181:246-248, 1973.

MITFORD, J. Experiments Behind Bars. Atlantic Monthly, 1972.

NUREMBERG CODE VS ADJUTANT GENERAL'S DEPARTMENT. Trials of war criminals before Nuremberg Military Tribunals under control council Law No. 10. The Medical Case, 2:181-185, 1947.

OPTON, E.M. & STENDER, F. A Clockwork Orange at UCLA. Mimeographed review of use of various 1972-1973 proposals in California to utilize prisoners for brain surgery and EBS experiments. Committee Opposing Psychiatric Abuse of Prisoners, 5406 Claremont Avenue, Oakland, California.

ORWELL, G. "1984". New York: Harcourt, Brace, Jovanovich Publishing Co., 1949.

PARADRINI, A. "Mind Study: "Front" or "Frontier"". Herald Examiner, Los Angeles, Sunday, April 15, 1973.

PRINCIPLES OF MEDICAL ETHICS (Pamphlet) AMA, 1957.

RANDEL, J. "Psychosurgery Trend Alarming". Washington Post, Feb. 1972.

RUSHMER, D.S. Testimony before House Human Resources Committee, Oregon, May 29, 1973.

SALPUKAS, A.   "Patient in Psychosurgery Ethics Case Says he has
     Changed Mind About Brain Operation to Alter Behavior".
     New York Times, Aguust 5, 1973, pp C26.
SCHMOCK, H.M., Jr.   "Mental Health Official Cautions Senate Panel
     on Psychosurgery".   New York Times, February 24, 1973.
SKINNER, B.F.   "Beyond Freedom and Dignity". New York: Alfred
     Knopf, 1971.
STOKES, L.   "Brain Surgery." Congress Rec., H1492, March 7, 1973.
VONNEGUT, K., Jr. "The Sirens of Titan".   New York: Dell, 1959.

APPENDIX 1.

Statement Presented by
Dr. Donald S. Rushmer
before the
House Human Resources Committee
on May 29, 1973

Re: SB-298, relating to psychosurgery and brain stimulation
in State institutions.

Mr. Chairman and Members of the Committee:

I am Donald Rushmer, Associate Director of the Laboratory
of Neurophysiology at Good Samaritan Hospital in Portland. I
hold a Ph.D. degree in Physiology and Neurobiology and spec-
ialize in the study of nervous system control of simple
movements.

Those of us in the neurosciences have used surgical and
electrical stimulation techniques as some of the most powerful
tools we have to explore the function of the nervous system.
I dare say that some one of us somewhere has made a lesion
in or electrically stimulated every possible brain structure in
animal experiments with the result that we have just begun to
reach a rudimentary understanding of how the brain functions
and a primative awareness of how the brain might control
behavior in animals such as cats, rats, and monkeys. But,
it is no understatement to say that we have barely scratched
the surface with our present knowledge of how even the
simple nervous system of the frog really works, let alone
how the billions of nerve cells in the human brain interrelate
to give the range of emotions, intellect and abilities we so
often take for granted. It is because I know firsthand the
limitations of our knowledge and the techniques we have
used for years, that I am very concerned indeed about any
suggestion that psychosurgical destruction or intracranial
brain stimulation be used in any other than the most extraordinary and controlled conditions. I am joined, I am sure,
by the vast majority of my colleagues in the outright con-
demnation of the use of psychosurgical and EBS techniques
to control human behavior under any other circumstances,
and certainly for any purpose other than to help the most

hopeless mental illness. We simply do not know enough, in my opinion, to make competent decisions about the use of such procedures.

But what of the future? In our continued quest for knowledge, we will no doubt make discoveries which would allow the total, if not arbitrary, control of emotion and indeed all facets of human behavior. It doesn't take much imagination to see that the horrors of the atom bomb are pale in comparison to the indiscriminate use of these procedures for political or other social aims to manipulate emotion, behavior and free thought. As a scientist involved in the study of the brain and as a possible contributor to these discoveries, it is my duty to do what is necessary to assure the responsible use of them for the good and the fredom of mankind and not to its detriment.

The pressures for the use of psychosurgical, EBS and other manipulations of brain in groups of prisoners, political radicals and others are growing. They have been recognized and discussed with some alarm by various of our professional organizations. Two sessions of the Winter Conference on Brain Research (January, 1973) were devoted to these issues, Science magazine; the journal of the American Association for the Advancement of Science has just published an article which condemns its indiscriminate use; the Society for Neurosciences has made these questions the emphasis for society discussions and symposia this year. Because the pressures from many sources will no doubt grow, it is imperative that responsible and carefully conceived legislation offering protection from the misuse of these techniques be established now.

In my original testimony to the Senate Human Resources Committee, I came out against SB-298 because I felt that in its original form it was a weak bill and would not achieve the purposes for which it was written. At that time, Dr. Robert Grimm, Mr. Hank Crawford of the OMA and myself were appointed to redraft the bill. We have spent a great deal of time with our council and legislature council in this task. We have sought, with advice from knowledgeable persons all over the United States to write a bill which will accomplish the following goals:

1) Acknowledge the fact that--and reading from the bill itself: "Whereas it is acknowledged that the human brain is the organ which gives man his unique qualities of thought and reason, personality and behavior, emotion and communication. And, indeed, is that unique structure importing to man his soul and ethical being; and, Whereas these things being so, the free and full use of brain is the absolute and inalienable right of each individual, a pre-requisite for making choices, possessing insight and judgment, and in health providing for the exercise of citizenship...."

2) To provide for the absolute protection from the use of these techniques for social or political ends.

3) To make it possible, however, for such techniques to be available for treatment of the sick as a course of last resort.

4) To guarantee the civil liberties and rights of any patient who might have such treatment.

I would like to acknowledge the work put in by Dr. Grimm, who unfortunately is in Boston this week, and Mr. Crawford who, although he did not lend active support for its passage, contributed many valuable suggestions which are incorporated here.

I feel that SB-298 accomplishes those goals mentioned above and will serve as model legislation throughout the country. I recommend that SB-298 be referred to the House of Representatives in its present form.

APPENDIX II.

OREGON LEGISLATIVE ASSEMBLY—1973 REGULAR SESSION

RE-ENGROSSED

Senate Bill 298

Ordered by the House June 18
(Including Amendments by Senate May 10 and by House Committee
on Human Resources June 8)

Sponsored by Senator HALLOCK

SUMMARY

The following summary is not prepared by the sponsors of the
measure and is not a part of the body thereof subject to consideration by the Legislative Assembly. It is an editor's brief
statement of the essential features of the measure.

Creates Psychosurgery Review Board to review, approve or disapprove
petition of licensed physician, institution or hospital intending to perform
psychosurgery or intercranial brain stimulation. Prescribes membership,
powers and duties of board. Requires hearing to determine if patient or
legal guardian has given voluntary and informed consent to such operation.
Prescribes hearing procedure. Requires board, subsequent to consent
hearing and prior to approving or disapproving operation, to determine if
treatment consented to has clinical merit and is appropriate for such patient. Requires petitioner and physician performing operation to submit
report of operation results to board. Provides for civil liability of person,
institution or hospital performing psychosurgery or intracranial brain
stimulation without obtaining permission of board.

Expands grounds for suspension or revocation of license to practice
medicine to include psychosurgery or intracranial brain stimulation performed without permission of Psychosurgery Review Board.

Declares emergency. Takes effect July 1, 1973.

NOTE: Matter in **bold face** in an amended section is new; matter [*italic and brack-
eted*] is existing law to be omitted; complete new sections begin with
SECTION.

Re-Eng. SB 298   [2]

1   A BILL FOR AN ACT

2 Relating to medical practices; creating new provisions; amending ORS

3   677.190; and declaring an emergency.

4   Whereas it is acknowledged that the human brain is the organ which

5 gives man his unique qualities of thought and reason, personality and

6 behavior, emotion and communication. And, indeed, is that unique structure

7 importing to man his soul and ethical being; and

8   Whereas these things being so, the free and full use of brain is the

9 absolute and inalienable right of each individual, a prerequisite for making

10 choices, possessing insight and judgment, and in health providing for the

11 exercise of citizenship; and

12   Whereas it is the policy of the State of Oregon that deliberate and

13 irreversible alteration of either the structure or function of brain to bring

14 about control of thoughts, emotional feelings, or behavior of a human

15 being shall not be considered except in the most extraordinary of situations

16 when such drastic procedures are proposed as a necessary course of last

17 resort to provide a person in need of special treatment with humane care;

18 now, therefore,

19   The intent of this Act is to provide the strictest possible control over

20 the advocacy and practice of operations specifically aimed at permanently

21 altering behavior.

22 **Be It Enacted by the People of the State of Oregon:**

23   **SECTION 1.** As used in sections 1 to 15 of this Act, unless the context

24 requires otherwise:

25   (1) "Electro-convulsive therapy" means a nonsurgical and generalized

26 electrical stimulation of the brain, designed to induce a convulsion.

27   (2) "Experimental" means a technique or procedure about which there

28 is not sufficient data to recommend it as a recognized treatment of choice,

29 or to predict accurately the outcome of its performance.

30   (3) "Intracranial brain stimulation" means the surgical implantation

31 of electrodes within the brain for the purpose of directly stimulating

32 specific brain structures to produce alteration of the thoughts, emotions,

33 or behavior in a human being. Intracranial brain stimulation does not in-

34 clude electro-convulsive therapy.

1   (4) "Operation" means psychosurgery or intracranial brain stimulation.

2   (5) "Patient" means any person upon whom psychosurgery or intra-
3 cranial brain stimulation is intended to be performed, including but not
4 limited to persons confined voluntarily or involuntarily in any state insti-
5 tutions or private hospitals.

6   (6) "Psychosurgery" means any operation designed to irreversibly
7 lesion or destroy brain tissue for the primary purpose of altering the
8 thoughts, emotions or behavior of a human being. "Psychosurgery" does not
9 include procedures which may irreversibly lesion or destroy brain tissues
10 when undertaken to cure well-defined disease states such as brain tumor,
11 epileptic foci and certain chronic pain syndromes.

12   (7) "Review board" means the Psychosurgery Review Board.

13   **SECTION 2.** No person, institution or hospital shall perform or cause
14 to be performed psychosurgery or intracranial brain stimulation on any
15 patient without complying with the provisions of this Act.

16   **SECTION 3.** (1) There is created the Psychosurgery Review Board
17 consisting of nine persons appointed by the Governor.

18   (2) The term of office of each member is four years, but a member
19 serves at the pleasure of the Governor. Before the expiration of the term
20 of a member, the Governor shall appoint a successor whose term begins
21 on July 1 next following. A member is eligible for reappointment. If
22 there is a vacancy for any cause, the Governor shall make an appointment
23 to become immediately effective for the unexpired term.

24   (3) Of the membership of the board:

25   (a) One shall be a physician licensed by the Board of Medical Ex-
26 aminers for the State of Oregon, practicing neurology, certified by the
27 American Board of Neurology and Psychiatry; and nominated pursuant to
28 section 4 of this Act;

29   (b) Two shall be physicians licensed by the Board of Medical Ex-
30 aminers for the State of Oregon, practicing neurosurgery, certified by the
31 American Board of Neurosurgery, and nominated pursuant to section 4
32 of this Act;

33   (c) Two shall be physicians licensed by the Board of Medical Ex-
34 aminers for the State of Oregon, practicing psychiatry, certified by the

Re-Eng. SB 298   [4]

1 American Board of Neurology and Psychiatry, and nominated pursuant to
2 section 4 of this Act;

3   (d) One shall be a clinical psychologist;

4   (e) One shall be a neuroscientist actively engaged in research on
5 the nervous system; and

6   (f) Two shall be members of the general public one of whom shall be
7 a member of the Oregon State Bar.

8   (4) All decisions of the review board shall be made by the affirmative
9 vote of not less than six members.

10   (5) No individual directly involved in conducting psychosurgery or
11 intracranial brain stimulation on human beings shall be a member of the
12 review board.

13   **SECTION 4.** Not later than June 1 of each year, the Oregon Medical
14 Association shall nominate three qualified physicians for each physician
15 member of the Psychosurgery Review Board whose term expires in that
16 year, and shall certify its nominees to the Governor. The Governor shall
17 consider these nominees in selecting successors to retiring board members.

18   **SECTION 5.** Notwithstanding the term of office specified by section 3
19 of this Act, of the members first appointed to the board:

20   (1) Two shall serve for terms ending June 30, 1974.

21   (2) Two shall serve for terms ending June 30, 1975.

22   (3) Two shall serve for terms ending June 30, 1976.

23   (4) Three shall serve for terms ending June 30, 1977.

24   **SECTION 6.** (1) Any institution, hospital or licensed physician intend-
25 ing to perform psychosurgery or intracranial brain stimulation for the
26 primary purpose of altering the thoughts, emotions or behavior of a human
27 being shall file a petition with the review board alleging that a patient is
28 in need of such treatment, that the patient or his legal guardian, if any,
29 has consented thereto, and that the proposed operation has legitimate
30 clinical value.

31   (2) Within 10 days of the filing of the petition under subsection (1)
32 of this section, the review board shall:

33   (a) Schedule a hearing to be held within 20 days to determine if the
34 patient or his legal guardian has given his informed, voluntary consent.

1   (b) Give notice of the hearing at least seven days prior thereto to
2 the patient, the legal guardian, if any, the legal counsel, if any, and the
3 petitioner.

4   (c) Conduct the consent hearing.

5   **SECTION 7.** (1) At the hearing held pursuant to subsection (2) of
6 section 6 of this Act, the review board shall determine whether or not the
7 patient or his legal guardian has given his voluntary and informed consent.

8   (2) For the review board to determine under subsection (1) of this
9 section that the consent given was voluntary and informed, it must ap-
10 pear that:

11   (a) A fair explanation was made of the procedures to be followed,
12 including an identification of those which are experimental;

13   (b) A description was given of the attendant discomforts and risks,
14 in any;

15   (c) A description was given of the benefits to be expected, if any;

16   (d) A disclosure was made of appropriate alternative treatments, if
17 any, that would be advantageous for the subject;

18   (e) An offer was made to answer any inquiries concerning the treat-
19 ment;

20   (f) Notice was given that the patient is free to withdraw his consent
21 and to discontinue the authorized treatment at any time;

22   (g) Disclosure was made of the relationship between the patient and
23 the institution, hospital or physician obtaining the consent; and

24   (h) Notice was given that the patient or his legal guardian, if any,
25 had a right to consult with and be advised or represented by legal counsel,
26 and if he could not afford one, legal counsel would be appointed for him
27 pursuant to subsection (2) of section 11 of this Act.

28   (3) If at any time during the hearing held under this section, the pa-
29 tient or his legal guardian requests an opportunity to consult or be repre-
30 sented by legal counsel, such a request shall be granted.

31   (4) At the conclusion of the hearing held under this section, the pa-
32 tient or his legal guardian, if any, shall be asked if he still consents to the
33 proposed psychosurgery or intracranial brain stimulation.

34   (5) If the patient appears to be incapable of giving an informed and

Re-Eng. SB 298 [6]

1 voluntary consent to the proposed operation, the necessary consent shall
2 be required to be given or withheld by the patient's legal guardian.

3 **SECTION 8.** (1) Subsequent to the hearing held under section 6 of
4 this Act, if the review board has found that the patient or his legal guard-
5 ian has given his voluntary and informed consent to the proposed operation
6 the review board shall review the proposed operation and make a deter-
7 mination of whether or not the operation has clinical merit and is an ap-
8 propriate treatment for the specific patient.

9 (2) In making its determination of whether or not the proposed oper-
10 ation has value in the specific clinical situation, the review board may
11 study pertinent literature, reports and legislation, conduct consultations
12 and interviews with persons knowledgeable in the field and conduct onsite
13 visitations. In the event the review board determines that the proposed
14 operation lacks clinical merit, the petition shall be denied and the petitioner
15 notified by registered mail.

16 (3) If the review board finds that the proposed operation has legiti-
17 mate clinical value, it shall review the clinical data of the patient pro-
18 posed for the psychosurgery or intracranial brain stimulation operation. The
19 review board shall determine whether or not such treatment is appro-
20 priate for the patient. In order for the review board to determine that
21 such an operation is appropriate, it must appear that:

22 (a) All conventional therapies have been attempted;

23 (b) The criteria for selection of the patient have been met;

24 (c) The operation offers hope of saving life, reestablishing health or
25 alleviating suffering; and

26 (d) All other viable alternative methods of treatment have been tried
27 and have failed to produce satisfactory results.

28 (4) The review board may undertake a specific diagnostic evaluation
29 as to the suitability of the patient for the proposed operation and the re-
30 view board may establish the procedure for such evaluation.

31 (5) The review board shall make a written order embodying its con-
32 clusions. The order shall specify whether or not the psychosurgery or in-
33 tracranial brain stimulation as requested in the petition may be performed.

1   (6) A copy of the order of the review board shall be served person-
2 ally or by registered mail on:

3   (a) The petitioner;

4   (b) The patient;

5   (c) The legal guardian, if any; and

6   (d) The patient's or legal guardian's legal counsel, if any.

7   **SECTION 9.** The review board may administer oaths, take depositions
8 and issue subpenas to compel the attendance of witnesses and the produc-
9 tion of documents or other written information necessary to carry out the
10 purposes of this Act. If any person fails to comply with a subpena issued
11 under this section or refuses to testify on matters on which he lawfully may
12 be interrogated, the procedure set out in ORS 183.440 shall be followed to
13 compel obedience.

14   **SECTION 10.** (1) If the patient does not have a legal guardian, and
15 the review board believes that the patient is incapable of giving an in-
16 formed and voluntary consent to the proposed operation, the review board
17 shall request that a legal guardian be appointed.

18   (2) Preference in appointment of a legal guardian under subsection
19 (1) of this section shall be in the following order:

20   (a) The patient's spouse.

21   (b) The patient's nearest next of kin.

22   (c) A personal friend of the patient.

23   (d) A public guardian if one exists in the county, under the provisions
24 of ORS 126.905 to 126.965.

25   (e) Any other person deemed appropriate by the court.

26   **SECTION 11.** (1) Any patient or legal guardian, if any, may be repre-
27 sented by legal counsel in the hearing held under section 7 of this Act.

28   (2) If the patient or legal guardian requests to be represented by
29 legal counsel but cannot afford one, the circuit court of the county in which
30 the patient resides shall appoint:

31   (a) The county public defender to represent him, when the office of
32 county public defender has been created under ORS 151.010 to 151.090.

33   (b) A member of the Oregon State Bar to represent him, when the
34 office of the county public defender has not been created.

Re-Eng. SB 298 [8]

1 (3) The fee of the legal counsel appointed under paragraph (b) of
2 subsection (2) of this section shall be paid out of funds appropriated by the
3 county for the payment of appointed counsel.

4 SECTION 12. Upon completion of the psychosurgery or intracranial
5 brain stimulation operation, the petitioner and any physician who per-
6 forms the operation shall make a written report of their results to the re-
7 view board.

8 SECTION 13. A member of the review board which permits psycho-
9 surgery or intracranial brain stimulation is presumed to be acting in good
10 faith. Unless it is alleged and proved that his action violated the standard
11 of reasonable professional care and judgment under the circumstances, he
12 is immune from civil or criminal liability that otherwise might be incurred.

13 SECTION 14. A person who relies on the review board's permission to
14 perform the psychosurgery or intracranial brain stimulation and performs
15 such treatment is presumed to be acting in good faith. Unless it is alleged
16 and proved that such person violated the standard of reasonable care and
17 judgment under the circumstances, he is immune from civil or criminal
18 liability that otherwise might be incurred.

19 SECTION 15. Any person, institution or hospital who performs psy-
20 chosurgery or intracranial brain stimulation without obtaining permission
21 of the Psychosurgery Review Board under section 2 to 14 of this Act
22 shall be subject to civil liability for any damages which the patient suffers
23 from the psychosurgery or intracranial brain stimulation.

24 Section 16. ORS 677.190 is amended to read:

25 677.190. The board may suspend or revoke a license to practice medi-
26 cine in this state for any of the following reasons:

27 (1) Unprofessional or dishonorable conduct.

28 (2) Conviction under ORS 435.455 or failure to comply with the pro-
29 visions of ORS 435.415 or 435.425.

30 (3) Employing any person to solicit patients for him.

31 (4) Representing to a patient that a manifestly incurable condition
32 of sickness, disease or injury can be cured.

33 (5) Obtaining any fee by fraud or misrepresentation.

34 (6) Wilfully or negligently divulging a professional secret.

1   (7) Conviction of any offense punishable by incarceration in a state
2 penitentiary or in a federal prison. A copy of the record of conviction,
3 certified to by the clerk of the court entering the conviction, shall be con-
4 clusive evidence.

5   (8) Habitual or excessive use of intoxicants or drugs.

6   (9) Fraud or misrepresentation in applying for or procuring a license
7 to practice in this state, or in connection with applying for or procuring
8 an annual registration.

9   (10) Making false or misleading statements regarding his skill or the
10 efficacy or value of the medicine, treatment or remedy prescribed or ad-
11 ministered by him or at his direction in the treatment of any disease or
12 other condition of the human body or mind.

13   (11) Impersonating another person licensed to practice medicine or
14 permitting or allowing any person to use his license or certificate of reg-
15 istration.

16   (12) Aiding or abetting the practice of medicine by a person not li-
17 censed by the board.

18   (13) Using his name under the designation "doctor," "Dr.," "D.O." or
19 "M.D." or any similar designation with reference to the commercial ex-
20 ploitation of any goods, wares or merchandise.

21   (14) Insanity or mental disease as evidenced by an adjudication or by
22 voluntary commitment to an institution for treatment of a mental disease,
23 or as determined by an examination conducted by three impartial psy-
24 chiatrists retained by the board.

25   (15) Gross negligence in the practice of medicine.

26   (16) Manifest incapacity to practice medicine.

27   (17) The suspension or revocation by another state of a license to
28 practice medicine, based upon acts by the licensee similar to acts de-
29 scribed in this section. A certified copy of the record of suspension or revo-
30 cation of the state making such suspension or revocation is conclusive
31 evidence thereof.

32   (18) Failing to designate the degree appearing on the license under
33 circumstances described in subsection (3) of ORS 677.184.

Re-Eng. SB 298   [10]

1   (19) Wilfully violating any provision of this chapter or any rule
2 promulgated by the board.

3   (20) Changing his location of practice as provided in ORS 677.170.

4   (21) Adjudication of or admission to a hospital for mental illness or
5 imprisonment as provided in ORS 677.225.

6   (22) Making a fraudulent claim.

7   **(23) Performing psychosurgery or intracranial brain stimulation with-**
8 **out obtaining permission of the Psychosurgery Review Board under sec-**
9 **tions 2 to 14 of this 1973 Act.**

10   SECTION 17. This Act being necessary for the immediate preservation
11 of the public peace, health and safety, an emergency is declared to exist,
12 and this Act takes effect on July 1, 1973.

————◇————

SUMMARY

I. S. Cooper, M. Riklan, and R. S. Snider

The invited participants agreed that several conclusions were warranted on the basis of evidence and data presented. Specifically, there was a clear consensus that cerebellar cortical stimulation can inhibit electrical and/or seizure activity induced in various cortical, subcortical and limbic system areas.

A. The experimental data presented in this Symposium indicated that cerebellar cortical stimulation can:

1. Alter the abnormal discharges in the primary penicillin induced seizure focus and arrest the major discharges in the mirror focus in the cat.

2. Arrest cobalt induced cortical seizures in the rat but not in the monkey.

3. Arrest or shorten electrically induced seizures arising in the neocortex, ventral thalamic nuclei, or the hippocampus in the monkey.

4. Alter or arrest photic induced Metrazol seizure discharges in the cat.

5. Reduce the amplitude and rate but not abolish the abnormal discharges due to chloralose medication in the cat.

6. Alter the frequency and amplitude of seizure discharges, and in some instances diminish seizures in the cat resulting from cobalt chloride applied to the hippocampus.

7. Suppress spontaneous and stimulus induced myoclonus.

8. Inhibit both photic and somatosensory evoked cerebral responses in cats.

Experimental data were also presented which suggested that the anti-epileptic action of diphenylhydantoin (Dilantin) may be related to augmentation of Purkinje cell discharge. Furthermore, sufficiently large lesions of the cerebellar cortex in monkeys were shown to produce docility in some previously aggressive animals.

B. The data on the human indicate that anterior or combined anterior and posterior cerebellar stimulation served to significantly reduce seizure activity in humans suffering from intractable seizure disorders of various etiologies. A surgical technique was described which involves exposing the cerebellum by approaching it through the tentorium cerebelli. A plate of silicon coated dacron mesh with 4 or 8 pairs of platinum electrodes affixed can thus be applied to the anterior or posterior cerebellar cortex. Chronic cerebellar cortex stimulation can be applied through an antenna fixed subcutaneously on the chest by means of a transepidermal coupling. In 7 patients undergoing this procedure, seizure activity was alleviated or reduced without any apparent untoward sensory or motor alteration, or noticeable damage to cerebellar neurons. These preliminary studies indicate that slow frequency stimulation (10 cycles per second) is most effective in arresting epileptiform seizures. In contrast, faster frequencies (100-200 cycles per second) are less effective and may be contraindicated. Effective arrest of seizures has continued up to one year at the present time. However, fast frequency stimulation (200 cycles per second) on anterior cerebellum significantly reduced intention myoclonus following cardiac arrest in a 39-year old female.

Psychological studies undertaken with 7 patients undergoing chronic cerebellar stimulation showed a pattern of verbal-motor facilitation for the group in contrast to decrements or slowing in visual-spatial perception. Intellectual functions tended to be maintained or improved during the course of chronic stimulation. The visual-spatial decrements tended to be lateralized and more closely associated with right cerebellar lobe stimulation and anterior placement. In most patients a reduction of subjectively felt anxiety, tension, and depression was reported. Reduction in aggressive behavior and improved emotional control was observed in several patients following chronic stimulation.

The preliminary nature of the clinical investigations was emphasized, as was the lack of any comprehensive theory concerning the exact mechanism of seizure reduction associated with cerebellar cortex stimulation. Suggestions were made for the continuation of electrophysiological, neurological, and psychological studies, as well as continuing long range assessment of patients subjected to this procedure by way

of a collaborative study among several institutions.   Interest was also
expressed in a variety of ethical considerations with respect to cerebellar stimulation as an innovative therapy in humans.